Treatment Resistant Depression

A ROADMAP FOR EFFECTIVE CARE

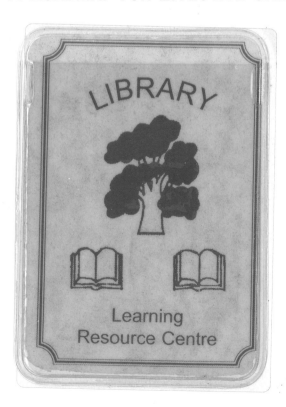

Treatment Resistant Depression

A ROADMAP FOR EFFECTIVE CARE

Edited by

John F. Greden, M.D.
Michelle B. Riba, M.D., M.S.
Melvin G. McInnis, M.D.

University of Michigan
Comprehensive Depression Center

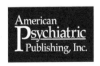

Washington, DC
London, England

Copyright © 2011 American Psychiatric Association
ALL RIGHTS RESERVED

Manufactured in the United States of America on acid-free paper
15   14   13   12   11   5   4   3   2   1
First Edition

Typeset in Adobe's Esprit and TradeGothic

American Psychiatric Publishing, Inc.
1000 Wilson Boulevard
Arlington, VA 22209–3901
www.appi.org

Library of Congress Cataloging-in-Publication Data
Treatment resistant depression : a roadmap for effective care / edited by John F. Greden, Michelle B. Riba, Melvin G. McInnis. — 1st ed.
    p. ; cm.
  Includes bibliographical references and index.
  ISBN 978-1-58562-409-6 (alk. paper)
  1. Depression, Mental—Treatment. I. Greden, John F., 1942– II. Riba, Michelle B. III. McInnis, Melvin G.
  [DNLM: 1. Depressive Disorder, Major—therapy. 2. Treatment Failure. WM 207]
  RC537.T7432 2011
  616.85′2706–dc22

                                                    2011000279

British Library Cataloguing in Publication Data
A CIP record is available from the British Library.

To purchase 25–99 copies of this or any other APPI title at a 20 % discount, please contact APPI Customer Service at appi@psych.org or 800-368-5777. If you wish to buy 100 or more copies of the same title, please e-mail us at bulksales@psych.org for a price quote.

Contents

CHAPTER
ONE

Contributors

Iyad Alkhouri, M.D.
Clinical Assistant Professor, Department of Psychiatry, University of Michigan, Ann Arbor, Michigan

Roseanne Armitage, Ph.D.
Professor of Psychiatry and Director, Sleep and Chronophysiology Laboratory, University of Michigan, Department of Psychiatry, Ann Arbor, Michigan

J. Todd Arnedt, Ph.D.
Assistant Professor of Psychiatry and Neurology, Sleep and Chronophysiology Laboratory, University of Michigan, Department of Psychiatry, Ann Arbor, Michigan

Virginia Barbosa, M.D.
Staff Psychiatrist, Cumberland River Behavioral Care Center, Lexington, Kentucky

Kirk J. Brower, M.D.
Professor of Psychiatry and Executive Director, University of Michigan Addiction Treatment Services (UMATS), Department of Psychiatry, University of Michigan, Ann Arbor, Michigan

Paul Burghardt, Ph.D.
Research Fellow, Molecular and Behavioral Neuroscience Institute, University of Michigan, Ann Arbor, Michigan

Simon Evans, Ph.D.
Assistant Research Professor, Department of Psychiatry, University of Michigan, Ann Arbor, Michigan

Heather A. Flynn, Ph.D.
Associate Professor and Director, Adult Psychotherapy Services, Department of Psychiatry, University of Michigan, Ann Arbor, Michigan

Neera Ghaziuddin, M.D., M.R.C.Psych.
Associate Professor, Department of Psychiatry, University of Michigan, Ann Arbor, Michigan

Rachel Lipson Glick, M.D.
Associate Chair for Clinical and Administrative Affairs and Clinical Professor, Department of Psychiatry, University of Michigan Medical School, Ann Arbor, Michigan

Mona Goldman, Ph.D.
Research Assistant Professor, Department of Psychiatry, University of Michigan, Ann Arbor, Michigan

David E. Goodrich, M.S., M.A., Ed.D.
Research Health Science Specialist, Ann Arbor VA HSR&D Center of Excellence, Center for Clinical Management and National Serious Mental Illness Treatment Research and Evaluation Center, Ann Arbor, Michigan

John F. Greden, M.D.
Rachel Upjohn Professor of Psychiatry and Clinical Neurosciences; Executive Director, University of Michigan Comprehensive Depression Center; and Research Professor, Molecular and Behavioral Neurosciences Institute, University of Michigan, Ann Arbor, Michigan; Chair, National Network of Depression Centers

Joseph Himle, Ph.D.
Associate Professor and Associate Director, Anxiety Disorders Program, Department of Psychiatry and School of Social Work, University of Michigan, Ann Arbor, Michigan

Victor Hong, M.D.
Outpatient and consultation-liaison psychiatrist, Contra Costa Health Services, Martinez, California

Helen C. Kales, M.D.
Associate Professor, Department of Psychiatry, University of Michigan; Director, Section of Geriatric Psychiatry; and Investigator, Health Services Research and Development Service, Serious Mental Illness Treatment Research Education and Clinical Center, Geriatric Research Education and Clinical Center, VA Ann Arbor Healthcare System, Ann Arbor, Michigan

Masoud Kamali, M.D.
Clinical Lecturer and Research Fellow, University of Michigan Depression Center, Ann Arbor, Michigan

Kevin Kerber, M.D.
Clinical Assistant Professor, Department of Psychiatry, University of Michigan, Ann Arbor, Michigan

Amy M. Kilbourne, Ph.D., M.P.H.
Associate Professor, Department of Psychiatry, University of Michigan, Ann Arbor, Michigan

Cheryl King, Ph.D.
Professor, Departments of Psychiatry and Psychology, University of Michigan, Ann Arbor, Michigan

Daniel F. Maixner, M.D.
Assistant Professor, Department of Psychiatry, University of Michigan, Ann Arbor, Michigan

Susan Maixner, M.D.
Clinical Assistant Professor; Director, Geriatric Psychiatry Clinic; and Director, Geriatric Psychiatry Fellowship Program, Department of Psychiatry, University of Michigan Health System, Ann Arbor, Michigan

Sheila M. Marcus, M.D.
Clinical Professor, Department of Psychiatry, University of Michigan, Ann Arbor, Michigan

Melvin G. McInnis, M.D.
Thomas B. and Nancy Upjohn Woodworth Professor of Bipolar Disorder and Depression; Professor of Psychiatry and Associate Director, University of Michigan Comprehensive Depression Center; and Section Director, Depression Center, University of Michigan, Ann Arbor, Michigan

Brian Mickey, M.D., Ph.D.
Assistant Professor of Psychiatry, University of Michigan, Ann Arbor, Michigan

Erin Miller, M.S.
Clinical Research Coordinator, Department of Psychiatry, University of Michigan, Ann Arbor, Michigan

Maria Muzik, M.D., M.Sc.
Assistant Professor and Director, Women's Perinatal Clinic and Parent-Infant-Program, Depression Center and Trauma, Stress and Anxiety Research Group (TSARG), Department of Psychiatry, University of Michigan; Assistant Research Scientist, Center for Human Growth and Development, University of Michigan, Ann Arbor, Michigan

John M. Oldham, M.D., M.S.
Senior Vice President and Chief of Staff, The Menninger Clinic; Professor and Executive Vice Chairman, Menninger Department of Psychiatry and Behavioral Sciences, Baylor College of Medicine, Houston, Texas

Parag G. Patil, M.D., Ph.D.
Assistant Professor, Department of Neurosurgery, University of Michigan Health System, Ann Arbor, Michigan

Paul Pfeiffer, M.D., M.S.
Clinical Lecturer, Department of Psychiatry, University of Michigan, Ann Arbor, Michigan

Michelle B. Riba, M.D., M.S.
Clinical Professor and Associate Director, Michigan Institute for Clinical and Health Research; Associate Director, University of Michigan Comprehensive Depression Center; and Associate Chair for Integrated Medical and Psychiatric Services, University of Michigan, Ann Arbor, Michigan

Kathryn Roeder, B.S.
Research Area Specialist Associate, Department of Psychiatry, University of Michigan, Ann Arbor, Michigan

Srijan Sen, M.D., Ph.D.
Assistant Professor of Psychiatry, University of Michigan Comprehensive Depression Center and University of Michigan Department of Psychiatry, Ann Arbor, Michigan

Todd Sevig, Ph.D.
Director, Counseling and Psychological Services, and Chair, Mental Health Work Group, University of Michigan, Ann Arbor, Michigan

Lisa S. Seyfried, M.D.
Clinical Assistant Professor, Department of Psychiatry, University of Michigan, Ann Arbor, Michigan

Claire Stano, M.A.
Research Area Specialist Associate, Department of Psychiatry, University of Michigan, Ann Arbor, Michigan

Kiran Taylor, M.D.
Assistant Professor, Department of Psychiatry, University of Michigan, Ann Arbor, Michigan

Stephan F. Taylor, M.D.
Professor, Department of Psychiatry, University of Michigan, Ann Arbor, Michigan

Jamie Travis, B.A.
Research Area Specialist Associate, Department of Psychiatry, University of Michigan, Ann Arbor, Michigan

Marcia Valenstein, M.D., M.S.
Associate Professor, Department of Psychiatry, University of Michigan, Ann Arbor, Michigan

Delia Vazquez, M.D.
Professor of Pediatrics and Communicable Diseases; Professor of Psychiatry, University of Michigan Medical School; and Research Professor, Center for Human Growth and Development, University of Michigan Medical School, Ann Arbor, Michigan

Heather Walters, M.S.
Research Coordinator, Department of Psychiatry, University of Michigan, Ann Arbor, Michigan

Robert Winfield, M.D.
Director, University Health Service, Division of Student Affairs, and Chief Health Officer, University of Michigan, Ann Arbor, Michigan

Kara Zivin, Ph.D.
Assistant Professor, Department of Psychiatry, University of Michigan; and Investigator, Department of Veterans Affairs, National Serious Mental Illness Treatment Research and Evaluation Center (SMITREC), Ann Arbor, Michigan

Disclosure of Interests

The following contributors to this volume have indicated a financial interest in or other affiliation with a commercial supporter, a manufacturer of a commercial product, a provider of a commercial service, a nongovernmental organization, and/or a government agency that could represent or could appear to represent a competing interest, as listed below:

Kirk J. Brower, M.D.—*Royalties:* Co-author of *BrainFit for Life,* a book for the lay public to promote lifestyle approaches to brain fitness.

Simon Evans, Ph.D.—*Royalties:* Co-author of *BrainFit for Life.*

Daniel F. Maixner, M.D.—*Research support (past):* Neuronetics.

Sheila M. Marcus, M.D.—*Fees:* Small remunerations from *Up-to-Date,* a division of Wolters Kluwer Health.

Melvin McInnis, M.D.—*Consulting:* Pfizer. *Speakers' Bureau:* Bristol-Myers Squibb, Janssen, Lilly, Merck.

Stephan F. Taylor, M.D.—*Grant support:* St. Jude Medical.

The following contributors indicated that they have no competing interests:

Iyad Alkhouri, M.D.
Roseanne Armitage, Ph.D.
J. Todd Arnedt, Ph.D.
Virginia Barbosa, M.D.
Paul Burghardt, Ph.D.
John F. Greden, M.D.
Heather A. Flynn, Ph.D.
Neera Ghaziuddin, M.D., M.R.C.Psych.
Rachel Lipson Glick, M.D.
Mona Goldman, Ph.D.
David Goodrich, M.S., M.A., Ed.D.
Joseph Himle, Ph.D.
Victor Hong, M.D.
Helen C. Kales, M.D.
Kevin Kerber, M.D.
Masoud Kamali, M.D.
Amy M. Kilbourne, Ph.D., M.P.H.
Cheryl King, Ph.D.
Susan Maixner, M.D.

Erin Miller, M.S.
Brian Mickey, M.D., Ph.D.
Maria Muzik, M.D., M.Sc.
Parag G. Patil, M.D., Ph.D.
Paul Pfeiffer, M.D., M.S.
Michelle B. Riba, M.D., M.S.
Kathryn Roeder, B.S.
Srijan Sen, MD, Ph.D.
Todd Sevig, Ph.D.
Lisa S. Seyfried, M.D.
Claire Stano, M.A.
Kiran Taylor, M.D.
Jamie Travis, B.A.
Marcia Valenstein, M.D., M.S.
Delia Vazquez, M.D.
Heather Walters, M.S.
Robert Winfield, M.D.
Kara Zivin, Ph.D.

Foreword

THE NATIONAL QUALITY FORUM recently hosted a conference on performance measurement in health care, entitled "Prioritization of High-Impact Medicare Conditions and Measure Gaps," in which the first task was to prioritize the 20 conditions that account for more than 95% of the Medicare costs of all medical disorders (National Quality Forum 2010). These 20 conditions included Alzheimer's disease, diabetes, ischemic heart disease, osteoporosis, stroke, lung cancer, breast cancer, and many other conditions, including major depression. The 20 conditions were prioritized based on the five dimensions of cost, prevalence, variability, improvability, and disparities. Preliminary rankings were developed based on a synthesis of the evidence. Congestive heart failure was ranked number 1, and major depression number 10. These rankings were reviewed by a group of experts, who first applied other considerations, such as risk factors and weighting of the five dimensions, and then followed a "multi-voting" procedure to reach agreement on a new prioritized list of conditions. The resulting final, prioritized list of high-impact Medicare conditions placed major depression at the top of the list, as the number 1 condition of concern. This recent exercise reinforced an earlier report by the National Quality Forum (2005), which identified screening for depression in acute medical settings as one of two "priorities for immediate action" (along with screening for alcoholism).

There has been a steady drumbeat of messages emphasizing the prevalent and disabling nature of major depressive disorder, particularly since the transformative report of the World Health Organization and the Harvard School of Public Health on the "Global Burden of Disease" (World Health Organization 2004), which identified major depression, among all medical conditions, as the number 1 cause of disability worldwide. The Institute of Medicine (2009) has also underscored the crucial public health need to identify and treat depression, recently recommending routine screening for depression in adolescents. These emerging findings, along with regular distressing headlines on the high rates of suicide in teens and in military and veteran populations, have focused public attention on the reality of depression as a critical social and public health problem.

Yet in spite of this evidence, it has been extremely difficult to erase the stigma that attaches to depression and to all psychiatric illness. At The Menninger Clinic, where I work, we have an inpatient treatment program called "Professionals in Crisis" where we help physicians, lawyers, nurses, corporate executives, and other professionals recover and get back on track. We explored the idea of establishing an "Officers in Crisis" program as a private, low-visibility treatment program for distressed active-duty military officers, with the goal of helping them recover and potentially return to duty if appropriate. So far, the program has not been developed; we were advised that officers would not volunteer for or agree to such treatment, fearing that doing so would end their careers. Efforts to combat such fears and perceptions are under way, including the National Institute of Mental Health's laudable campaign "Real Men, Real Depression" and the first report on mental illness ever issued from the Office of the Surgeon General. In that report, David Satcher emphasized that mental disorders are real illnesses, and he suggested that the best antidote for stigma is the existence of effective treatments for psychiatric conditions.

Research has taught us a great deal about the mainstream medical nature of depression—for example, that it is an independent risk factor for cardiac death, that it involves suppression of the immune system and hyperactivation of the stress hormone system, and that it can even involve neuronal damage. Our colleagues in medicine, primary care, pediatrics, family medicine, and many other areas are eager to partner with psychiatry in the fight to overcome depression, recognizing that depression destabilizes and complicates the course of many co-occurring medical conditions such as diabetes and heart disease. The National Network of Depression Centers (NNDC), modeled on the National Cancer Center Network, is a welcome and highly visible national effort to move depression from being viewed as a shameful sign of weakness and failure to being understood as a heritable biological illness that can be prevented or overcome.

So how effective are our treatments for depression? The good news about depression is that many effective treatments exist, including medication, psychotherapy, and electroconvulsive therapy, and that new treatments are emerging—such as transcranial magnetic stimulation, vagus nerve stimulation, and deep brain stimulation—that offer hope and promise. These treatments are reviewed eloquently by the experts who have authored this outstanding and badly needed volume, *Treatment Resistant Depression: A Roadmap for Effective Care.* John Greden, senior editor, is well known for his pioneering role in the crusade against depression and for being the founder of the first Depression Center that stimulated the development of the NNDC. His initiative in organizing and serving as senior editor of this new book represents another significant contribution to the campaign to overcome depression.

What is unique about this book is that it focuses on the not-so-good news about depression—the surprising number of patients with depression who do not respond well to known effective treatments. Shining the spotlight on the problem of "refractory depression" or "treatment-resistant depression" is now an urgent need, and this book represents the single best source of knowledge about the magnitude of this problem and the hard work under way to reach those who need individualized and nonroutine treatment intervention. New findings are emerging rapidly, and there is every reason to be optimistic. With the help of the dedicated researchers and clinicians whose voices emerge from the pages of this book, depression, like cancer, will be transformed in the public eye from a shameful secret to a curable illness for which people seek treatment and from which people recover.

John M. Oldham, M.D.

References

Institute of Medicine: Preventing Mental, Emotional, and Behavioral Disorders Among Young People: Progress and Possibilities. March 12, 2009. Available at: http://www.iom.edu/Reports.aspx. Accessed December 6, 2010.

National Quality Forum: Integrating Behavioral Healthcare Performance Measures Throughout Healthcare: Workshop Proceedings. Edited by Power EJ, Zadrozny S, Nishimi RY, et al. Washington, DC, National Quality Forum, 2005. Available at: http://www.qualityforum.org/Publications/2005/05/Behavioral_Health_full.aspx. Accessed November 30, 2010.

National Quality Forum: Prioritization of High-Impact Medicare Conditions and Measure Gaps. NQF Measure Prioritization Advisory Committee. Washington, DC, National Quality Forum, May 2010. Available at: http://www.qualityforum.org/projects/prioritization.aspx?section = MeasurePrioritizationAdvisoryCommitteeReport2010-05-24. Accessed November 30, 2010.

World Health Organization: The Global Burden of Disease. 2004. Available at: http://www.who.int/healthinfo/global_burden_disease/2004_report_update/en/index.html. Accessed November 30, 2010.

Preface

I'm not sad, Doc; I'm *sick*. This depression thing is wrecking my life. There *must* be some treatments out there that could make me feel the way I once did.

47-year-old businessman with
treatment-resistant major depressive disorder

Major depressive disorder (MDD) contributes to more disability and diminution of quality of life than almost all other diseases in the world. The treatment resistance associated with MDD is a significant reason for its huge burdens. Its public health dimensions are staggering—MDD afflicts more than 300 million citizens of the world at some point in their lifetime, and treatment resistance occurs in 30%–40% of those who are fortunate enough to receive care.

Treatment Resistant Depression (TRD) is painfully linked with suicides, broken marriages and relationships, job losses, bankruptcy claims, impaired physical health, stressed families, and financially strained health systems. An estimated 4%–5% of all Americans struggle at some time with TRD, and worldwide, treatment resistance in major depression is a key determinant of burgeoning health care costs. These individuals, their families, and their clinicians are joined in the businessman's search for "some treatments out there that could make me feel the way I once did." This book provides a comprehensive review of the progress made in that search and the strategies most likely to achieve that goal.

The principles that inform this roadmap are gleaned from the experiences of the University of Michigan Comprehensive Depression Center's Treatment Resistant Depression Program and the array of clinical research advances from other programs throughout the world. What are these principles?

First, we must identify depressive illnesses earlier and seek to stop illness progression "in its tracks." Our roadmap must assist clinicians, patients, and families in finding and diagnosing these disorders earlier in life by focusing on childhood, when these disorders begin, and treating them more effectively and preventing the recurrences and chronicity that otherwise follow in later decades. This goal is parallel to what specialists in diabetes and cardiovascular disease have long emphasized: earlier prevention and treatment equate with better outcomes. In the following chapters, the authors describe how to screen; the best approaches for early treatment to wellness; when to combine or augment; the vital role of evidence-based psychotherapies; how to use complementary treatments; and updated assessments of the effectiveness of new treatments such as transcranial magnetic stimulation, deep brain stimulation, and ketamine infusions.

Second, the roadmap provides guidance for treating depressive illness as the chronic disorder that it is rather than continuing to focus on only the acute stage. Clinical depression is most often an episodic, recurrent lifetime disorder, so by necessity, our roadmap formalizes a lifetime perspective that seeks to attain *and maintain* wellness.

Third, in components of this book we seek to integrate long-term, participatory, and self-management treatment approaches from the first clinical visit onward. These aspects include how to incorporate strategies of health care management, exercise, and nutrition; how to best treat co-occurring substance abuse; and how to address the special issues encountered by pregnant women, children, those who have sleep disturbances, the elderly, and the medically ill.

Fourth, our current treatment portfolio remains inadequate. Clinical depression is not a single entity, so no single treatment will ever suffice. We really are dealing with "depressions," so our roadmap must assist in promoting development of new, personalized, and predictive biomarkers to deliver more targeted treatment strategies. We hope that readers will emerge with a sense of how far we have come, how far we have to go, and how to move forward now with the still incomplete knowledge we have.

Fifth, the roadmap must aid us in transforming public policy. Goals are to overcome stigma with forthright explanations (appropriate language is suggested); change our policies for sharing information so we can finally expand our knowledge base with large-scale research studies comparable to those so effectively completed by our colleagues in cancer and heart disease (programs of the National Network of Depression Centers are described); export treatment toolkits to aid self-management (a link to the Depression Center's "Toolkit" is provided in the book); and guide us toward more assertive treatment with the newest strategies for patients who have already developed treatment resistance. The interdisciplinary experts at the University of Michigan Comprehensive Depression Center address each of these issues in understandable language that crosses traditional interdisciplinary boundaries.

The University of Michigan Comprehensive Depression Center was established to foster and integrate interdisciplinary research, clinical translation, education, and public policy pertaining to depression, bipolar illnesses, and related disorders. The center's mission also included launching the previously referenced National Network of Depression Centers (www.NNDC.org), with its goals of having a Center of Excellence and satellite clinics within 200 miles of every citizen in America. As advances are made by this collaborating network, we will strive to translate them rapidly and to educate—anyone and everyone—so that we can attack as a team of thousands rather than in small, isolated pockets. We passionately believe that stigma will fade as we make this journey, just as it has faded for cancer.

This book is written for clinicians and clinical investigators, with the focus on practical and clinically oriented approaches in a variety of treatment settings. At the same time, we have sought to make the material informative for patients who struggle to achieve and sustain wellness, for their families and friends seeking to enhance their own knowledge so that they can better assist their loved ones, and for policy makers who must address this costly disorder. We offer a special thanks to Robert Hales, M.D., M.B.A., for his vision and leadership and to all our colleagues, patients, and families who made this book and this journey possible.

John F. Greden, M.D.
Michelle B. Riba, M.D., M.S.
Melvin G. McInnis, M.D.

Dedication and Acknowledgements

This book is dedicated to the magnanimous individuals and foundations whose generous gifts helped support the efforts to conquer Treatment Resistant Depression:

The Noble Foundation
Waltraud E. Prechter–World Heritage Foundation–Prechter Family Fund
Phil F. Jenkins
Edwin E. and Mary Upjohn Meader
Thomas B. and Nancy Upjohn Woodworth
Todd Ouida Children's Foundation
Jack L. Berman, M.D., and Barbara A. Berman, Ph.D.
The Cohen Family Fund
Jonathan and Therese Miller

The Richard Scott Noble Memorial Fund has graciously provided support to distribute copies of this book to University of Michigan psychiatry residents and postdoctoral students. The editors and authors have agreed to donate royalties to support the Treatment Resistant Depression program at the University of Michigan Comprehensive Depression Center.

Drs. Greden, Riba, and McInnis are profoundly grateful to their family members who have contributed passion, zeal, encouragement, and support for these important endeavors over many years. They would also like to extend appreciation to Linda Gacioch, Cindy Ellis, and Heidi Butz for their excellent administrative, technical, and editorial assistance in the preparation of this book.

CHAPTER ONE

Treatment Resistant Depression

Overview of the University of Michigan Depression Center Roadmap

John F. Greden, M.D.
Michelle B. Riba, M.D., M.S.
Melvin G. McInnis, M.D.
Srijan Sen, M.D., Ph.D.

Definition of Treatment Resistant Depression

Treatment Resistant Depression (TRD) is an ambiguous term used to describe major depressive disorder (MDD) in individuals who have not yet responded to at least two courses of evidence-based antidepressant treatment approaches of adequate dose and duration (Berman et al. 1997; Fava and Davidson 1996). Clinicians, researchers, patients, and families often seem to struggle with the meaning of the term, perhaps because of the absence of an agreed-upon definition, but its usage has become entrenched (Greden 2001a). The most common criteria for TRD and our recommended criterion are summarized in Table 1–1.

In this book, we generally define treatment resistance as failure to achieve remission after two evidence-based antidepressant treatment courses known to have been of acceptable dose and duration. We emphasize that the term *treatment resistance* should never be used to imply that the individuals battling depression are resistant to improvement or that their depressive illness cannot be treated.

Clinical Vignette

(In this speculative clinical vignette, we encourage readers to note the causal roles of multiple episodes; to realize the importance of thorough clinical and laboratory evaluations, adherence, self-management, and long-term maintenance; and to assume that perhaps by 2015, new treatment and preventive advances will have become a routine part of approaches commonly used by clinicians.)

A 37-year-old married woman gives birth to her third child. Tragically, 1 month later, her grandmother, who raised her, dies unexpectedly. The new mother has 11 months of progressively worsening depression and 5 months of unsuccessful treatment trials of two different selective serotonin reuptake inhibitors (SSRIs), one serotonin-norepinephrine reuptake inhibitor (SNRI), sedative-hypnotics, and antianxiety agents. She is functioning poorly. Her husband tells her: "This reminds me of your three prior episodes of depression—the one in college, the one after Joey was born, and then the one 2 years ago before you become pregnant. But now they're happening more frequently and lasting so long! I'm very worried about you. Sweetheart, our baby's not doing so well, and our other two kids miss the Mom they know."

The primary care physician arranges a consultation with a psychiatrist and her team. A comprehensive evaluation is completed, including a genome-wide sequencing scan (cost in 2014 $550, reimbursed by insurance carrier); stress-neuroendocrine-glucocorticoid, inflammatory (e.g., interleukin-10 [IL-10], C-reactive protein, tumor necrosis factor alpha), and neurotrophin measures (e.g., brain-derived neurotrophic factor, nerve growth factor); sleep and chronophysiology laboratory assessment; 1 week of actigraph measures at home to assess sleep phase patterns; functional magnetic resonance imaging with a stress challenge; and a thorough medical evaluation. Afterward, the psychiatrist states, "You appear to have what we call a treatment resistant depression. That doesn't mean it can't be treated; it is just more difficult. We are steadily developing a kind of a 'fingerprint' of depression and bipolar disorders to help us select the best treatments for each person, and your genotyping provides some understanding of why you had so much trouble with weight gain and sexual side effects when you took your antidepressant last time. But recent studies of new antidepressant approaches have been completed in a large network of depression centers, and results make me confident in saying

TABLE 1–1.	Common definitions and descriptions of Treatment Resistant Depression

Various criteria for Treatment Resistant Depression

Posttreatment decrease in a depression rating scale score of less than 50% from baseline

Posttreatment depression rating scale score remains higher than an established cutoff on a certain measure, even after a specified treatment time (e.g., a 17-item Hamilton Rating Scale for Depression [Ham-D] score >16 after 8–12 weeks of treatment)

Failure to achieve remission after one, two, or three adequate clinical treatment courses

Evidence of clinical response but failure to regain functional performance

Combinations of the above

Recommended criterion for Treatment Resistant Depression

Failure to achieve remission after two well-established antidepressant treatment courses known to have been of evidence-based acceptable dose and duration

---

that we can get you better without these same severe side effects. But remember, all treatments have some side effects. You will need to tolerate these so we can get you better. Second, your sleep laboratory results identified sleep apnea that is treatable, and addressing this will help counteract your depression."

The physician continues, "Just as importantly, the antidepressant and other medications we give you may require 2–4 months to work, so let's get ready for that now. Second, I am reassured that you and your husband are both here today. Family involvement is so important, so please plan to continue joint visits whenever possible. We also are going to be using new adaptations of cognitive-behavioral therapy (CBT) or interpersonal therapy (IPT) for addressing the recent stresses you encountered. Psychotherapy is very important, so please make those appointments right away. Next, we are adding additional medications—what we commonly call augmenting agents—because those same large-sample studies showed that for some people these medications may make it possible for your main treatments to work more effectively in the brain. A quick summary is that I would like you to take a multivitamin, omega-3, methylfolate, and vitamin D. This Depression Center 'Toolkit' pamphlet I am handing you explains why. Please, please don't take any other over-the-counter herbal or nutritional substances because they sometimes interfere with the medicines we will prescribe. In fact, I would prefer that you check with me before you take any other medicines, even things such as cold medicines. Continuing on, we are going to prescribe 'exercise.' To explain, physical exercise itself changes your brain's chemistry, specifically your neurotrophins, sometimes called 'plant foods of the brain.' So we are referring you to our exercise physiologist."

"Now, perhaps most important for you personally, we're confident you will improve. Should it not occur immediately, we have other options. But starting now, we must also think long term and focus on preventing you from getting another of these episodes. To do so, you almost certainly need to continue indefinitely the treatments that make you better to prevent future recurrences. Difficult as it might be to hear that, it is so important. A deal? Great! Believe me, it will be worth it."

Consequences of Major Depressive Disorder and Major Contributors to Treatment Resistance

MDD by itself generates one of the greatest burdens of all diseases worldwide, accounting for almost 11% of the burden of the 100 presumably most significant diseases (World Health Organization data [Lopez et al. 2006]). MDD, often colloquially referred to as "clinical depression," also is routinely found to be the second most costly disorder in the U.S. population (costs range from $81 billion to an estimated $130 billion annually). Of the estimated 30,000–35,000 suicides in the United States each year, 80%–90% are associated with clinical depression. Untreated clinical depression also is associated with earlier death from other medical causes.

A key element for clinicians is that perhaps 40% of these huge burdens, disabilities, and costs are attributable to TRD. Chief contributors to the burdens of MDD are summarized in Figure 1–1.

Major Contributors to Burdens of Major Depressive Disorder

Major contributors to burdens of MDD are interactive. To begin with, MDD is a prevalent, early-onset, genetically influenced disorder that commonly remains unrecognized, undiagnosed, and untreated. Episodes are often precipitated and accentuated by stress, especially for the earlier episodes, and tend to worsen and become more difficult to treat over time. Prevention of recurrence can be quite successful (Geddes et al. 2004), sustaining wellness in about 70%; yet much less emphasis is placed on such prevention with MDD than with bipolar disorder. Stigma, poor adherence, misinformation, and side effects commonly interfere with maintenance of wellness once it is achieved. Changes in neurogenesis (the processes by which new nerve cells are generated and others are maintained), brain circuitries (Sapolsky 2000), and brain morphology associated with multiple

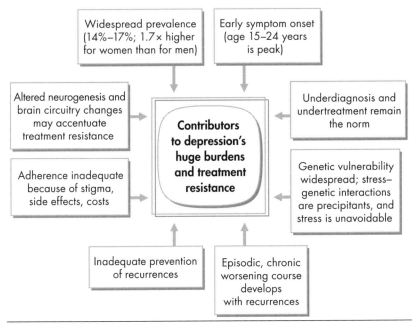

FIGURE 1–1. Contributors to depression's huge burdens.

Source. Adapted from Greden 2001b. Burdens summarized in Murray and Lopez 1996.

episodes or development of chronicity begin to occur and may make the individual's symptoms even less likely to respond to routine antidepressant treatments. Early awareness and interventions to counteract contributors to the ensuing disability are key parts of the roadmap for clinicians planning strategies for the treatment and prevention of TRD.

The major contributors to TRD (Table 1–2) are milestones or target areas in the roadmap for its effective treatment or prevention.

TABLE 1–2.   Major contributors to Treatment Resistant Depression (TRD)

Inadequate screening during younger years and among high-risk patients

Difficulties in achieving remission with current treatment approaches

Increasing risk of relapses or recurrences for those not achieving remission

Brain alterations of genomic expression, stress, neurotrophins, and circuitry changes associated with recurrences and chronicity may predispose to TRD

Poor adherence, often associated with stigma

Failure to use long-term or indefinite maintenance treatment among those with multiple prior episodes of TRD

Inadequate Screening During Younger Years and Among High-Risk Patients

MDD afflicts an estimated 14%–17% of people in their lifetime (bipolar disorder strikes 3%–5%). Symptom onset is most common during younger years for both disorders, peaking between ages 15 and 24 (Greden 2001a), as illustrated in Figure 1–2 (Zisook et al. 2007).

A prevailing misconception is that clinical depression is predominantly a disease with onset in elderly persons. The more characteristic pattern is that episodes develop during the youthful years but are milder in severity during early episodes and remain commonly undiagnosed or attributed to other causes, such as "adjustment reaction of adolescence." This diagnosis may actually derail early treatment for some who would benefit. Diagnoses tend to be made only years after onset, and by then many have developed the classic, more-severe profile following multiple episodes.

Early onset cries out for earlier screening and interventions because depression and bipolar disorder are most treatable in their earlier, milder stages (Judd et al. 2000). Screening is also advised at any age among those at high risk for MDD, such as individuals with cancer, diabetes, and cardiovascular disease, and geriatric patients.

Difficulties in Achieving Remission With Current Treatment Approaches

Currently used "first-line" interventions for TRD are not routinely effective in producing remission in most patients. The Sequenced Treatment Alternatives to Relieve Depression (STAR*D) study confirmed that most did not achieve remission in a large-sample database designed to assess the effectiveness of various single or combined antidepressant medications and evidence-based cognitive-behavioral therapy (CBT) for depressed outpatients (Insel and Wang 2009; Rush et al. 2006).

To summarize, the first phase of STAR*D treatment began with an SSRI (citalopram; Trevedi et al. 2006). At the conclusion of an adequate trial, only between 35% and 40% of the patients with MDD had achieved remission, depending on the criteria used. The remaining two-thirds, perhaps best considered as those with "early hints of treatment resistance," at least to SSRIs, were transitioned to another level in the STAR*D trial and were given combinations of antidepressants, augmenting agents, or CBT. The "big picture" showed that only an additional 30% of those with initial resistance at the first level achieved remission at the second level. Thus, after two sustained courses of antidepressant treatment, approxi-

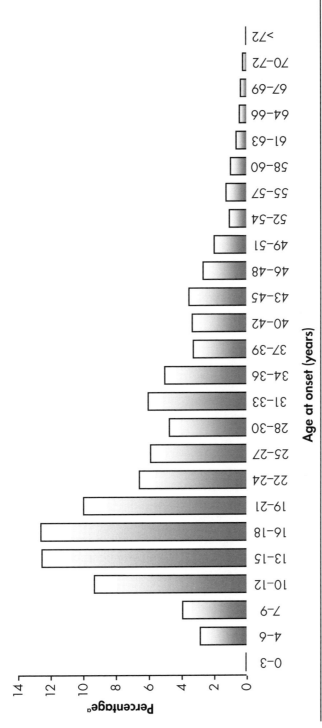

FIGURE 1–2. Onset of symptoms of first major depressive disorder episode.

Symptom onset peaks during younger years (Sequenced Treatment Alternatives to Relieve Depression study; *N* = 1,500). Diagnosis usually occurs years later.

[a]Percentage of individuals with eventual major depressive disorder who experienced onset of symptoms at respective ages.

Source. Adapted from Zisook et al. 2007.

mately 60 % of the total depressed group had achieved wellness, but 40 % were still "treatment resistant." Even after two additional—four total— treatment levels almost a full year later, approximately 30 % of those with MDD still had not achieved remission. A simple metric for remembering that progressively smaller percentages are likely to achieve remission during each of the four levels of treatment in STAR*D is "35–30–13–13." TRD is not as responsive to current first-line antidepressant approaches.

Treatment resistance to current first-line antidepressant approaches can arguably be perceived as having begun after the second failed attempt at achieving remission. Earlier recognition and earlier determination of those at risk for TRD, followed by more effective courses of treatment, are necessary. Such personalized treatment approaches remain elusive, however, so we must use the available modalities more effectively, and perhaps earlier and in different combinations.

For clinicians who plan "next steps" for those who are medication resistant in early stages: It appeared to make little difference in STAR*D whether unresponsive depressed patients were switched after one treatment failure to another SSRI (sertraline), to an SNRI (venlafaxine), or to bupropion; remission rates remained smaller than those achieved during the first treatment, ranging between 17.6 % and 24.8 % (differences not significant) (Rush et al. 2006). For those receiving augmentation agents (bupropion or buspirone), the remission rates were 29.7 % and 31.1 %, respectively. For those still not achieving remission, Fava and colleagues (2006) described random assignment to another 14 treatment weeks with nortriptyline (with dosing up to 200 mg/day) or mirtazapine (ranging up to 60 mg/day). Remission rates remained lower than in prior treatment attempts: 19.8 % and 12.3 %, respectively. Lithium (maximum dose of 900 mg/day) or triiodothyronine (T_3; maximum dose of 50 µg/day) also was given to 142 STAR*D individuals. T_3 produced improvements in 24.7 % and lithium in 15.9 %; these differences did not achieve statistical significance. In the final phase of STAR*D, McGrath et al. (2006) evaluated the combination of venlafaxine plus mirtazapine or tranylcypromine, a monoamine oxidase inhibitor (MAOI). Remission rates remained disappointing (13.7 % and 6.9 %, respectively), but it must be recognized that remission already had failed to occur in multiple prior treatment trials in these patients.

So what is the clinician to do when encountering those who have not responded to repetitive prior treatment attempts? Thase (2008) reviewed comparative studies between SSRIs and SNRIs and pointed out that few individual studies found any significant differences in outcome when these agents were compared. Meta-analyses previously indicated that the SNRI venlafaxine may produce modest improvement of 5 %–10 % in re-

---

TABLE 1–3.   Clinical barriers to achieving remission among patients with Treatment Resistant Depression

Pathophysiologies or genetic polymorphisms among some patients that make them unresponsive to traditional medication or psychotherapy treatments

Misdiagnosed etiologies

Pharmacogenetic metabolism patterns that prevent adequate treatment levels despite apparently adequate dosages and duration

Brain changes, produced by chronic depressed states, that make individuals progressively more treatment resistant

Combinations of these and other variables

---

mission rates, although no advantages were identified when venlafaxine was contrasted with the SSRI escitalopram.

In essence, modestly large-sample naturalistic studies such as STAR*D, randomized controlled trials (RCTs), and meta-analyses all appear to indicate collectively that no known one or two antidepressant medications routinely lead to remission among those receiving first-line treatments, no automatic next step is known to produce remission for those who have failed to respond to the initial SSRI, and remission is more difficult to achieve with each treatment failure (Figure 1–3). Although we do not know for any given individual the underlying reasons for lack of response to established antidepressant treatments, likely clinical barriers are summarized in Table 1–3.

Despite the prevalence and the disabling consequences of TRD, an important message for patients is that persistence is rewarded. If response to medication is partial but incomplete, optimization of dosage is indicated. Switching is not the first recommended step. Augmentation is the next choice for patients who continue to have partial but incomplete response to the initial medication. Augmentation should be routinely used in starting treatment for anyone with prior TRD.

In STAR*D, each new treatment combination produced incremental remission. It is important to remind patients and family members of this pattern. Sustaining hope for those with a disorder that has hopelessness as a core feature is vital.

Increased Risk of Relapses or Recurrences for Those Not Achieving Remission

When untreated, episodes are generally characterized by a recurrent, worsening course progressing over decades, with episodes becoming more frequent, more chronic, and less strongly linked with severe stressors, as schematically illustrated in Figure 1–4 (Greden 2001b).

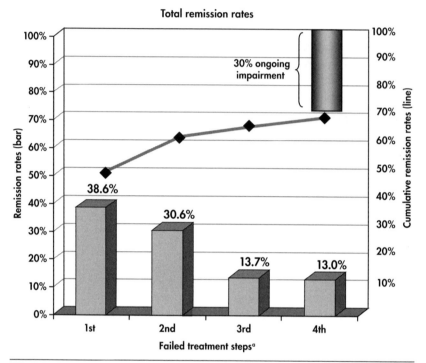

FIGURE 1–3. **Increased difficulty of achieving remission with repeated treatment failures.**

Treatment resistance to first-line antidepressant treatments is common and remission harder to achieve with each treatment failure. After four optimized, well-delivered treatments, approximately 70% of patients achieve remission. However, an estimated 30% continue to experience significant impairment even after four levels of treatment. With each prior treatment failure, remission rates decrease, and relapse rates increase.

[a]Percentages reflect approximate remission rates per level.

Source.   Adapted from Greden 2001b.

The relapse rate for those with MDD steadily climbed in STAR*D after each failure to achieve and sustain remission, starting at 58% if remission was achieved after the first treatment level and jumping to 68%, 76%, and 83% after the second, third, and fourth steps, respectively (Warden et al. 2007). This pattern is sometimes referred to as brain *sensitization* or *kindling* when it follows prior episodes. Increasing rates of recurrences with each new episode further explain why earlier sustainability of wellness is an essential goal for those who get better. It is not known what pathophysiologies underlie these greater risks for recurrence.

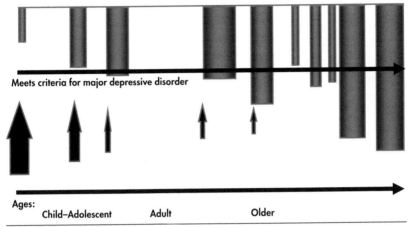

FIGURE 1–4. Course of untreated depression.

Untreated clinical depression generally has an episodic, recurrent lifetime course. Stressors (designated by *vertical arrows*) lessen in importance as more episodes (designated by *gray bars*) occur.

Source. Adapted from Greden 2001b.

Not surprisingly, as unresponsiveness becomes more evident, total health costs increase with each depression medication regimen change, essentially doubling from $600 per month in the first level to $1,200 per month in the fourth level of STAR*D. Improving and *maintaining* individuals' health is both clinically and fiscally wise (Kamlet et al. 1995).

Neuroscience Factors That May Predispose to TRD

This chapter is not designed to address in detail the incredible neuroscience advances that are enabling better understanding of depression or bipolar disorder. However, these are so clearly linked with TRD treatment options that a few highlights are necessary.

First, genomic mechanisms underlie patterns of depression and bipolar disorder and are steadily being unveiled. Second, stress is a known precipitant of depressive episodes and causes chronically elevated glucocorticoids or "stress hormones"; these actions appear to reduce brain neurotrophins (sometimes referred to as "plant foods" of the brain). Such brain alterations in chronically depressed patients endanger neurons or brain cells, alter neuroplasticity and cell proliferation, and appear to contribute to morphological changes in the brain (Sapolsky 2000; Sheline et al. 1996). Third, neurotransmitter circuitry functions are altered. Fourth, these changes may combine to produce not only the classic signs and symptoms of MDD but also modest cognitive impairments, alterations in insulin resistance and other biochemical pathways that may contribute to metabolic syndromes, and increased risk of diabetes and hyperlipidemia.

Within the past 15 years, we have learned that the more episodes or days of depression one has (Sheline et al. 1996) and the longer one struggles with severe symptoms, the more likely it becomes that adverse morphological brain changes may develop. Although no causal link has been proven, the parallel correlation of these developments with clinical course and treatment response strongly hints that the cumulative brain changes in those with multiple episodes of depression may be a key contributing step to development of treatment resistance. If depression is untreated for prolonged periods, the depressed person's brain and other parts of his or her body pay a price.

Importantly, effective treatment of depression may reverse this pattern. It has been known for some years that antidepressants (Dranovsky and Hen 2006), environmental enrichment, exercise (van Praag 2009; van Praag et al. 1999), and learning (Leuner et al. 2004) stimulate neurogenesis. It is promising that Boldrini et al. (2009) recently presented the first evidence that antidepressants increase neural progenitor cells in the human hippocampus. Future studies will seek to determine whether these effects have relevance for treating TRD; it is reasonable to infer that they will.

A formulation supported by emerging clinical and neuroscience observations is that we are dealing with "depressions" rather than "depression"; that MDDs are episodic, recurrent, chronic disorders that characteristically need to be managed over one's lifetime rather than "cured" after a single episode; and that "personalized" treatment adherence and maintenance are required to address the unique pathophysiologies of each individual. However, we still lack knowledge about which specific treatment works for which individual, so until research fills the void, we need to make better use of all the treatment strategies we have. If individuals with MDD are converted to wellness as early as possible in their lifetime course and wellness is sustained, a significantly smaller percentage may develop multiple episodes and treatment resistance. The roadmap aims to help identify and promote such preventive practices.

Frequent Association of Stigma and Poor Adherence

Adherence to antidepressant medications, psychotherapy, and other treatments tends to diminish steadily over the first 6 months after initiation of treatment. By then, fewer than half of patients are adhering to the recommended treatment course. Poor adherence is a huge obstacle to a good outcome.

Stigma is one of the more powerful contributors to development of poor adherence and thus to TRD (see Figure 1–1). It deters individuals from seeking, entering, and adhering to treatments. Even when effective treatments are administered and produce improvements, and even when clinicians promote adherence to maintenance treatment because it is effective, many resist because of side effects, cost, stigma, or misinformation. When individuals discontinue their treatment prematurely, especially if they have had multiple prior episodes, relapses tend to occur within several years. Approximately two-thirds of those with multiple prior episodes will relapse within several years after switching to placebo or no treatment unless effective maintenance treatment is provided (Geddes et al. 2003). These long-term data failed to receive adequate attention in recent, controversial meta-analysis reports suggesting that antidepressant effectiveness varies with severity and may be only modestly more effective than placebo for those with mild symptoms (Fournier et al. 2010). These analyses neglect the perspective that to prevent greater severity and TRD from developing, MDD must be treated as a characteristically chronic long-term illness.

Misguided concepts reinforce stigma (Golberstein et al. 2008). Most Americans now recognize that depression is a brain illness, but 22% still report perceiving it as a sign of "personal weakness." Only 3% identify the same for cancer and 4% for diabetes.

As we search for better answers, stigma also stands in the way of procuring support for conducting and translating new research into new public health programs. Mental health research receives approximately one-eighth the funding provided to cancer research, even though more people in the United States are affected by depression and bipolar illness than by cancer, and the total medical costs are higher (American Cancer Society 2008; Horner et al. 2006; Kessler et al. 2005).

Stigma can be conquered. Cancer, once saddled with its own stigma, serves as a prototype. The "war on cancer" was launched in the 1970s to find better treatments, earlier recognition, and prevention strategies (Rehemtulla 2009). The cancer initiative sought to establish comprehensive cancer centers within several hundred miles of every U.S. resident, and today there is a national network of cancer centers supported by the National Cancer Institute as well as an ancillary network promoting clinical translation and guidelines. Using the gains made in these National Institutes of Health "crown jewels," National Cancer Institute research initiatives from 1975 to 2005 drove an increase in the 5-year survival rate for cancer from 50.1% to 67.8% during this 30-year period. No similar improvements in depression outcomes or reductions in suicide rates have occurred during the past 40 years. Efforts to conquer depression are likely to benefit from following the same strategies used in the cancer initiative (as well as in cardiovascular, diabetes, Parkinson's, and other disorders). Such efforts are under way (www.NNDC.org).

Roadmap for Effective Treatment of Treatment Resistant Depression

The contributors to TRD are milestones on the roadmap for treating and maintaining wellness among TRD patients. The roadmap is schematically illustrated in Figure 1–5.

1. Screen with self-rating scales and schedule weekly to monthly monitoring. The roadmap starts with screening. The high prevalence and disease burden of depression described earlier support more widespread screening for those within peak ages at onset or those at high risk because of other medical diseases. Evidence supports screening (Wang et al. 2007). In 2009, the Institute of Medicine and National Research Council strongly endorsed mental health screening as accurate and effective for identifying adolescent depression. Yet more than two-thirds of primary care clinicians and many psychiatrists and mental health clinicians do not use routine screening for adolescent patients (Ozer et al. 2009). The same patterns appear to prevail equally for patients of all ages; screening also favorably affects workplace outcomes (Wang et al. 2007). Depression screening is well accepted in primary care by patients, parents, and providers (Zuckerbrot et al. 2007). Screening without follow-up treatment is obviously not helpful, so treatment or referral networks should accompany screening strategies. When a screening questionnaire indicates that an individual has "clinical risk," clinicians should respond proactively by monitoring more closely, repeating rating scales, treating earlier to prevent long-term chronicity, and making referrals if indicated.

We strongly encourage adoption of one standardized, validated screening and severity scale so that numbers can be understood by all, similar to hearing that someone has a temperature of 103°F and understanding the implications. Our recommended options for screening and monitoring are listed in Table 1–4. Schools, colleges, obstetric clinics, and facilities in high-risk medical settings should develop special strategies for screening (Ozer et al. 2009). These "vital signs" of psychiatry and mental health care deserve far more widespread dissemination.

2. Identify and respond earlier to risks for TRD. Clinical warning signs of TRD are summarized in Table 1–5.

1. Screen patients with self-rating scales and repeat with weekly to monthly monitoring.
2. Identify and respond earlier to clinical warning signs of TRD: Prior failure to respond to a single course of antidepressant of adequate dose and duration; multiple prior episodes; family history of mood disorders; prior alcohol or drug abuse; rapid mood changes; significant anxiety; suicidal thoughts, acts, or plans; or overt reluctance to enter or maintain treatment.
3. Conduct thorough medical and comprehensive laboratory evaluation.
4. Educate thoroughly before treatment and recommend a "toolkit" to aid self-management.
5. Combine evidence-based psychotherapy with psychopharmacological medications and ensure adequate dose and duration.
6. Make initial selection of psychopharmacological medications.
   a. Restart previously used effective antidepressant if the recurrence developed primarily because patient stopped medication.
   b. Consider SNRIs, TCAs, and MAOIs as "first line" for TRD if prior failed trials were of SSRIs.
   c. Combine chosen antidepressant(s) with atypical antipsychotic (quetiapine or aripiprazole).
   d. Combine two antidepressants from different classes than were previously used.
7. Augment routinely for those with TRD.
   a. Lithium, thyroid (T_3, T_4) or both.
   b. Omega-3, vitamin D, methylfolate.
8. Start exercise and nutrition program to enhance brain neurotrophins and counteract metabolic syndrome.
9. Counsel patients to avoid herbal medications and tramadol, to inquire beforehand about any new medication (e.g. antihistamines), and to avoid Internet suggestions without consultation.
10. Counteract stigma and emphasize self-management to enhance adherence.
11. Refer for consultation if no remission after one or two additional trials.
12. Initiate pharmacogenetic testing for those who repeatedly do not respond to adequate high doses, for those who cannot tolerate even modest doses, and possibly to predict personalized treatment responsivity.
13. Refer for consultation and/or neuromodulation if no response after several additional treatment failures.
    a. Electroconvulsive therapy
    b. Repetitive transcranial magnetic stimulation
    c. Vagus nerve stimulation
14. Consider research strategies if still no improvement:
    a. Deep brain stimulation
    b. Ketamine infusion or other glutamate modulation strategies
    c. Antiglucocorticoid therapy
15. Establish indefinite maintenance with treatments that achieved remission.

FIGURE 1–5. Roadmap for effective treatment of Treatment Resistant Depression (TRD).

MAOIs = monoamine oxidase inhibitors; SSRIs = selective serotonin reuptake inhibitors; SNRIs = serotonin-norepinephrine reuptake inhibitors; TCAs = tricyclic antidepressants.

TABLE 1–4. Recommended screening and severity rating scales to promote standardization for depression and related conditions ("vital signs")

Condition/scale	Reference
Depression	
Quick Inventory of Depressive Symptomatology— Self-Report (QIDS-SR)	Rush et al. 2003
Patient Health Questionnaire–9 (PHQ-9)	Spitzer et al. 1999
Co-occurring alcohol/addictions	
CAGE (**C**ut down, **A**nnoyed, **G**uilty, **E**ye-opener)	Allen et al. 1995
Co-occurring pain	
Brief Pain Inventory (BPI); co-occurring chronic pain	Keller et al. 2004
Suicide risk	
Concise Health Risk Tracking (CHRT) scale	Trivedi et al. 2010
Columbia Suicide-Severity Rating Scale (C-SSRS)	Posner et al. 2007

For individuals who are reluctant to pursue treatment, or for those who have a history of poor adherence, motivational interviews that make use of family or other supporters, coaches, religious leaders, or selected Web videos should be encouraged. The goal is to enhance mental health and neuroscience literacy. The overall messages are that "you are not alone, these are treatable illnesses, treatment works, and it is a sign of real strength to seek treatment." Patients with other medical risks warrant special consideration, closer monitoring, and earlier consideration of more assertive treatment to prevent TRD *before* multiple episodes have occurred.

3. Conduct thorough medical and comprehensive laboratory evaluations. A clinically significant but numerically unknown number of cases of TRD are attributable to co-occurring medical etiologies, including hypothyroidism, cancer, multiple sclerosis, diabetes, and many others. Truly thorough medical and laboratory profiles are recommended whenever possible for adequate assessment. Appropriate assessments may include serum or salivary cortisol level or, preferably, the combined dexamethasone/corticotropin-releasing hormone test (Heuser et al. 1994); thyroid measures; inflammatory cytokine assessments (e.g., IL-1, IL-6; IL-18); and vitamin D and folate levels (Stahl 2007). Alterations of each have been linked with TRD cases, but more research is needed to know how commonly these occur.

Sleep apnea is an important and overlooked contributor to TRD. Children have an estimated 2%–8% prevalence of apnea, but adults older than 55 have startling 30%–60% prevalence rates (Giles et al. 2006). Ob-

TABLE 1–5.   Clinical warning signs of Treatment Resistant Depression

Prior failure to respond to a single course of antidepressant or psychotherapy treatment of adequate dose and duration

Multiple prior episodes

Family history of mood disorders or treatment resistance

Prior alcohol or drug misuse, abuse, or dependency

Rapid mood changes

Significant anxiety

Suicidal thoughts or prior suicide attempts

Overt reluctance to enter treatment despite evident mood symptoms

structive sleep apnea and increased depression scores are estimated to be associated between 25% and 40% of the time. Cases of TRD may be exacerbated or even caused by unrecognized and untreated sleep apnea. Too few studies have been conducted to determine whether treatment of sleep apnea tends to resolve MDDs in general, and even fewer assessments have been conducted for TRD, but common sense dictates that if sleep apnea is present, it should be treated concomitantly with any depression. The primary treatment currently used is continuous positive airway pressure (Giles et al. 2006), but other evidence-based approaches are available.

To address other sleep issues efficiently and inexpensively, actigraph wrist or ankle devices are now available to measure activity and light exposure on a 24-hour, 7 days a week basis for 1- to 2-week intervals (Hedner et al. 2004). If sleep phase shifts are present, such as staying up until early morning hours and then sleeping until late morning or even afternoon hours, phase shifting should be arranged gradually. Patients also should be instructed to avoid late-night exposure to computer screens and advised to put red lights in bathrooms to avoid bright-light exposure that might meaningfully alter sleep patterns. Behavioral sleep programs are described further by Armitage and Arnedt in Chapter 9 of this book.

4. Educate patients and families thoroughly before treatment and provide a "toolkit" to promote self-management.   Informed patients and families are crucial partners for overcoming TRD. Education must start before treatment. Patients can and should be informed with a supportive, optimistic approach about the likelihood that 8–12 weeks, and sometimes longer, will be required before concluding that treatments are not working and that once better, they are entering a lifetime approach to treatment.

Education at the initial stage should dramatize the need to avoid alcohol, drugs, and over-the-counter medications and to do one's best to tolerate predictable side effects of the antidepressant treatments. It may be beneficial to explain that side effects indicate that the medications are having their anticipated actions in the brain and elsewhere. Treatment switches every several weeks do *not* produce good outcomes, so patience and cooperation from the depressed individual and family, partners, or friends are essential if clinicians are to avoid multiple requests such as "let's try a new treatment since this one doesn't seem to be working." Self-management approaches are wisely being recommended by many clinicians in the form of "toolkits" (www.depressiontoolkit.org), and referral to a source may pay long-term dividends.

5. Combine evidence-based psychotherapy with psychopharmacological medication for depressive illnesses whenever possible.   Combinations of CBT or IPT and appropriate psychopharmacological medication have repeatedly been reported to be more effective for TRD. Flynn and Himle review this topic in Chapter 10 of this book. Such combined treatments are effective even in younger patients. Brent et al. (2008) reported that among adolescent depressed patients who failed to respond to an SSRI, 54.8% of those who subsequently received CBT along with a different antidepressant responded, compared with 40.5% of those who took the medication alone ($P = 0.009$). March and colleagues (2004) observed that the combination appeared beneficial in preventing adolescent suicide attempts or death by suicide. This pattern has been confirmed in adults and geriatric patients as well, as reviewed in subsequent chapters.

If therapy is to be provided by a separate clinician, desired therapist qualifications include experience (a growing number of CBT and IPT therapists are being certified); willingness to collaborate closely and share information with other clinicians; willingness to involve family members, close friends, or partners in the treatment program; and commitment to support the need for combination medications when indicated (Riba and Balon 2008). If therapist unavailability or financial constraints make psychotherapy unfeasible, brief CBT manuals or online CBT programs should be recommended for patients and family members (Wright et al. 2010).

6. Make the initial selection of psychopharmacological medications. Initial selection of psychopharmacological medications is addressed by Sen and colleagues in greater detail in Chapter 2 of this book. SSRIs are valuable and widely used medications; however, they have become mainstays of first-line treatment primarily because of safety and side-effect benefits, not because they are significantly more effective (Thase 2008).

Several guidelines deserve emphasis. First, all treatment options should be considered for those with TRD. Second, documented prior response to a specific medication or a family history of favorable response to a specific drug (less well established) may be a promising predictor. Lifestyle modifications are indicated as well as medications and psychotherapy. Simply prescribing a different course of medication or another course of psychotherapy is much less likely to be effective for those who have not responded to prior treatments. Prescribing a *comprehensive* approach is analogous to planning an effective treatment plan for diabetes mellitus. Third, we now recognize that it may take longer than the previously accepted 3–4 weeks to judge treatment response; thus, if patients are showing slow but steady improvement on rating scales, continuation of the ongoing treatment for another 3–4 weeks may be appropriate. Generally, if no improvements or minimal improvements have occurred by 8 weeks, other steps are required. This judgment should be supported by serial ratings of severity with the nine-item depression scale of the Patient Health Questionnaire (PHQ-9) or Quick Inventory of Depressive Symptomatology–Self-Report (QIDS-SR). Fourth, for those whose symptoms do not respond after several well-established combinations and augmentations and adequate time duration, consideration and discussion of nonmedication alternatives such as newer neuromodulation treatments (repetitive transcranial magnetic stimulation [rTMS] or vagus nerve stimulation [VNS]) or electroconvulsive treatments are indicated. Although such treatments are less favorably perceived by many and evoke expressions of concern, they may be necessary to break the treatment-resistant pattern and perhaps could be even lifesaving. Achieving remission sooner is preferable to having patients remain in a state of chronic depression for additional months or years.

Inadequate standardized data for TRD make it impossible to recommend one standardized treatment approach that applies for all. The following recommendations are a blend of the evidence-based reports and clinical experiences of those who work with TRD patients.

a. Restart the previously used effective antidepressant if the patient's recurrence developed primarily because maintenance medications were stopped or dosages reduced. "Newer is not always better" when selecting an antidepressant. If a specific treatment has worked for one or more prior episodes of MDD and a new episode of depression has developed primarily because the patient stopped taking the medication or significantly reduced the dosage, the same antidepressant can justifiably be considered as the first-line agent, or the dosage can be reinstated to prior levels as soon as tolerated.

Ruhé and colleagues (2006) pointed out that little evidence indicates increasing the dose of an SSRI improves response for those who are not improving. However, anecdotally, increasing SSRI dosage is observed to be beneficial among those who have shown partial, steady response but not remission, perhaps because they are metabolizing the medications rapidly.

Brent and colleagues (2008) concluded that if depression in an adolescent does not respond to an initial SSRI, a different antidepressant should be used, and combined CBT is preferable to prescribing a second antidepressant in isolation.

b. Consider SNRIs, tricyclic antidepressants, and MAOIs as first-line agents for TRD.   If only SSRIs have been tried and have failed, SNRIs can be considered first-line agents. Tricyclic antidepressants (TCAs) and MAOIs have unfortunately been discarded by too many prescribers for individuals with TRD. If not used previously, they also should be considered first line if symptoms have not responded to several courses of SSRIs or SNRIs. All antidepressants appear to have approximately equal efficacy in published studies, but clinicians should recall that such data emerge from large samples, and each person likely has "personalized" underlying neurobiology or pharmacogenetic mechanisms that make his or her symptoms respond to the additional mechanistic actions associated with antidepressants of a different class than previously used.

c. Combine selected antidepressant with atypical antipsychotic medication. For those whose TRD is based on repeated failures to respond to a traditional first-line agent, the selected antidepressant can be combined with an atypical antipsychotic to procure different mechanisms of action or different pathways of drug metabolism. The fact that some of these atypical antipsychotics incorporate partial dopaminergic and unique serotonin receptor agonist activities may have usefulness for some individuals. Selection should begin with a quick review to determine that there are no known drug-drug interactions or competing metabolic pathways with other medications or over-the-counter products being used.

As early as 1999, Ostroff and Nelson reported that risperidone augmented SSRI treatment of major depression, and Ghaemi and Katzow (1999) observed that quetiapine seemed to do the same for those with TRD. A positive placebo-controlled trial of olanzapine for TRD followed in 2001 (Shelton et al. 2001). Papakostas et al. (2005) reported that aripiprazole improved outcomes when coupled with SSRIs in SSRI-resistant MDD, and other atypical antipsychotics also have been studied. Suppes et al. (2009) compared the combination of quetiapine with additional medications and quetiapine with placebo and showed that quetiapine plus lithium or divalproex significantly reduced the time to recurrence of *any* mood event, whether depression or mania. Data for adolescents are modest, but scattered studies have shown benefit (Pathak et al. 2005). Quetiapine and aripiprazole have been approved by the U.S. Food and Drug Administration (FDA) for treatment of TRD.

Patients at any age who begin taking second-generation antipsychotics or certain antidepressants must be monitored closely by periodically assessing weight and abdominal girth measures for metabolic syndrome, diabetes, hyperlipidemia, and associated concerns. Atypical antipsychotics and antidepressant medications are effective for some but are documented to induce weight gain and probably modifications in insulin resistance and lipid metabolism. SSRIs occasionally cause short-term weight loss but also are associated with long-term weight gain. All patients receiving these treatment regimens should be enrolled in exercise programs if their health permits.

7. Augment routinely for those with significant TRD. As illustrated by the STAR*D study design and results, augmentation strategies currently recommended most frequently include thyroid (T_3 or T_4), lithium, bupropion, or another antidepressant of a different class. The only agents that have been studied enough to generate some evidence-based efficacy as augmenting medications are lithium, thyroid, and atypical antipsychotics.

When receiving lithium and thyroid agents, however, as illustrated in the STAR*D study results, most patients fail to respond. Nevertheless, for those with significant TRD, these and other augmenting strategies can be recommended as soon as TRD is diagnosed. Most such strategies appear to be relatively safe with careful monitoring. Trials that increase response rate by an additional 10%–20% may appear to represent modest gains, but such seemingly small improvements may well represent one of the few avenues to remission.

Additional augmentations to consider include a multivitamin, methylfolate (7.5–15 mg/day), omega-3 (500–1,000 mg/day), and vitamin D (1,000 IU/day) (Berk et al. 2007; Papakostas et al. 2004). For depressed patients with prior weight loss, inactivity, cardiac issues, or other medical problems, such interventions might be recommended from the onset. The rationale for methylfolate is that folate deficiency in the brain has been associated with greater risk of depression and may reduce the action of antidepressants, possibly attributable to genetic polymorphisms in some individuals (Stahl 2007). Antidepressant improvements have been noted in some when folic acid, folinic acid, or L-methylfolate (active in the brain) is added as an augmenting agent, presumably because of folate's trimonoamine modulator actions that enhance synthesis of dopamine, serotonin, and norepinephrine (Coppen and Bailey 2000; Stahl 2007). These should be continued for 3–4 months before it is concluded they are not

beneficial. Additional studies are needed. Data are similarly modest for vitamin D supplementation, but the literature is growing (Berk et al. 2007).

Anecdotal reports suggest that pindolol, dopaminergic agonists, stimulants, modafinil, estrogen, testosterone, and others may be successful in
augmenting, but data are sketchy and largely unsubstantiated.

**8. Start an exercise and nutrition program to enhance brain neurotrophins
and counteract metabolic syndrome.**   Exercise and nutrition have been
anecdotally perceived as relevant to mood regulation for centuries. Until
recently, documentation of effectiveness and of possible mechanisms for
any improvement has been lacking. Evidence, however, is growing rapidly,
and even though exercise and nutritional programs should not be considered sufficient as isolated treatments, they arguably should be considered
necessary accompaniments of pharmacotherapy, stress management, psychotherapy, sleep interventions, and other fundamental elements of a
treatment roadmap for anyone with depression or bipolar illnesses, analogous to treatment of diabetes and cardiovascular diseases. To illustrate
the importance of exercise and nutrition, a dedicated chapter is provided
in this text (see Evans and Burghardt, Chapter 12).

**9. Counsel patients to avoid herbal medications, inquire beforehand about
starting any new medication, and avoid following Internet suggestions without discussion.** Millions of herbal medication users appear unaware that
many or most such medications have minimal or no documented evidence
of effectiveness; some may be harmful for certain individuals. Many
herbal medications are metabolized through the same cytochrome P450
pathways as other medications being prescribed, and their interactions
may interfere with crucial medical actions, produce unwanted side effects
leading to poor adherence, or actually precipitate harmful medical consequences. It is appropriate to recommend that patients not start herbals or
any other prescribed or over-the-counter medications without first checking with their clinician.

Clinicians are further advised to caution TRD patients about altering
treatments unilaterally on the basis of anecdotal Internet or Internet blog
recommendations that they may have read. Consultation with clinicians
is again important. Because effective self-management is beneficial, referral to a trusted Web site of a well-referenced self-management toolkit,
such as www.depressiontoolkit.org, is recommended.

**10. Counteract stigma and emphasize self-management to enhance adher-
ence.**   Stigma lessens adherence to depression treatments and thus promotes relapse or recurrence (Melfi et al. 1998). Stigma is reported to be
greater among males, elderly patients, minorities, those with lower socio-

economic status, and those without familiarity with mental health services. Lin and colleagues (2003) and Ludman and associates (2003) showed that interventions to improve adherence produced positive changes, including improvements in depression symptom scores.

Clinicians should proactively combat misguided perceptions with appropriate messages and attitude, categorizing depression and bipolar disorder as treatable brain illnesses comparable to other medical illnesses. When coupled with effective literature, this helps counteract the prevailing impression among some that these remain signs of "weakness."

Words count. Euphemisms and phrases such as "let's try this for awhile" should be avoided. When presented as a medical condition, the phrase *clinical depression* has become quite understandable, and stigma is fading for its use. Involvement of family members, exposure to toolkits, alignment of dates of all the patient's medication prescriptions so they become due on the same date, periodic telephone calls, and refill reminders also enhance adherence (Valenstein et al. 2009). Availability of accurate literature and involvement in advocacy groups such as the Depression and Bipolar Support Alliance (DBSA) are important steps.

11. Refer for consultation if no remission occurs after one or two additional trials. If the previously discussed strategies have not succeeded in producing improvement after adequate duration, referrals should be sought. If the patient is geographically or financially constrained, telemedicine options should be explored.

12. Initiate pharmacogenetic testing for those whose symptoms repeatedly fail to respond to adequate high doses or who cannot tolerate even modest doses, and to predict personalized treatment responsivity. Most clinical trials involve comparisons of an active agent with placebo, and few have explored pharmacogenetic assessments adequately. It is highly probable that an unknown number of participants in trials have not responded because they were ultrarapid metabolizers and never achieved effective plasma and brain levels. Conversely, a small number may have discontinued medications because they were poor metabolizers and side effects developed. Clinicians currently rely on clinical judgments for such determinations. For those whose symptoms have repeatedly failed to respond to seemingly adequate dosages or who were unable to tolerate repetitive treatment trials, pharmacogenetic testing can be recommended. As prices decline, such testing predictably will become routine for those with TRD and perhaps, as suggested in the introductory vignette, for *all* patients with MDD.

Common genetic variants are reported to be associated with antidepressant response (McMahon et al. 2006; Perlis et al. 2008), but predictive strength is still modest at best; in the future, combinations of genetic variants most likely will be developed and become part of a personalized treatment approach.

Perlis et al. (2008) provided an early example of this strategy. They linked outcomes over 3 years with a pharmacogenetic test result from the STAR*D study reported to indicate greater likelihood of SSRI response (serotonin hydroxytryptamine variation) and compared responses to an SSRI and to bupropion. Their analyses of cost-effectiveness and societal benefit suggested that such testing is likely to become cost-effective for improving quality-adjusted life-years as the price for the test declines. It is hoped that will occur soon, but more studies and less-expensive lab tests are both needed.

13. Consider neuromodulation if still no response after several additional treatment failures.   If remission has not yet been achieved after one or two additional trials, it is time to consider more assertive treatment steps and/or referral to specialty centers providing such treatments. Currently available neuromodulation treatments include electroconvulsive therapy (ECT), rTMS, and VNS. The FDA has approved these for TRD and other medical conditions. ECT, rTMS, and VNS are addressed in detail by Taylor and colleagues in Chapter 11 of this book.

A widespread perception about rTMS and VNS is that their seemingly low response and remission rates indicate their lack of or lesser effectiveness when compared with medications. In our view, this is a premature and perhaps an erroneous conclusion. These treatments were tested on those with TRD whose symptoms had not responded to one or more treatment trials, and outcome results for rTMS, for example, appeared comparable to those for traditional pharmacological or psychotherapeutic augmentation or combination strategies from STAR*D and other trials when used for the same severely ill patients. In fact, few pharmacological agents have been approved for TRD by the FDA. For some, such as those with diabetes, cardiovascular disease, or ongoing suicide risk, neuromodulation treatments may produce fewer significant adverse events than do complex polypharmacy regimens. Although these techniques cannot yet be considered to have proven effectiveness for TRD, the evidence may be as compelling as for many medications. This commentary simply illustrates the pressing need for greater research.

14. Consider research strategies if still no improvement.   There arguably have been no major breakthroughs in psychopharmacology for mood disorders for more than 20 years (Berton and Nestler 2006; Mathew et al. 2008). New treatment strategies are being sought for TRD. Sen and Sanacora

(2008) and Mathew et al. (2008) summarized evidence supporting neurotransmitter systems as new targets for antidepressants, agents that act more promptly, or those with new mechanisms. There is some reason for optimism. Sample strategies include glutamate modulation using ketamine infusions and riluzole; *S*-adenosylmethionine (SAM-e); antiglucocorticoid therapy; and combinations of medications with other new approaches, such as rTMS, magnetic stimulation treatment (MST), or DBS. These and other topics are addressed briefly by Sen and colleagues in Chapter 2 of this volume (Brennan et al. 2010; Zarate et al. 2004, 2006).

Deep brain stimulation (DBS) is a research tool and has been studied for those with TRD in small samples only, but results to date have been encouraging. In the years ahead, DBS conceivably could become as widely used for individuals with severe TRD as it is for those with medication-refractory Parkinson's disease (Goodman and Insel 2009). The next 5 years predictably will witness increased focus on this modality, a trend that is already evident (Holtzheimer 2010).

A great deal of treatment development and research translation remain to be done before any of these techniques are usable in routine clinical practice, but knowing that future options are being evaluated promises additional hope for those struggling with or treating TRD.

15. Continue indefinite maintenance with treatments that achieved remission.   Greden (2001a, p. 15) suggested that "clinicians need to shift their emphasis to prioritizing the *prevention* of recurrences and using all methods shown to make a difference." Nothing has changed. Multiple studies confirm that ongoing medication maintenance is significantly superior to discontinuation of treatment or placebo in preventing recurrences among those who have had prior episodes.

Geddes and colleagues (2003) showed in a large meta-analysis covering 31 trials and 4,410 patients with multiple episodes that the medication class that results in remission—whether this be noradrenergic reuptake inhibitors, monoamine oxidase inhibitors, tricyclic antidepressants, SSRIs, or other—is meaningfully superior in sustaining wellness when compared with placebo crossovers ($P = 0.0001$ in pooled odds ratio). An estimated 70% maintain wellness. Although the data sets are not yet as large, as illustrated in a subsequent chapter in this book, standardized psychotherapies such as CBT and IPT aid in preventing recurrences.

Because of the paucity of large-sample follow-up studies, clinicians continue to struggle with identifying those patients who should be routinely considered candidates for maintenance. Clinically based but still inadequately studied guidelines for selecting such patients are listed in Table 1–6.

TABLE 1–6.	Guidelines for identifying patients who need indefinite antidepressant treatment for recurrent major depressive disorder (MDD)

Three or more previous episodes of MDD

Two or more previous episodes of MDD, plus one of the following:

   Family history of MDD with at least one family member affected

   More than 120 days spent depressed during lifetime

One or two previous severe episodes of MDD, plus two or more of the following:

   Early age at onset

   Family history of MDD with at least one family member affected

   More than 120 days spent depressed during lifetime

   Treatment Resistant Depression (TRD)

   Psychosis

   Prompt relapse or recurrence following previous discontinuation of treatment

   Previous suicide attempt or persistent suicidal ideation during depressive episodes

   Current severity of episode (e.g., PHQ-9 score >9 or 17-item Hamilton Rating Scale for Depression score >18)

   Concurrent medical illnesses or personal or occupational circumstances that make any future depressive recurrence truly "hazardous"

   Presence of one or more of the following selected laboratory variables:

      Persistent abnormalities of stress hormone regulation, with elevated glucocorticoids or abnormal hypothalamic-pituitary-adrenal measures

      Magnetic resonance brain imaging evidence of hippocampal or amygdala atrophy not attributable to other causes

Summary

Depression and bipolar illnesses are collectively the most burdensome and costly disorders in all health care; better treatments are sorely needed, and dissemination to the millions of underserved is essential. In addition to drug discovery initiatives to expedite breakthroughs and clinical translations, the nation's goals for the next decade surely must include a strong public health preventive program, development of biomarkers to forge individualized "fingerprints" for diagnosis, better treatments, and more rapid clinical translations into routine clinical practice. Federal agencies (e.g., National Institutes of Health, Substance Abuse and Mental Health Services Administration, Department of Veterans Affairs, Agency for Healthcare Research and Quality), private foundations, and academic institutions must be key partners. Large standardized trials must be conducted—and sustainable collaborative networks will be essential for this to occur, following the remarkably successful pathways established by the cancer, cardiovascular, and diabetes networks. Collaborative care will be a required component. A start has been made with the formation of the National Network of Depression Centers, a collection of academic institutions with expertise in depression, bipolar disorder, and related diseases.

Meanwhile, it is time to better use the knowledge we have to attack treatment resistance. It is time to accelerate our journey as we seek to aid the millions struggling with TRD.

Key Clinical Concepts

- *Treatment Resistant Depression* (TRD) is a term for failure to achieve wellness or remission after two complete courses of evidence-based antidepressant treatment. TRD develops in more than 30% of those with initial major depressive disorder (MDD).

- The best ways to prevent and treat TRD include

  - Treat as early as possible. MDD generally has an age at onset between 15 and 24 years, usually starts with mild symptoms, and is often overlooked during early stages then worsens with each episode. Screen with rating scales to detect early.

  - No medication has been shown to be superior to others for preventing or treating TRD. The "roadmap" provides guidance for initial selection of antidepressant medications.

  - Optimize the patient's current medication regimen. This is the first recommended step in the management of MDD with inadequate response.

  - Augmentation is the next choice if patients have partial but incomplete response to the initial medication. Augment routinely when starting treatment for anyone with prior TRD.

  - Treat to wellness. "Better but not well is not good enough." The roadmap provides clues for attaining and maintaining recovery.

  - Openly counteract stigma to optimize treatment adherence; stigma often leads to discontinuation of medication, and discontinuation leads to recurrences.

  - Prescribe exercise and nutrition programs for all depressed patients; avoid herbal medications.

■ Patient-rated clinical scales (PHQ-9, QIDS-S) are the "vital signs" for clinical depression practice. They are remarkably helpful in monitoring response to treatment. Use weekly or at least monthly.

■ The combination of antidepressant medications and cognitive-behavioral therapy or interpersonal psychotherapy is more effective than either in isolation.

■ Atypical antipsychotics improve response in TRD but commonly cause weight gain, hypercholesterolemia, and metabolic syndrome.

■ The clinician should consider neuromodulation (electroconvulsive therapy, transcranial magnetic stimulation, vagus nerve stimulation) for those whose symptoms do not respond after several additional treatments. If still no response, refer for newer treatment strategies.

■ Continue indefinite maintenance with treatments that achieved remission; emphasize long-term wellness.

References

Allen JP, Maisto SA, Connors GJ: Self-report screening tests for alcohol problems in primary care. Arch Intern Med 155:1726–1730, 1995

American Cancer Society: Cancer Facts and Figures, 2008. Estimated New Cancer Cases and Deaths by Sex, U.S, 2008. Atlanta, GA, American Cancer Society, 2008, p 4

Berk M, Sanders KM, Pasco JA, et al: Vitamin D deficiency may play a role in depression. Med Hypotheses 69:1316–1319, 2007

Berman RM, Narasimhan M, Charney DS: Treatment-refractory depression: definitions and characteristics. Depress Anxiety 5:154–164, 1997

Berton O, Nestler EJ: New approaches to antidepressant drug discovery: beyond monoamines. Nat Rev Neurosci 7:137–151, 2006

Boldrini M, Underwood MD, Hen R, et al: Antidepressants increase neural progenitor cells in the human hippocampus. Neuropsychopharmacology 34:2376–2389, 2009

Brennan BP, Hudson JI, Jensen JE, et al: Rapid enhancement of glutamatergic neurotransmission in bipolar depression following treatment with riluzole. Neuropsychopharmacology 35:834–836, 2010

Brent D, Emslie G, Clarke G, et al: Switching to another SSRI or to venlafaxine with or without cognitive behavioral therapy for adolescents with SSRI-resistant depression: the TORDIA randomized controlled trial. JAMA 299:901–913, 2008

Coppen A, Bailey J: Enhancement of the antidepressant action of fluoxetine by folic acid: a randomized, placebo controlled trial. J Affect Disord 60:121–130, 2000

Dranovsky A, Hen R: Hippocampal neurogenesis: regulation by stress and antidepressants. Biol Psychiatry 59:1136–1143, 2006

Fava M, Davidson KG: Definition and epidemiology of treatment-resistant depression. Psychiatr Clin North Am 19:179–200, 1996

Fava M, Rush AJ, Wisniewski SR, et al: A comparison of mirtazapine and nortriptyline following two consecutive failed medication treatments for depressed outpatients: a STAR*D report. Am J Psychiatry 163:1161–1172, 2006

Fournier JC, DeRubeis RJ, Hollon SD, et al: Antidepressant drug effects and depression severity. JAMA 303:47–53, 2010

Geddes JR, Carney SM, Davies C, et al: Relapse prevention with antidepressant drug treatment in depressive disorders: a systematic review. Lancet 361:653–661, 2003

Geddes JR, Burgess S, Hawton K, et al: Long-term lithium therapy for bipolar disorder: systematic review and meta-analysis of randomized controlled trials. Am J Psychiatry 161:217–222, 2004

Ghaemi SN, Katzow JJ: The use of quetiapine for treatment-resistant bipolar disorder: a case series. Ann Clin Psychiatry 11:137–140, 1999

Giles TL, Lasserson TJ, Smith B, et al: Continuous positive airways pressure for obstructive sleep apnoea in adults. Cochrane Database of Systematic Reviews 2006, Issue 3. Art. No.: CD001106. DOI: 10.1002/14651858.CD001106.pub3.

Golberstein E, Eisenberg D, Gollust SE: Perceived stigma and mental health care seeking. Psychiatr Serv 59:392–399, 2008

Goodman WK, Insel TR: Deep brain stimulation in psychiatry: concentrating on the road ahead. Biol Psychiatry 65:263–266, 2009

Greden JF: The burden of disease for treatment-resistant depression. J Clin Psychiatry 62 (suppl 16):26–31, 2001a

Greden JF (ed): Treatment of Recurrent Depression (Review of Psychiatry Series; Oldham JM and Riba MB, series eds.). Washington, DC, American Psychiatric Press, 2001b

Hedner J, Pillar G, Pittman SD, et al: A novel adaptive wrist actigraphy algorithm for sleep-wake assessment in sleep apnea patients. Sleep 27:1560–1566, 2004

Heuser I, Yassouridis A, Holsboer F: The combined dexamethasone/CRH test: a refined laboratory test for psychiatric disorders. J Psychiatr Res 28:341–356, 1994

Holtzheimer PE III: Focal neuromodulation for the treatment of depression. Biol Psychiatry 67:95–96, 2010

Horner MJ, Ries LAG, Krapcho M (eds): Table 2.18: "Estimated United States Cancer Prevalence Counts on January 1, 2006," All Cancer Sites (Invasive): prevalence within past 5 years. SEER Cancer Statistics Review, 1975–2006, National Cancer Institute. Bethesda, MD, based on November 2008 SEER data submission, posted to the SEER Web site, 2009. Available at: http://seer.cancer.gov/csr/1975_2006. Accessed September 15, 2010.

Insel TR, Wang PS: The STAR*D trial: revealing the need for better treatments. Psychiatr Serv 60:1466–1467, 2009

Judd LL, Paulus MJ, Schettler PJ, et al: Does incomplete recovery from first lifetime major depressive episode herald a chronic course of illness? Am J Psychiatry 157:1501–1504, 2000

Kamlet M, Paul N, Greenhouse J: Cost utility analysis of maintenance treatment recurrent depression. Control Clin Trials 16:17–40, 1995

Keller S, Bann CM, Dodd SL, et al: Validity of the brief pain inventory for use in documenting the outcomes of patients with noncancer pain. Clin J Pain 20:309–318, 2004

Kessler RC, Chiu WT, Demler O, et al: Prevalence, severity and comorbidity of twelve-month DSM-IV disorders in the National Comorbidity Survey Replication (NCS-R). Arch Gen Psychiatry 62:617–627, 2005

Leuner B, Mendolia-Loffredo S, Kozorovitskiy Y, et al: Learning enhances the survival of new neurons beyond the time when the hippocampus is required for memory. J Neurosci 24:7477–7481, 2004

Lin EH, Katon W, Von Korff M, et al: Effect of improving depression care on pain and functional outcomes among older patients with arthritis: a randomized controlled trial. JAMA 290:2428–2429, 2003

Lopez AD, Mathers CD, Ezzati M, et al: Global and regional burden of disease and risk factors, 2001: systematic analysis of population health data. Lancet 367:1747–1757, 2006

Ludman E, Katon W, Bush T, et al: Behavioural factors associated with symptom outcomes in a primary care-based depression prevention intervention trial. Psychol Med 33:1061–1070, 2003

March J, Silva S, Petrycki S, et al: Fluoxetine, cognitive-behavioral therapy, and their combination for adolescents with depression: Treatment for Adolescents With Depression Study (TADS) randomized controlled trial. JAMA 292:807–820, 2004

Mathew SJ, Manji HK, Charney DS: Novel drugs and therapeutic targets for severe mood disorders. Neuropsychopharmacology 33:2080–2092, 2008

McGrath PJ, Stewart JW, Fava M, et al: Tranylcypromine versus venlafaxine plus mirtazapine following three failed antidepressant medication trials for depression: a STAR*D report. Am J Psychiatry 163:1531–1541, 2006

McMahon FJ, Buervenich S, Charney D, et al: Variation in the gene encoding the serotonin 2A receptor is associated with outcome of antidepressant treatment. Am J Hum Genet 78:804–814, 2006

Melfi CA, Chawla AJ, Croghan TW, et al: The effects of adherence to antidepressant treatment guidelines on relapse and recurrence of depression. Arch Gen Psychiatry 55:1128–1132, 1998

Murray CJL, Lopez AD: The Global Burden of Disease: A Comprehensive Assessment of Mortality and Disability From Disease, Injuries, and Risk Factors in 1990 and Projected to 2020, Vol 1. Cambridge, MA, World Health Organization/Harvard University Press, 1996

Ostroff RB, Nelson DJ: Risperidone augmentation of selective serotonin reuptake inhibitors in major depression. J Clin Psychiatry 60:256–259, 1999

Ozer EM, Zahnd EG, Adams SH, et al: Are adolescents being screened for emotional distress in primary care? J Adolesc Health 44:520–527, 2009

Papakostas GI, Petersen T, Mischoulon D, et al: Serum folate, vitamin B12, and homocysteine in major depressive disorder; part 1: predictors of clinical response in fluoxetine-resistant depression. J Clin Psychiatry 65:1090–1095, 2004

Papakostas GI, Petersen TJ, Kinrys G, et al: Aripiprazole augmentation of selective serotonin reuptake inhibitors for treatment-resistant major depressive disorder. J Clin Psychiatry 66:1326–1330, 2005

Pathak S, Johns ES, Kowatch RA: Adjunctive quetiapine for treatment-resistant adolescent major depressive disorder: a case series. J Child Adolesc Psychopharmacol 15:696–702, 2005

Perlis RH, Moorjani P, Fagerness J, et al: Pharmacogenetic analysis of genes implicated in rodent models of antidepressant response: association of TREK1 and treatment resistance in the STAR(*)D study. Neuropsychopharmacology 33:2810–2819, 2008

Posner K, Oquendo MA, Gould M, et al: Columbia Classification Algorithm of Suicide Assessment (C-CASA): classification of suicidal events in the FDA's pediatric suicidal risk analysis of antidepressants. Am J Psychiatry 164:989–991, 2007

Rehemtulla A: The war on cancer rages on. Neoplasia 11:1252–1263, 2009

Riba MB, Balon R: Combining psychotherapy and pharmacotherapy, in The American Psychiatric Publishing Textbook of Psychiatry, 5th Edition. Edited by Hales RE, Yudofsky SC, Gabbard GO. Washington, DC, American Psychiatric Publishing, 2008, pp 1279–1301

Ruhé HG, Huyser J, Swinkels JA, et al: Switching antidepressants after a first selective serotonin reuptake inhibitor in major depressive disorder: a systemic review. J Clin Psychiatry 67:1836–1855, 2006

Rush AJ, Trivedi MH, Ibrahim H, et al: The 16-item Quick Inventory of Depressive Symptomatology (QIDS), clinician rating (QIDS-C), and self-report (QIDS-SR): a psychometric evaluation in patients with chronic major depression. Biol Psychiatry 54:573–583, 2003

Rush AJ, Trivedi MH, Wisniewski SR, et al: Bupropion-SR, sertraline, or venlafaxine-XR after failure of SSRIs for depression. N Engl J Med 354:1231–1242, 2006

Sapolsky RM: The possibility of neurotoxicity in the hippocampus in major depression: a primer on neuron death. Biol Psychiatry 48:755–765, 2000

Sen S, Sanacora G: Major depression: emerging therapeutics. Mt Sinai J Med 75:204–225, 2008

Sheline YI, Wang PW, Gado MH, et al: Hippocampal atrophy in recurrent major depression. Proc Natl Acad Sci USA 93:3908–3913, 1996

Shelton RC, Tollefson GD, Tohen M, et al: A novel augmentation strategy for treating resistant major depression. Am J Psychiatry 159:155–156, 2001

Spitzer R, Kroenke K, Williams J: Validation and utility of a self-report version of PRIME-MD: the PHY Primary Care Study. JAMA 282:1737–1744, 1999

Stahl SM: Novel therapeutics for depression: L-methylfolate as a trimonoamine modulator and antidepressant augmenting agent. CNS Spectr 12:739–743, 2007

Suppes T, Vieta E, Liu S, et al: Maintenance treatment for patients with bipolar I disorder: results from a North American study of quetiapine in combination with lithium or divalproex (trial 27). Am J Psychiatry 166:476–488, 2009

Thase ME: Are SNRIs more effective than SSRIs? A review of the current state of the controversy. Psychopharmacol Bull 41:58–85, 2008

Trivedi MH, Rush AJ, Wisniewski SR, et al: Evaluation of outcomes with citalopram for depression using measurement-based care in STAR*D: implications for clinical practice. Am J Psychiatry 163:28–40, 2006

Trivedi MH, Morris DW, Wisniewski SR, et al: Concise Associated Symptoms Tracking (CAST) Scale and Concise Health Risk Tracking (CHRT) Scale: brief self and clinician ratings of suicidality and associated symptoms. Poster presented at NCDEU 50th anniversary meeting, Boca Raton, FL, June 15, 2010

Valenstein M, Kavanagh J, Lee T, et al: Using a pharmacy-based intervention to improve antipsychotic adherence among patients with serious mental illness. Schizophr Bull Nov 21, 2009 [Epub ahead of print]

van Praag H: Exercise and the brain: something to chew on. Trends Neurosci 32:283–290, 2009

van Praag H, Kempermann G, Gage FH: Running increases cell proliferation and neurogenesis in the adult mouse dentate gyrus. Nat Neurosci 2:266–270, 1999

Wang PS, Simon GE, Avorn J, et al: Telephone screening, outreach, and care management for depressed workers and impact on clinical and work productivity outcomes: a randomized controlled trial. JAMA 298:1401–1411, 2007

Warden D, Rush AJ, Trivedi MH, et al: The STAR*D project results: a comprehensive review of findings. Curr Psychiatr Rep 9:449–459, 2007

World Health Organization: The Global Burden of Disease 2004 Update. 2008. Available at: http://www.who.int/healthinfo/global_burden_disease/en. Accessed September 16, 2010.

Wright JH, Sudak DM, Turkington D, et al. (eds): High-Yield Cognitive-Behavior Therapy for Brief Sessions: An Illustrated Guide. Washington, DC, American Psychiatric Publishing, 2010

Zarate C Jr, Payne JL, Quiroz J, et al: An open-label trial of riluzole in patients with treatment-resistant major depression. Am J Psychiatry 161:171–174, 2004

Zarate CA Jr, Singh JB, Caarlson PJ, et al: A randomized trial of an N-methyl-D-aspartate antagonist in treatment-resistant major depression. Arch Gen Psychiatry 63:856–864, 2006

Zisook S, Lesser I, Stewart JW, Wisniewski SR, et al: Effect of age at onset on the course of major depressive disorder. Am J Psychiatry 164:1539–1546, 2007

Zuckerbrot RA, Maxon L, Pagar D, et al: Adolescent depression screening in primary care: feasibility and acceptability. Pediatrics 119:102–108, 2007

CHAPTER TWO

Psychopharmacological Roadmap for Treatment Resistant Depression

Srijan Sen, M.D., Ph.D.
Brian Mickey, M.D., Ph.D.
John F. Greden, M.D.

ANTIDEPRESSANT MEDICATIONS currently are the primary treatments used to resolve major depressive disorder (MDD). Reliance on them began to grow following the introduction of the monoamine oxidase inhibitors (MAOIs) and the tricyclic antidepressants (TCAs) in the 1950s, and by 2008, antidepressants had become the third most commonly prescribed class of all drugs in the United States (Consumer Reports Health 2010). Medications are relatively easy to disseminate, reasonably safe, widely available, heavily promoted, generally reimbursed by payers, and quite effective for some but not all individuals. Although antidepressant medications are used for depressions of all severities, they are the mainstay in the initial and ongoing management of Treatment Resistant Depression (TRD). Nevertheless, antidepressant medications have important limitations for many individuals with clinical depression, including those with TRD. As summarized by Greden et al. in Chapter 1 of this text, recent real-world effectiveness trials such as the Sequenced Treatment Alternatives to Relieve Depression (STAR*D) study and meta-analyses of clinical trials indicate that antidepressants produce remission for only about 30%–40% of individuals in the first stages and a lessening percentage following each additional treatment failure.

Goals for Antidepressant Pharmacotherapy

Ideal goals for antidepressant medications include early response, achievement of remission (wellness), prevention of recurrences, prevention of chronicity, and return to previous functioning. Unfortunately, medication treatments commonly fail to achieve these admirable goals. Response is delayed for many. Most patients do not achieve remission (wellness) during the initial course of treatment with a single antidepressant. With each pharmacological failure, the chance of remission during the next trial diminishes. These medications do prevent recurrences for perhaps 70% of those whose symptoms have responded. Whenever any of the abovementioned goals for antidepressant medications fail to be met, the likelihood of TRD becomes increasingly a reality (Gaynes et al. 2008).

In this chapter, we use a sequential decision-making model to provide additional details about use of antidepressant psychopharmacological medications for those whose symptoms have not responded to an initial antidepressant. This model builds on the roadmap presented by Greden and colleagues in Chapter 1 of this book. The focus is on psychopharmacology, but several newer neurostimulation treatments are included.

Pharmacological Roadmap for Major Depressive Disorders

Initial Steps

Selective serotonin reuptake inhibitors (SSRIs) are the most common first-choice antidepressants. An array of SSRI medications is available.

Most SSRI agents have been considered relatively equivalent in the percentage of responders or remitters produced, but a multiple-treatments meta-analysis of 117 trials recently compared the newer generation of antidepressants and reported that sertraline may have a slightly superior combination of efficacy, side effects, and cost (Cipriani et al. 2009). Unfortunately, in the general population, 65%–80% of patients still do not achieve full remission with an SSRI such as sertraline (Fava and Davidson 1996).

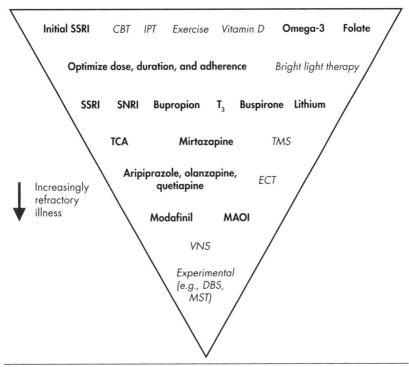

FIGURE 2–1. Sequential steps to be taken for those with Treatment Resistant Depression.

Boldface and *italic* type indicate pharmacotherapy and nonpharmacotherapy options, respectively. CBT = cognitive-behavior therapy; DBS = deep brain stimulation; ECT = electroconvulsive therapy; IPT = interpersonal psychotherapy; MAOI = monoamine oxidase inhibitor; MST = magnetic stimulation treatment; SNRI = serotonin-norepinephrine reuptake inhibitor; SSRI = selective serotonin reuptake inhibitor; T_3 = triiodothyronine; TCA = tricyclic antidepressant; TMS = transcranial magnetic stimulation; VNS = vagus nerve stimulation.

Treatment Steps When Symptoms Fail to Respond to Initial Antidepressant Treatment

The early descent toward "treatment resistance" begins when symptoms do not respond to the initial treatment trial. Clinicians' goals after initial failures include moving the patient toward recovery as quickly as possible, preventing progression to TRD, and sustaining wellness. For purposes of illustration, we use a triangle that summarizes steps to be taken for those with refractory illness (Figure 2–1).

One important step in this process that is worth special mention is the initiation of an early discussion about electroconvulsive therapy (ECT).

Many patients are unfamiliar with (or ill-informed about) ECT, so education about the procedure, its effectiveness, and common side effects is particularly important. (Discussion of repetitive transcranial magnetic stimulation may also be introduced at this point, although the role of this treatment in clinical practice is less well defined.) ECT is indicated particularly for patients with severe functional impairment, dangerous suicide risk, or psychotic or catatonic features. However, even in the absence of these signs, ECT should be considered in addition to pharmacological treatment to prevent progression of the episode beyond 6 months. Once a decision has been made to proceed with ECT, pharmacological management during and immediately after ECT should be planned with the goal of preventing relapse following the course of ECT. This aspect of medication management lies outside the scope of this chapter. However, note that medications that were ineffective or not tolerated before ECT (during a severe phase of the illness) may be effective and tolerated after ECT when symptoms have markedly improved. We recommend initiating a discussion about ECT after the second failed medication trial.

Optimization

Assuming that some improvement has occurred and that side effects are tolerable, the first recommended step in the management of an inadequate response to an antidepressant is the optimization of the patient's current medication regimen. A large proportion of depression medication trials never use the maximum tolerable dose, and although good large-sample data are not readily available for TRD patients, some of those who are believed to have TRD are better considered as inadequately treated. This outcome may occur because patients do not fully adhere to recommended doses, are rapid metabolizers, or have a particular type of depression that is not completely responsive to this medication. Nevertheless, partial response represents an important clue for the clinician. Inadequate doses not only reduce the likelihood of achieving a response in patients but also can create difficulties in future treatment decisions.

Ideally, for each medication tried, the dose should be increased to the maximum tolerable level. Furthermore, the maximum dose should be maintained for at least 6 weeks before the trial is considered a failure. As mentioned, an additional and underappreciated issue related to ensuring that a patient has received an adequate trial is medication adherence. Explicit evaluations of adherence, along with medication event monitoring, ideally should include periodic telephone calls. Use of care managers, pill diaries, and pill count strategies all help in monitoring adherence (compliance).

Complementary Adjunctive Treatments

Ensuring an optimal trial of the first-choice medication is an important initial step in the management of depression; however, a substantial proportion of patients will require further intervention. Consideration of other medications for many of these patients may ultimately be necessary, but it may be worthwhile first to consider a set of underused interventions that have shown efficacy for some with little risk of increased side effects. The most important of these interventions is evidence-based psychotherapy. Multiple studies have shown that the combination of antidepressant medications and cognitive-behavioral therapy (CBT) or interpersonal psychotherapy (IPT) is generally more effective than either in isolation. Furthermore, both CBT and IPT provide sustained effects that last beyond the conclusion of therapy sessions (Petersen 2006). When individual psychotherapy is not available to patients, alternatives such as online psychotherapy modules and group therapy can be considered. Unfortunately, even when evidence-based psychotherapy is made available, many patients choose not to take part or cannot do so for practical reasons.

In addition to psychotherapy, other nonpharmacological complementary treatments have proven efficacy as adjunctive treatments for depression. For instance, meta-analyses support the use of light therapy augmentation of SSRI treatment for some patients, especially targeting those with seasonal affective disorder or seasonal accentuations of major depression. Various forms of exercise therapy are increasingly being studied and showing efficacy as a component of depression treatment, analogous to the role of exercise in individuals following an acute coronary event.

Complementary oral supplements also have been studied extensively as adjunctive treatments for depression. In this class, omega-3 fatty acids, S-adenosylmethionine (SAM-e), and folate have consistently shown efficacy as adjuncts to SSRI medications, with few side effects (Freeman et al. 2010; Papakostas et al. 2010).

Clinical Vignette 1:
When Should ECT Be Introduced?

A 52-year-old man presented with a history of recurrent depression since early adulthood and onset of the latest episode 6 months ago, triggered by job-related stress. Family history was significant for depression in multiple family members. Two second-degree relatives had committed suicide. He had some past benefit from fluoxetine, but it made him feel "numb." A recent trial of venlafaxine, 150 mg/day for 2 months, was ineffective, and he discontinued it because it made him feel "more aggressive." He was started on a course of nortriptyline, titrated to 125 mg/day, and this was augmented by CBT. Although the patient had verified therapeutic blood levels of the drug, he experienced little improvement.

Given the persistence of substantial depressive symptoms (score of 22 on the nine-item depression scale of the Patient Health Questionnaire [PHQ-9]) and the failure of two medication trials, the possibility of ECT as a treatment option was raised. The patient initially declined ECT and preferred to try additional medication trials. As a result, the decision was made to add lithium, starting slowly at 150 mg/day, to the patient's regimen. Unfortunately, he developed stomach upset and worsening anxiety with the lithium and was unable to tolerate increased doses of the medication. ECT was discussed again, and the patient was more open to the idea but preferred to try additional medication trials. Nortriptyline was switched to bupropion, but over the course of the next 2 months, the patient experienced no improvement in his depressive symptoms. Eventually, the patient became more pessimistic, his sleep worsened, his suicidal ideation intensified, and he was forced to take a leave of absence from work. Because of his symptomatic and functional deterioration, ECT was strongly recommended. The patient agreed to a consultation and began ECT as an outpatient. (ECT, one of the possible neuromodulation treatments available, is discussed by Taylor and colleagues in Chapter 11 of this book.) The patient showed improvement after the fourth treatment and achieved a PHQ-9 score of 7 after eight treatments. Maintenance medication strategies were then implemented.

Switching, Combining, or Augmenting Medications

When optimization of an initial SSRI and the addition of benign adjunctive treatments are ineffective, clinicians must decide whether to switch from the initial antidepressant to a new medication or to combine the initial antidepressant with an additional agent (this strategy is considered *combination therapy* if the second agent is an antidepressant, and *augmentation* if it is not an antidepressant). Table 2–1 details the primary agents to consider for switching or augmentation after failure of an initial SSRI.

If the patient had no response to the initial medication or experienced intolerable side effects, switching medications may be the best choice.

Augmentation or combination therapy may be the optimal choice when patients have had a measurable but incomplete response to the initial medication. However, combining agents may increase the cost of treatment and requires extra attention to pharmacological interactions and adverse effects because the coadministered agents may share side effects or metabolic pathways. If the agents have shared pathways, plasma and brain levels of the initial antidepressant may be increased or decreased.

Given the large number of individual agents, countless combinations are possible. To make this decision, clinicians should weigh multiple factors, including effectiveness, patient preference, medication tolerance, past personal or family member experiences with the medication, symptom profile, family history, and medical and psychiatric comorbidities.

TABLE 2–1.   Grades of effectiveness and tolerability for augmentation
             therapy and antidepressant switching after SSRI failure

Agent	Effectiveness	Tolerability	Special patient populations
Augmentation/ combination			
Lithium	A–	B–	Bipolar spectrum
Triiodothyronine (T$_3$)	A	B +	Hypothyroidism
Atypical antipsychotics	A	C	Bipolar spectrum, anxiety, and underweight
Mirtazapine	B +	B	Insomnia and anorexia
TCA, trazodone	C +	B–	Insomnia and pain
Bupropion	B–	A	Fatigue, nicotine dependence, and antidepressant-associated sexual dysfunction
Modafinil	B	A	Sleepiness or fatigue
Omega-3 fatty acids	B–	A	
Folate	B	A	Excessive alcohol use; women
Buspirone	D	A–	
S-adenosylmethionine (SAM-e)	B	A	
Antidepressant switch			
TCA	A–	B	Melancholic or endogenous depression
MAOI	A	C	
SNRI	A	B +	
Mirtazapine	A	B	Insomnia and anorexia
Bupropion	B	A	Sexual dysfunction, increased weight, and fatigue
SSRI	B	A	

Note. MAOI = monoamine oxidase inhibitor; SNRI = serotonin-norepinephrine reuptake inhibitor; SSRI = selective serotonin reuptake inhibitor; TCA = tricyclic antidepressant.

    Almost all of the commonly used agents have shown augmentation ef-
ficacy in case series and open-label studies. The evidence from randomized controlled trials (RCTs) varies considerably between agents. We
focus heavily on the evidence from RCTs and the STAR*D effectiveness
trial on the most common combination and augmentation strategies.

Once a choice is made, a trial of at least 4 weeks at a therapeutic dose is generally necessary to assess effectiveness. Such time periods seem inordinately long for suffering patients and families but are required.

Lithium.   Lithium augmentation has been used for decades, and its use is well supported. A meta-analysis of nine placebo-controlled studies found that lithium augmentation resulted in a 27% increased response rate, with a number needed to treat (NNT) of 3.7. An NNT of 4 or less is generally considered to be of high clinical relevance. However, lithium was tested at the third level of the STAR*D study, with disappointing results (15.9% remission rate) (Nierenberg et al. 2006). Some have attributed this low remission rate to the relatively low dose of lithium used in STAR*D and the reluctance of clinicians to increase the dose. This finding underscores that lithium should be used only when the clinician is familiar with its use and is available for close monitoring of blood levels and side effects. If these conditions are met, however, lithium is among the best and most underused augmenting agents. Lithium carbonate may be dosed at 600–900 mg/day, or dosage can be guided by serum levels with a target level of 0.6–1.0 mEq/L. Lithium is well tolerated when titrated slowly from 150 mg. Patients with symptoms on the bipolar spectrum may be most appropriate. Perhaps this represents another reason for the reported low response in the STAR*D trial, because most of those with bipolar disorder were eliminated from trial participation.

Lithium is contraindicated in pregnancy.

Triiodothyronine (T_3, liothyronine).   Triiodothyronine is another older agent with an extended history of evidence as an augmentation agent for depression. Although most of the evidence involves augmentation for TCAs, newer studies suggest that T_3 is also an effective augmenting agent for SSRIs. Two augmentation RCTs have been performed, with a large RCT showing a significant effect of T_3 and a much smaller RCT finding no effect. Furthermore, open-label studies have reported a significant effect of T_3. The most notable finding was that in the third level of the STAR*D trial, T_3 augmentation resulted in a remission rate of 23.3%, a nonsignificant improvement in response rate from the lithium comparator and a relatively high rate considering the level of treatment resistance present in the subjects who remained in that stage of the trial.

At present, evidence is insufficient to estimate the effect size of T_3 augmentation or whether some proposed biomarkers (e.g., baseline thyrotropin) are useful predictors of T_3 response. Some evidence suggests that the mechanisms may relate to modifications in receptor affinities rather than to resolution of any underlying thyroid abnormalities. One important advantage of T_3 is that its side-effect profile is relatively benign. T_3 can be started at a dose of 25 µg/day and increased to 50 µg/day if no side effects are reported. T_3 is contraindicated in patients with recent myocardial infarction, thyrotoxicosis, or adrenal insufficiency (Shelton et al. 2010).

Atypical antipsychotics.   Over the past few years, pharmaceutical companies have conducted several trials with low-dose atypical antipsychotics in efforts to obtain U.S. Food and Drug Administration (FDA) indications for depression augmentation. A meta-analysis of 16 RCTs found evidence that atypical antipsychotic augmentation had efficacy for depression (odds ratio = 1.69) compared with placebo. The study also found that compared with placebo, atypical agents resulted in a fourfold increase in the likelihood of medication discontinuation because of side effects (Nelson and Papakostas 2009). A recent Cochrane review (Komossa et al. 2010) suggests that atypical antipsychotics likely improve response in TRD but also come with serious and relatively common long-term side effects (weight gain, hypercholesterolemia, and metabolic syndrome).

Olanzapine.   Olanzapine has been studied almost exclusively in combination with fluoxetine. A meta-analysis of 5 RCTs found a 10%– 15% better response rate for olanzapine plus fluoxetine compared with fluoxetine alone. The safety meta-analysis by the same group, however, found that combination treatment resulted in increases in weight, random blood glucose levels, low-density lipoprotein cholesterol levels, and QT interval. Other studies have shown that over the course of 1.5 years, the addition of olanzapine resulted in an average increase of 12 pounds in weight and 6.2 mg/dL in random blood glucose levels. The olanzapine-fluoxetine combination has received FDA approval for treatment-refractory depression.

Aripiprazole and quetiapine.   Another FDA-approved medication in this class is aripiprazole. Three RCTs have been published to date, and all have found significant evidence of efficacy. Similarly, three RCTs have assessed quetiapine for depression augmentation and found evidence for efficacy. For both aripiprazole and quetiapine, however, the trials suggested that serious side effects include weight gain, sedation, and akithisia. Although direct comparison studies are still lacking, indirect evidence suggests that aripiprazole and quetiapine may have smaller effect sizes than olanzapine but also a lower rate of serious side effects. Both aripiprazole and quetiapine have received FDA approval for depression augmentation.

Other atypical antipsychotics.   In contrast to olanzapine and aripiprazole, the evidence for the other atypical antipsychotics is mixed or lacking. Although open-label trials of risperidone and ziprasidone generally have been favorable, strong evidence from RCTs is lacking. Specifically, for risperidone, two of the four published trials have been positive. For quetiapine, one of the two published trials has been positive. For ziprasidone, no RCTs have yet been published in peer-reviewed journals. Thus, more data are necessary before we can determine what role these agents should play in the treatment of TRD. In general, atypical antipsychotics may be most appropriate for patients with weight loss, those with symptoms on the bipolar spectrum (Philip et al. 2010; Shelton et al. 2010), and those with no family history of hypercholesterolemia or diabetes.

Although the dyskinesias traditionally associated with antipsychotics in the past are considerably lessened with the newer atypical antipsychotics, they do develop in some, and clinicians need to monitor for such symptoms.

Bupropion.   Bupropion is one of the most popular augmenting medications used in combination with SSRIs and serotonin-norepinephrine reuptake inhibitors (SNRIs). The popularity of bupropion is likely a result of its side-effect profile. In particular, the relative absence of sexual side effects and weight gain are attractive to many patients. The results from the second level of the STAR*D trial also provided some support for the use of bupropion as an augmenting agent. Compared with buspirone, bupropion used as an augmenting medication resulted in fewer depressive symptoms and had greater tolerability. Note, however, that no published RCTs have assessed augmentation with bupropion compared with placebo. Given the lack of RCTs, it may be that bupropion is used as an augmenting agent more frequently than is supported by the current evidence. We believe bupropion augmentation should be used mainly for patients with relatively mild depressive symptoms or additional symptoms such as fatigue, antidepressant-associated sexual dysfunction, or significant weight gain. Bupropion is contraindicated for patients with eating disorders or epilepsy.

Mirtazapine.   Mirtazapine is another antidepressant often combined with SSRIs and SNRIs. The only RCT conducted to date was small but found a significant effect of mirtazapine augmentation. This conclusion is supported by a series of open-label trials. The disadvantages of using mirtazapine are the side effects of substantial weight gain, sedation, and sexual dysfunction. Typically, the medication is more sedating at starting doses (7.5–15 mg/day) than at target doses (30–45 mg/day). With the significant side effects, mirtazapine is most appropriate for patients with insomnia or weight loss.

Tricyclic and heterocyclic antidepressants.   Other older generic medications that have been used to augment SSRIs include the tricyclic and heterocyclic antidepressants. Several open-label studies and case series reports supported the efficacy of nortriptyline, amitriptyline, and trazodone. Two randomized trials have been published to date; one found evidence for TCA efficacy, and the other reported no effect. As with many of the other older agents, more large RCTs are needed to evaluate the efficacy and effect size of TCA augmentation in depression. TCAs are better tolerated when titrated slowly and may be particularly helpful for patients with insomnia or chronic pain. For individuals with suspected ultrahigh metabolism, serum level monitoring can be useful to verify an adequate dose. These agents are contraindicated among patients with recent myocardial infarction.

Modafinil. Modafinil is a wakefulness-promoting agent with novel pharmacology. A pooled analysis of the two published depression augmentation RCTs found a small but significant effect of modafinil in the subset of patients with substantial baseline somnolence. Most studies to date suggest that the side-effect profile of modafinil is relatively benign; the most common complaints include headache, nausea, and dry mouth. Although studies in the general TRD population are still lacking, modafinil may have an important role as an augmentation agent for patients with prominent fatigue or daytime sleepiness or those with sleep apnea or narcolepsy.

Serotonin type 1A receptor agonists. Buspirone and pindolol are serotonin type 1A receptor agonists that have been used to augment SSRIs in depression. Buspirone was not significantly worse than bupropion in the primary clinician-rated effectiveness outcome in the second level of the STAR*D trial, but it was found to be inferior on the patient-rated scales and side-effect profiles. Furthermore, the two published augmentation RCTs found no evidence that buspirone is superior to placebo.

Some smaller early studies supported the efficacy of pindolol augmentation, but two more recent and well-powered RCTs in TRD patients found no evidence that pindolol augmentation was superior to placebo. Thus, the current evidence does not support a major role for buspirone or pindolol as an augmentation agent in TRD.

Other agents. Numerous other agents have been used in augmentation or combination strategies, with weak or anecdotal support. These agents include dopaminergic agonists (pergolide, amantadine, pramipexole, ropinirole), perhaps indicated only for those with co-occurring restless legs syndrome; psychostimulants (methylphenidate, amphetamines); selective norepinephrine reuptake inhibitors (atomoxetine, reboxetine);

the nicotinic antagonist mecamylamine; the melatonin agonist agomelatine; anticonvulsants; inositol; opiates; sedative-hypnotics; and ste-
roid hormones (estrogen, dehydroepiandrosterone, testosterone). In
general, these approaches are not yet supported by evidence from large
RCTs and meta-analyses. Future studies may provide additional evidence
supporting use of these agents, and they may prove useful for particular
situations or patients. All uses described here are off label except adjunctive aripiprazole and olanzapine-fluoxetine.

Clinical Vignette 2: Which Augmentation or Combination Strategy to Use?

A 40-year-old woman presented with gradual onset of clinical depression
that worsened over 2 years. She was uncertain about prior episodes. Comorbidities included overweight status (body mass index = 27), corrected
hypothyroidism, and recurrent binge eating. Both parents reportedly had
problematic eating behaviors as well.

She was started on a course of paroxetine, titrated up to 40 mg/day.
After 2 months, the patient had experienced a marked improvement in
compulsive eating symptoms but only a slight improvement in depressive
symptoms. She started omega-3 fatty acid supplementation and began
seeing a cognitive therapist, which she found somewhat helpful after
6 weeks. However, the depression persisted and was still affecting her
work and relationships, so she inquired about other medication strategies.
Given the partial response and the patient's preference, augmentation was
deemed preferable to switching primary medications. Lithium augmentation was avoided because of mild hypothyroidism, and bupropion combination was avoided because of the comorbid eating disorder. Low-dose
atypical antipsychotic medications and combination therapy with mirtazapine and TCAs were avoided because of concern for weight gain. After
the clinician checked the patient's thyrotropin and found it to be in the
normal range (4.9 mIU/L; reference range = 0.3–5.5), the patient started
taking liothyronine, 25 µg/day. After 8 weeks, she reported no compulsive
eating symptoms and only minor residual depressive symptoms.

Following failure of an antidepressant trial, clinicians commonly switch
to another agent. Switching after short, uncomplicated trials of inadequate
doses is not advisable. Switching antidepressants makes the most sense
when the current medication is ineffective, minimally effective, or not well
tolerated, because the patient in that situation routinely believes that he or
she has "nothing to lose" by discontinuing the current medication.

In general, if a clinician has decided to switch medications after SSRI
failure, six options are commonly considered: 1) another SSRI, 2) an
SNRI, 3) a TCA, 4) an MAOI, 5) mirtazapine, or 6) bupropion. Common
sense suggests that changing to an antidepressant in a class distinct from

the first agent (interclass switch) may be more effective than changing to an agent in the same class (intraclass switch). A recent meta-analysis of RCTs supports this hypothesis, finding that after the failure of an initial SSRI, switching to a non-SSRI was modestly more effective (NNT = 22) than switching to another SSRI (Papakostas et al. 2008). Most of the individual studies that have made direct comparisons among different agents, however, showed no significant difference, potentially because of insufficient power. Because the direct comparison trials provide little guidance, there is scant basis to make evidence-based recommendations on switching medications after SSRI failure. Nonetheless, we summarize the evidence to date and the few general principles that emerge from the evidence.

SNRIs, mirtazapine, and bupropion. A meta-analysis of three RCTs that compared venlafaxine (an SNRI) with a new SSRI after an initial SSRI failure found a small but significant advantage for venlafaxine (NNT = 13) (Weinmann et al. 2008). Another RCT comparing a switch to a new SSRI with mirtazapine found no evidence of a difference between the groups. Additional switching comparison studies come from levels 2, 3, and 4 of the STAR*D trial. After citalopram failure, the second level of the STAR*D trial showed no difference in efficacy between sertraline (an intraclass switch) and bupropion or venlafaxine (interclass switches). Similarly, at the third level of the STAR*D trial, no difference in response was seen between the patients switched to mirtazapine and those switched to nortriptyline. At the fourth level, a nonsignificant trend toward a better response was reported among patients switched to mirtazapine combined with venlafaxine than among patients switched to tranylcypromine (an MAOI) alone (Gaynes et al. 2008).

TCAs and MAOIs. Most modern RCTs may be designed to favor newer agents or to show equivalency of newer and older agents. Consequently, the available literature is problematic for drawing conclusions about the differential effectiveness of TCAs, SSRIs, and MAOIs in real-world TRD. SSRIs have replaced TCAs and MAOIs as first-line treatments, probably because of better overall tolerance and effective pharmaceutical marketing. However, evidence indicates that SSRIs may be more disruptive to sleep architecture, and less effective overall, for patients with refractory depression. In particular, TCAs appear to be more effective than SSRIs for traditional "endogenous or melancholic" illness. For patients with symptoms of insomnia, a sedating agent such as nortriptyline, amitriptyline, or imipramine may be appropriate. If a nonsedating agent is preferred, desipramine is a good choice. These drugs are more noradrenergic and anticholinergic than SSRIs. In theory, each agent's somewhat distinct receptor pharmacology might

TABLE 2–2.   Research strategies being evaluated for Treatment Resistant Depression

Target system	Promising compounds	Probability of clinical availability in next decade	Probability of substantial efficacy beyond current antidepressants
Neurotrophic factors	PDE4 inhibitors (rolipram), GSK-3 inhibitors	+	+ + + +
Glutamate modulation	NMDA antagonists (ketamine, riluzole)	+ + +	+ + + + +
GABA	GABA$_A$ receptor inhibition (eszopiclone)	+ +	+ +
Hypothalamic-pituitary-adrenal modulation (e.g., CRH antagonist)	CRF antagonists, vasopressin V$_{1b}$ receptor antagonists, glucocorticoid receptor antagonists	+ + +	+ + + + +
Immune modulation	TNF-α antibodies	+ +	+ + + + +
Neurokinins	NK-1 receptor antagonists (aprepitant)	+ +	+ +
Monoaminergic	Triple reuptake inhibitors	+ + + + +	+
Cholinergic modulation	Nicotinic receptor antagonists (mecamylamine)	+ + +	+ + +
Neuromodulation	Deep brain stimulation	+ + +	+ + + +

Note.   CRF = corticotropin-releasing factor;   CRH = corticotropin-releasing hormone; GABA = γ-aminobutyric acid; GABA$_A$ = GABA type A; GSK-3 = glycogen synthase kinase 3; NMDA = N-acetyl-D-aspartate; NK-1 = neurokinin 1; PDE4 = phosphodiesterase type 4; TNF-α = tumor necrosis factor alpha.

Source.   Adapted from Sen and Sanacora 2008.

underlie their differential effectiveness. In practice, optimal use of TCAs requires, first, remembering to use them and, second, slow titration from a low starting dose (e.g., typically 10–20 mg/day for desipramine).

MAOIs represent a unique class of antidepressant that has been even more neglected than TCAs, mainly because of safety concerns related to medication and food interactions. MAOIs can be safely used by most patients, however, and should be routinely considered after the third failed medication trial. Among the MAOIs, tranylcypromine (starting dose = 10 mg/day; target dose = 30–60 mg/day) tends to have the greatest stimulant-like effect, which is often desirable. Alternatively, phenelzine (target dose = 45–90 mg/day) or isocarboxazid (target dose = 20–60 mg/day) may be used. For patients who experience gastrointestinal side effects with oral MAOIs, transdermal selegiline may be used (target dose = 9–12 mg/24 h). While taking MAOIs, some dietary restrictions are necessary to avoid the tyramine reaction, but these restrictions are not as difficult to abide by as traditionally feared and are easily met by most patients. Likewise, frequent assessment for potential drug interactions is necessary to avoid a hypertensive reaction, but these interactions are predictable, and most patients easily avoid them.

Other research strategies. Because glutamatergic abnormalities may play key roles in those with bipolar disorder and TRD, glutamate-modulating medications are receiving more attention (Brennan et al. 2010; Zarate et al. 2004, 2006). The focus has been predominantly on agents that produce alterations in glutamate circuitry, such as ketamine and riluzole; studies have shown promise, but data are very early. Nevertheless, for individuals with severe TRD, when "approved" alternatives appear to be disappointing in their results, referral to programs conducting research trials with glutamate-altering agents, neuromodulation, or other strategies can be recommended. This referral pattern closely parallels that which occurs with cancer patients being referred to comprehensive cancer centers.

Table 2–2 portrays a set of research strategies adapted from Sen and Sanacora 2008, accompanied by our subjective estimates of their probable clinical availability within the next decade and the likelihood of their substantial efficacy beyond the efficacy of current antidepressants.

Key Clinical Concepts

▮ Agents that are not antidepressants, including dietary and vitamin supplements (vitamin D, omega-3, folate), should be considered as augmenting medications throughout the course of a depressive illness.

▮ Psychotherapy may be helpful early in the course of the illness, and psychotherapy-medication combinations, when available, appear to be the most effective approaches.

▮ Electroconvulsive therapy (ECT) and other forms of neuromodulation may be useful, and even lifesaving, for those with severe

Treatment Resistant Depression (TRD) and prior treatment failures. When an initial antidepressant fails, it may be best to augment when the patient has a partial response to the original medication, and switch when the patient has no response or intolerable side effects.

■ For severely depressed patients with TRD, ECT should be discussed with the patient and family as an option after the second failed trial. Many are unfamiliar with or ill-informed about ECT, so education is particularly important. ECT is indicated particularly for patients with severe functional impairment, dangerous suicide risk, psychotic or catatonic features, or inability to tolerate psychopharmacological agents.

■ If a decision is made to proceed with ECT, pharmacological management during and immediately after ECT should be planned to achieve the difficult goal of preventing relapse following the course of ECT. Note that medications that were ineffective or not tolerated before ECT during a severe phase of the illness may be effective and tolerated after ECT when symptoms have markedly improved.

References

Brennan BP, Hudson JI, Jensen JE, e al: Rapid enhancement of glutamatergic neurotransmission in bipolar depression following treatment with riluzole. Neuropsychopharmacology 35:834–846, 2010

Cipriani A, La Ferla T, Furukawa TA, et al: Sertraline versus other antidepressive agents for depression. Cochrane Database of Systematic Reviews 2010, Issue 4. Art. No.: CD006117. DOI: 10.1002/14651858.CD006117.pub4.

Consumer Reports Health: Best Buy Drugs: The Antidepressants. October 2010. Available at: http://www.consumerreports.org/health/resources/pdf/best-buy-drugs/Antidepressants_update.pdf. Accessed February 8, 2011.

Fava M, Davidson KG: Definition and epidemiology of treatment-resistant depression. Psychiatr Clin North Am 19:179–200, 1996

Freeman MP, Mischoulon D, Tedeschini E, et al: Complementary and alternative medicine for major depressive disorder: a meta-analysis of patient characteristics, placebo-response rates, and treatment outcomes relative to standard antidepressants. J Clin Psychiatry 71:682–688, 2010

Gaynes BN, Rush AJ, Trivedi MH, et al: The STAR*D study: treating depression in the real world. Cleve Clin J Med 75:57–66, 2008

Nelson JC, Papakostas GI: Atypical antipsychotic augmentation in major depressive disorder: a meta-analysis of placebo-controlled randomized trials. Am J Psychiatry 166:980–991, 2009

Nierenberg AA, Fava M, Trivedi MH, et al: A comparison of lithium and T(3) augmentation following two failed medication treatments for depression: a STAR*D report. Am J Psychiatry 163:1519–1530 [quiz: 1665], 2006

Papakostas GI, Fava M, Thase ME: Treatment of SSRI-resistant depression: a meta-analysis comparing within- versus across-class switches. Biol Psychiatry 63:699–704, 2008

Papakostas GI, Mischoulon D, Shyu I, et al: S-adenosyl methionine (SAMe) augmentation of serotonin reuptake inhibitors for antidepressant nonresponders with major depressive disorder: a double-blind, randomized clinical trial. Am J Psychiatry 167:942–928, 2010

Petersen TJ: Enhancing the efficacy of antidepressants with psychotherapy. J Psychopharmacol 20 (suppl 3):19–28, 2006

Philip NS, Carpenter LL, Tyrka AR, et al: Pharmacologic approaches to treatment resistant depression: a re-examination for the modern era. Expert Opin Pharmacother 11:709–722, 2010

Sen S, Sanacora G: Major depression: emerging therapeutics. Mt Sinai J Med 75:204–225, 2008

Shelton RC, Osuntokun O, Heinloth AN, et al: Therapeutic options for treatment-resistant depression. CNS Drugs 24:131–161, 2010

Weinmann S, Becker T, Koesters M: Re-evaluation of the efficacy and tolerability of venlafaxine vs SSRI: meta-analysis. Psychopharmacology (Berl) 196:511–522, 2008

Zarate CA Jr, Payne JL, Quiroz J, et al: An open-label trial of riluzole in patients with treatment-resistant major depression. Am J Psychiatry 161:171–174, 2004

Zarate CA Jr, Singh JB, Carlson PJ, et al: A randomized trial of an N-methyl-D-aspartate antagonist in treatment-resistant major depression. Arch Gen Psychiatry 63:856–864, 2006

CHAPTER THREE

Treatment Resistant Depression in Adolescents

Neera Ghaziuddin, M.D., M.R.C.Psych.
Virginia Barbosa, M.D.
Cheryl King, Ph.D.

A SIGNIFICANT NUMBER of adolescents experience depression that does not respond to conventional evidence-based treatments. However, no systematic studies have examined the prevalence of Treatment Resistant Depression (TRD) in adolescents or determined when depression in adolescence should be labeled as TRD. Although depression that does not respond to an antidepressant or a psychotherapy trial may be considered treatment resistant, clinicians are more likely to label depression as treatment refractory when it does not respond to "multiple" antidepressant trials with documented adequate dosage and duration, combined with psychotherapy. In this chapter, we consider definitional issues and review studies pertinent to TRD in children and adolescents. We then present and discuss recommendations, based on the evidence currently available, for the assessment, treatment, and management of what would be regarded as TRD in adolescents by most clinicians. A flowchart is included in this chapter (see p.68) as a suggested guideline and is based on the currently available treatments.

The Problem of Nonresponse: Untreated and Treatment Resistant Depression

Inadequately treated or unremitted depression is burdensome for both the individual and society. A well-known association exists between adolescent major depressive disorder (MDD) and poor self-esteem, disrupted family relationships, increased use of alcohol and street drugs, failure to reach full potential, recurrent self-injurious behaviors, and completed suicide (Emslie et al. 2003; Giaconia et al. 2001). Moreover, depression that fails to remit can interfere with adolescent development because adolescence is a time-limited phase with complex psychosocial milestones to be completed. It has been shown that adults who fail to achieve remission of depression are also more likely to experience lifetime relapses (Thase 2001). On the basis of the adult literature and published and unpublished adolescent data, it would be reasonable to speculate that the already known high relapse rate of 69 % over a 5-year period for children and adolescents with MDD (Rao et al. 1995) and the high rates of reported dysfunction (Emslie et al. 2003; Giaconia et al. 2001) are further increased among adolescents who have TRD.

Evidence Base for Treating Depression in Children and Adolescents

Ample evidence indicates that selective serotonin reuptake inhibitors (SSRIs) and certain types of psychotherapy are at least modestly effective for many—but not all—depressive disorders in children and adolescents. This is a critical starting point for clinicians dealing with these individuals. More than a decade ago, Botteron and Geller (1997) attempted to summarize the status of TRD. They concluded that inadequate data regarding treatment response among children and adolescents, in addition to high placebo response rates, suggested that childhood depression may respond in a nonspecific manner. That is, without the evidence for definite treatment response, it was not possible to discuss treatment resistance in a meaningful way. Fortunately, many more randomized controlled treatment trials have been conducted since, and the field is significantly further along in its understanding of treatment for our child and adolescent population.

Pharmacotherapy

Monotherapy with an SSRI is often the first-line pharmacological treatment of moderate to severe depression, usually in combination with psychotherapy. Six of the seven published randomized controlled studies of the efficacy of SSRIs in children and adolescents report significant differences on some measures, indicating more favorable outcomes for those taking SSRIs (Emslie et al. 1997; Keller et al. 2001; March et al. 2004; Wagner et al. 2003, 2004). For instance, relatively large placebo-controlled trials have confirmed the efficacy of fluoxetine (March et al. 2004), sertraline (Wagner et al. 2003), and paroxetine (Keller et al. 2001) among adolescents. Although relatively high placebo response rates are incorporated into these numbers, trials of SSRIs among adolescents show an approximate 60% response to either an antidepressant alone or an antidepressant in combination with cognitive-behavioral therapy (CBT).

Not all symptoms respond, however. In clinical practice, failure to respond to one or two SSRIs is usually followed by treatment with a second-generation antidepressant. However, information specific to adolescents regarding the use of these agents is limited. For instance, bupropion has been studied in only a small number of adolescents with comorbid attention-deficit/hyperactivity disorder (ADHD) or substance abuse disorders. One such study found a 58% response rate among adolescents with a diagnosis of comorbid depression and ADHD (Daviss et al. 2001), and improvement in both depression and substance abuse was noted when the two conditions were co-occurring (Solhkhah et al. 2005). Information about venlafaxine is limited because of open-label study design. An early study failed to find a clear response to this agent (Mandoki et al. 1997); a more recent open-label study found a reduction in depression scores (Emslie et al. 2007). Literature pertaining to duloxetine is limited to three case reports (Delgado et al. 2007; Meighen 2007), which all found that this agent may be useful in children. No publications are available, at this writing, on the use of mirtazapine in patients younger than 18 years.

Pharmacological augmentation is often the next step when the response to monotherapy with one or two antidepressants is inadequate or absent. However, no systematic studies are specific to this age group. Frequently used strategies are the addition of an antipsychotic, a stimulant, lithium, mirtazapine, or bupropion. Adult studies suggest that augmentation with an atypical antipsychotic may have a favorable outcome. One study in adults found enhanced remission and response rates after the addition of risperidone in patients who were already receiving an antidepressant (Rapaport et al. 2006). Experience with aripiprazole, again based on adult studies, is somewhat sparse and is limited to one small, uncontrolled study (Hellerstein et al. 2008). Similarly, no controlled studies of augmentation with a stimulant or lithium have been done among adolescents with TRD. However, a placebo-controlled study in adults found a higher number of responders among participants who received an extended-release formulation of methylphenidate in addition to their pre-existing antidepressant (Patkar et al. 2006). Data regarding lithium augmentation in adolescents whose symptoms have not responded are limited to a single case report (Walter et al. 1998).

Psychotherapy

Research generally suggests that depressive disorders in children and adolescents respond in modestly positive ways to differing "active" psychosocial interventions (Brown 2007). The two specific types of psychotherapy with the most proven efficacy in children or adolescents are CBT and interpersonal psychotherapy for adolescents (IPT-A). The usefulness of psychotherapy for TRD in adolescents, however, has only recently been examined in a scientifically rigorous clinical trial. In the Treatment of Resistant Depression in Adolescents (TORDIA) trial, symptoms that had failed to respond to an initial trial of an SSRI improved significantly when treated with a combination approach of CBT and a different antidepressant, compared with a different antidepressant alone (Brent et al. 2008).

CBT for depression is a time-limited, here-and-now, collaborative approach that focuses on cognitive and behavioral factors related to the youth's presenting symptoms. Therapy goals commonly include 1) reducing negative, maladaptive cognitions; 2) improving problem-solving and coping skills; and 3) increasing involvement in healthy, pleasurable activities (Lewinsohn et al. 1990). Clinical trials have incorporated different variations of CBT, with some emphasizing cognitive restructuring (Brent et al. 1997) and others emphasizing behavioral activities and skills training (Lewinsohn et al. 1990).

Randomized controlled trials comparing CBT with either no treatment or relaxation training have generally found CBT to be superior (Clarke et al. 1999; Wood et al. 1996). More recent trials have included active control conditions such as systemic family therapy (Brent et al. 1997), IPT (Rossello and Bernal 1999), a life skills/tutoring intervention (Rohde et al. 2004), and SSRIs (March et al. 2004). CBT was associated with more positive initial recovery rates than were systemic family therapy and supportive therapy (Brent et al. 1997); however, remission, recovery, relapse, and recurrence rates did not differ across a 2-year follow-up. In contrast, CBT was not significantly better than placebo in the Treatment for Adolescents With Depression Study (TADS), which may reflect the severity of depression required for inclusion in this study, the particular form of CBT, or a combination of factors. Nevertheless, the combination treatment of SSRI plus CBT was associated with the most positive outcomes in the TADS, and CBT seemed to have a protective effect against suicidal thoughts and behaviors (March et al. 2004), resulting in the highest risk-benefit ratio. Suicidal thoughts and behaviors clearly have become a major concern for clinicians since the U.S. Food and Drug Administration included a warning on antidepressants for use in youths and young adults, even though not a single participant died by suicide during any of the SSRI trials (Bridge et al. 2007).

IPT-A is a modification of the IPT originally developed for depressed adult outpatients by Klerman et al. (1984). It uses a focused, time-limited approach to address interpersonal issues common during adolescence (i.e., role transitions, challenges of stepparent families) (Mufson et al. 1993). In two randomized controlled trials, one comparing IPT-A with clinical monitoring and one comparing IPT-A with treatment as usual from school-based health clinicians, patients who received IPT-A reported a greater reduction in depressive symptoms and more substantial improvement in social functioning (Mufson et al. 2004).

In this section, we have underscored that empirically based pharmacological and psychotherapeutic treatments are available and effective for many adolescents with clinical depression.

The Problem of Nonresponse: Treatment Resistant and Treatment Refractory Depression

Unfortunately, a significant minority of children and adolescents have depression that does not respond to these treatments, especially during their initial treatment trials. As is evident in the cases presented in the following section, such a failure to respond is often associated with increasingly compromised developmental trajectories and downward spirals of psychosocial functioning. Recurrent episodes accompanied by morbidity are often pronounced.

Clinical Vignettes of Cases Involving Use of Electroconvulsive Therapy

The following case raises questions about the somewhat haphazard use of antidepressants among adolescents whose depression fails to respond and the need to diagnose TRD in a timely manner whenever possible.

This patient, for instance, was prescribed hormones to treat depression (although no evidence supports this treatment), and unsuccessful treatment with sertraline was followed by failed trials of duloxetine and lamotrigine (relatively less well studied agents in this age group).

Vignette 1

Alice, a 17-year-old girl, had a 3-year history of TRD and school phobia with adequate premorbid functioning. She had several features often noted among adolescents with TRD: unremitting depression spanning several years, multiple failed medication trials in combination with psychotherapy, comorbidity with severe anxiety, and severe functional impairment.

Alice was referred to a university child and adolescent psychiatry clinic for evaluation and treatment after her treating psychiatrist told her that he could no longer treat her because "all known treatments have been exhausted." Her symptoms included daily crying spells, suicidal ideation (wanted to die to end her pain), initial insomnia, fatigue, and loss of interest in previously enjoyed activities (ballet, saxophone, and diving). She first noted depression at age 14 years and was given a contraceptive pill by her pediatrician, in the hope that "hormones may regularize periods and improve mood." Subsequently, she underwent unsuccessful treatment with sertraline, duloxetine, escitalopram, and lamotrigine, with each agent administered in adequate dose and duration. A brief trial of lithium was discontinued for unknown reasons. She received psychotherapy for several months, without any significant improvement. She could not recall any significant period when she had been free of symptoms.

In addition to the mood symptoms, Alice had gradually developed an intense fear of attending school. On most school days, she would follow a routine of getting ready but would end up staying at home. However, she continued to complete her school assignments, which were brought to her. She had no history of any medical disorder, substance or alcohol use, abuse or any other trauma, or behavior problems. She was described by her parents as a good child with no problems before age 14. Her birth and developmental histories were noncontributory. A positive history of depression was reported in a second-degree relative. Thyroid function test results were normal.

After the evaluation, Alice was diagnosed with TRD, severe, without psychotic features, and school phobia. She was advised to increase the dose of selegiline patch, which she was already receiving, and quetiapine was continued. In addition to CBT for depression, behavior modification with exposure and response prevention was added to treat the school phobia. Because of the lack of response to these treatments, Alice eventually received electroconvulsive therapy (ECT) over 3 months, with moderate success. Alice was able to start college while she continued taking fluoxetine and aripiprazole, which had been added toward the end of the ECT course. She refused to participate in continued psychotherapy.

In the following case, comorbid pervasive developmental disorder (PDD) likely contributed to the lack of treatment response and overall psychosocial failure in a youth with preadolescent-onset TRD.

Vignette 2

Brian, a 16-year-old boy, was referred after his depression failed to respond to multiple medication trials in combination with psychotherapy over the past 7 years. Severe symptoms had led to the inability to attend school, for the most part, since sixth grade. Presenting symptoms included severe depression, anxiety, initial insomnia and frequent awakenings, poor concentration, anhedonia, not being able to get out of bed on most days, daily suicidal ideation but no suicide attempts, no change in appetite but a long-standing history of food fads (such as inability to tolerate certain textures), severe hopelessness, and reduced motivation. Symptoms were worse when he was alone or in a public place, when he would experience panic attacks accompanied by feeling dizzy, nauseous, and fearful that he might pass out.

Brian had no history of abuse or trauma, use of alcohol or illicit drugs, fighting, running away, involvement with the legal system, or any other behavior problems. Family history was positive for depression in father, mother, and several maternal relatives. A family history of completed suicide was reported (in a maternal aunt when she was in her 20s).

At the time of his referral, Brian was receiving lamotrigine, aripiprazole, clonazepam, bupropion, propranolol for migraine headaches, amantadine for extrapyramidal symptoms, and amitriptyline to augment antidepressant treatment. Psychiatric history included hospitalizations at ages 9 and 12 and a 4-month stay at a residential facility at age 13. Past unsuccessful pharmacotherapy trials included fluoxetine, paroxetine, risperidone, valproate, mirtazapine, omega-3 fatty acids, lorazepam, and venlafaxine. Brian had been in weekly psychotherapy of unspecified type since he was 7 years old, with little or no benefit, despite good rapport with his therapist.

Pregnancy, birth, and early development were normal until excessive sensitivity to change, difficulty with transitions, and early development of language was noted (spoke like an adult, per mother). Early play was stereotyped, with restricted interests (lining up toys, excessive interest in toy weapons; later developed preoccupation with military paraphernalia). Despite having an advanced vocabulary, Brian had difficulty understanding humor or social cues.

On the basis of this presentation, he was diagnosed with severe depression without psychotic symptoms, generalized anxiety disorder (GAD), and PDD: Asperger's disorder. Brian received ECT with a moderately positive outcome. He experienced remission in suicidal ideation, was able to attend school, and graduated from high school. However, he continued to be impaired as a result of symptoms related to social awkwardness and feeling isolated. Subsequent treatments included lamotrigine, quetiapine, and supportive psychotherapy.

The following case highlights that severe anxiety or anxiety syndromes may precede TRD and are possible risk factors.

Vignette 3

Cindy, a 16-year-old girl, had anxiety since age 10 years followed by depressed mood for the past 2 years. Her symptoms included fatigue, anhedonia, daily suicidal ideation, hopelessness, poor appetite, and initial insomnia. She had made three suicide attempts by overdosing on ibuprofen and admitted engaging in self-cutting to relieve anxiety. She reported preoccupation with her appearance and was often unable to leave home because she felt "ugly" or her hair did not "look just right." Cindy had been hospitalized on three occasions and began taking antidepressants at age 14 years. Antidepressant trials had been made of fluoxetine, sertraline, escitalopram, clomipramine, and venlafaxine, administered alone or in combination with mood stabilizers. Medications were administered in adequate dose and duration. Augmentation agents used without success were oxcarbazepine, carbamazepine, aripiprazole, amphetamine, and methylphenidate. Cindy also had received unspecified psychotherapy since age 10 and regular CBT during the previous 7 months. She reported transient relief following some medications but had continued to experience significant symptoms, including inability to attend school on most days. Following evaluation, she was given the diagnoses of TRD, GAD, and obsessive-compulsive disorder (OCD).

Cindy was euthymic after treatment with ECT over 14 months. Complete remission of symptoms was maintained at 3 months post-ECT with ongoing treatment with fluoxetine, aripiprazole, and CBT.

In the following case, a youth with TRD and catatonia developed bipolar disorder.

Vignette 4

David, a 17-year-old boy, lived with both biological parents and was in regular education. He first presented to a university psychiatry outpatient clinic with symptoms of depression during the previous 10 months and failure to respond adequately to multiple treatment trials combined with weekly psychotherapy. A previous episode experienced at age 13 years had resolved with psychotherapy alone, and David had remained well until 10 months earlier.

Presenting symptoms included academic decline and inability to attend school, tearfulness and irritability, anhedonia, anergia, worthlessness, psychomotor retardation, loss of appetite, sleeping 16–23 hours per day, poor concentration, and poor motivation. He had dropped out of all activities and ceased communication with his peers. A moderately severe stressor was failing to qualify for an "extreme scouting trip." David did not report problems with anxiety, OCD, inattention, psychosis, elevated mood, grandiosity, risk-taking behaviors, or perceptual disturbances. He denied history of suicidality, trauma, or illicit substance use aside from experimenting with marijuana twice. He was diagnosed with MDD with catatonic features (immobility, reduced speech, and reduced food and fluid intake). His Global Assessment of Functioning (GAF) Scale score at the time of the hospitalization was 25.

David's medical history was significant for headaches and recurrent otitis media as a child. His developmental history was positive for delayed speech, but he had no subsequent communication deficits. Premorbid personality was normal, with age-appropriate social relationships. A family history of bipolar disorder was reported (involving multiple second-degree maternal relatives).

Past medication trials included fluoxetine, sertraline, venlafaxine, bupropion, and augmentation with divalproex, methylphenidate, and tri-iodothyronine. All agents were administered in adequate dosage and duration. Additionally, David received CBT, with unsatisfactory response.

Consultation with neurology, endocrinology, and infectious disease services did not identify any significant findings. Thyrotropin and free thyroxine were within the normal range. David received a diagnosis of TRD, which was successfully treated with ECT. Eighteen months later, he developed additional symptoms and was given the diagnosis of bipolar disorder II. However, he continued to function well, and his symptoms were well controlled with monotherapy with aripiprazole. David declined to participate in psychotherapy, however.

Defining and Characterizing Treatment Resistant Depression

A few studies have unsuccessfully attempted to define adolescent TRD, but no widely accepted definition exists (Botteron and Geller 1997). Kratochvil et al. (2005) attempted to define TRD by inviting a panel of experts to discuss the management of adolescent depression that had not responded to two adequate trials of SSRIs. Brent and Birmaher (2006) reviewed TRD and proposed that the condition appears to exist on a continuum, and the failure to respond to even a single adequate trial, in some instances, may constitute TRD. More recently, Brent et al. (2008) compared treatment options for adolescent depression that had failed to respond to an initial trial of an SSRI. Although Kratochvil et al. (2005) and Brent and Birmaher (2006) have attempted to address the management of adolescent depression that fails to respond to treatment, a precise definition and treatment guidelines remain far from clear.

Kratochvil et al. (2005) invited three experts in the field to discuss the management of a first episode of major depression in a 13-year-old boy. The depression had not responded to sertraline 200 mg/day and had partially responded to combined treatment with fluoxetine 60 mg/day and

CBT. Each treatment was administered over 12 weeks. The patient's father had a diagnosis of depression, and a paternal aunt had a diagnosis of bipolar disorder. After receiving the combined treatment with fluoxetine and CBT, the patient was no longer suicidal; academic and social functioning had improved; and insomnia, energy, and appetite had normalized. However, he continued to experience anhedonia, guilt, and poor concentration. The opinion of the experts regarding the management of residual symptoms included ruling out comorbid conditions such as posttraumatic stress disorder (PTSD), ADHD, substance abuse, and bipolar disorder; ruling out medical conditions; and identifying psychosocial stress. Reconsidering the primary diagnosis, such as schizophrenia or bipolar disorder, also was recommended. Treatment strategies suggested were switching to a different class of antidepressant and augmentation with a stimulant, an atypical antipsychotic, or lithium. The experts noted, however, that data specific to adolescents are lacking in regard to several antidepressants and augmentation strategies. Also, the investigators disagreed as to whether the patient's symptoms met criteria for TRD because of the partial, versus absent, response to fluoxetine combined with CBT.

In the TORDIA multicenter clinical trial, Brent et al. (2008) compared treatment options for adolescent depression that had not responded to an initial trial of an SSRI. In a randomized controlled design, adolescents (12–18 years) were assigned to one of four different treatments over a 12-week period: an SSRI alone (citalopram, sertraline, or fluoxetine), an SSRI combined with CBT, venlafaxine alone, or venlafaxine combined with CBT. Participants who received either antidepressant in combination with CBT did equally well, with a 50% response rate. No differences in the treatment effects in terms of depression severity or suicidal ideation and behavior were seen; however, side effects such as elevated blood pressure or rashes were more likely among those who received venlafaxine. This was the first large-scale empirical study to examine the relative efficacy of multiple treatment options following a failed initial antidepressant trial. Even though this study defined treatment resistance as the failure to respond to a single 12-week antidepressant trial, it was one step on a continuum toward understanding the treatment for adolescent TRD.

Another important source of information about the definition of TRD, and data regarding its treatment, is the literature on ECT. By no means does this suggest that ECT is the only treatment for TRD; however, depressed adolescents who receive ECT invariably have severe treatment resistance, by guideline requirements (Ghaziuddin et al. 2004), and are a noteworthy source of understanding.

Several reports on adolescents with TRD who are given ECT have been published. The main drawback of these studies is that they are characterized by small sample sizes; nevertheless, they are an important source of information for the presentation, comorbid conditions, and complications of a highly treatment-refractory group. Moreover, they are important to our understanding of TRD because in the United States two or three child psychiatrists must reach consensus that an adolescent indeed has refractory depression before he or she can receive ECT. Therefore, despite limitations, this literature is an important source of consensus regarding the definition of TRD.

In one such study, Ghaziuddin et al. (1996) described 11 patients with depression who later received ECT. Nine subjects were diagnosed with MDD, one with bipolar depression, and one with depression secondary to a medical condition (brain tumor). The 9 subjects in the MDD subgroup had received 24 unsuccessful antidepressant trials, in addition to 1–2 augmentation trials each (usually a mood stabilizer and/or an antipsychotic agent). Comorbid Axis I diagnoses were common—an anxiety disorder or dysthymia was diagnosed in 5 of 9 participants. Similarly, Cohen et al. (1997) described a group of 10 adolescents (mean age = 17 years) with TRD and concomitant psychotic symptoms. Seven of the 10 patients were experiencing their first depressive episode, 3 had a positive psychiatric history, and 7 had a positive family history of depression.

The following discussion presents unpublished data on 33 adolescents (females = 19; males = 14), all of whom received ECT, over a 20-year period at the University of Michigan Department of Psychiatry and the University of Michigan Comprehensive Depression Center. These data (displayed in Table 3–1) were collected after obtaining approval from the institutional ethics committee.

Outcome immediately following ECT showed that 30 patients were improved to very much improved. One patient did not experience any change, and the records for two patients could not be located. Clearly, these data are evidence for a severe form of depression among adolescents with clinical characteristics that far exceed those generally considered essential for labeling a patient with TRD (i.e., failure to respond to two to three medication trials combined with psychotherapy). This group lends unequivocal support to the existence of a highly disabling form of TRD and provides information about severity, duration, and details of past psychiatric treatment.

A noteworthy finding in this group was the frequent co-occurrence of other Axis I disorders; comorbid anxiety disorders were found among 39%, PDD among 21%, catatonia among 15%, disruptive behavior disorders among 24%, and eating disorders among 6%. High comorbidity with anxiety disorders has been reported previously among adults with TRD compared with non-TRD patients (Petersen et al. 2001). Addition-

TABLE 3–1.   **Characteristics of 33 adolescents with depression who received electroconvulsive therapy**

Variable	Mean±SD
Mean age of group in years	15.8±1.5
Child Depression Rating Scale–Revised score	67±17
GAF Scale score	20±8
Number of psychotropic medications tried	8.2±4.2
Number of SSRI trials	2.2±1
Number of non-SSRI trials	1.7±1.3
Number of antipsychotic trials	1.7±1.3
Number of mood stabilizer trials	1.1±1.3
Duration of psychotherapy in weeks	127±144
Number of hospitalizations	3.5±2
Number of lifetime suicide attempts	2.1±2.2

Note.   GAF = Global Assessment of Functioning; SD = standard deviation; SSRI = selective serotonin reuptake inhibitor.

ally, 52% of the group had engaged in self-injurious behaviors, 88% had severe academic or school-related issues, and 65% had disturbed family or peer problems. The majority of adolescents denied ever ingesting alcohol (69%) or using illicit drugs (75%), which was a counterintuitive finding.

Assessment and Management

Definition

On the basis of the current state of knowledge, adolescent TRD may be best defined as the failure to respond to two *adequate* antidepressant trials combined with psychotherapy. Psychotherapies shown to be effective for the treatment of adolescent depression are CBT and IPT. Adequate antidepressant treatment should be assessed in terms of dose and duration. An adequate dose of an SSRI may vary in relation to the drug under consideration. However, adequate duration of antidepressant treatment is at least 8 weeks, with at least 4 weeks at an equivalent dose of fluoxetine (20 mg).

Absence of class I data on adolescents for several commonly prescribed antidepressants is one likely obstacle in defining adolescent TRD. Antidepressants that are relatively understudied in this age group include bupropion, mirtazapine, and duloxetine. The use of augmentation strategies with lithium, atypical antipsychotics, or stimulants is also based on anecdotal reports. Therefore, at this time augmentation strategies cannot be included in defining adolescent TRD.

General Consideration for Assessment

A complete diagnostic evaluation is essential before a patient is determined to have TRD. A biopsychosocial conceptual approach is necessary for the assessment of individual psychiatric, medical, and personality factors; family functioning and interaction styles; family psychiatric history; and details of past treatment. Clinical variables such as longer episodes, greater illness severity, psychosis, suicidality, and sleep disturbance are associated with poorer outcome and chronicity (Emslie et al. 2003).

Comorbid Axis I Psychiatric Disorders

Comorbid psychiatric conditions are common and may precede or coexist with TRD. Although many of the disease management steps remain the same, age-related modifications of the "roadmap" described by Greden and colleagues in Chapter 1 are indicated. Assessment and treatment must evaluate for anxiety disorders, school refusal, PDD, disruptive behavior disorders, such as ADHD, oppositional defiant disorder and conduct disorder, dysthymia, and catatonia. Comorbidity with PDD or catatonia is less frequently recognized. PDD is more likely to be overlooked in the presence of normal IQ. For the diagnosis of PDD, careful history should identify social and communication deficits accompanied by restricted or stereotyped interests. Semistructured diagnostic interviews such as the Autism Diagnostic Interview—Revised (Rutter et al. 2003), observation schedules such as the Autism Diagnosis Observation Schedule (Lord et al. 2000), standardized rating scales such as the Social Communication Questionnaire (Rutter et al. 2003), and neuropsychological testing should be completed. As in adults, difficulties in differentiating between unipolar and bipolar depression may be a factor underlying poor response. Confusion between the two diagnoses may occur because bipolar II disorder and bipolar disorder not otherwise specified are more likely to present with depression or irritability as the intake affective episode, unlike bipolar I disorder, which is more likely to present with elated mood (Masi et al. 2007). Therefore, appropriate treatment may be implemented after revising the diagnosis.

Comorbid Axis II Psychiatric Disorders

Developmental learning and speech disorders should be explored. Mild mental retardation or borderline intelligence may be overlooked in some cases and can be a contributing reason for gaps in treatment response. In our unpublished data, a quarter of the subgroup (24 %) had a learning disability diagnosis, and 17 % had a developmental speech disorder. Learning disability and developmental speech disorders may be diagnosed with the help of standardized tests such as the Wide Range Achievement Test (Jastak et al. 1984) and the Clinical Evaluation of Language Fundamentals—4 (Semel et al. 2003), respectively.

Comorbid Axis III Medical Disorders

Adolescents with TRD must receive a comprehensive medical evaluation to identify comorbid medical conditions that may complicate the treatment of both psychiatric and medical disorders. Basic laboratory investigations (complete blood count, urinalysis, urine toxicology, metabolic panel, thyroid and liver function tests) may be followed by additional tests, if necessary. Although rare, brain tumors can present as depression in children and adolescents (Oreskovic et al. 2007). Therefore, careful history and examination are essential, and computed tomography or magnetic resonance brain imaging may be necessary. A large study among children found an overall association between depression and medical disorders, especially immunological conditions (Cohen et al. 1998). Consistent with this literature, youths with type 1 diabetes are more likely to have more protracted and recurrent depression (Kovacs et al. 1997).

Psychosocial Functioning

Careful assessment of psychosocial functioning and rehabilitation is necessary as part of successful treatment outcome. Chronic TRD, lasting over months or years, is likely to have interfered with engagement in age-appropriate peer relationships and extracurricular activities, and this is unlikely to resolve without specific intervention. CBT and IPT can be particularly helpful.

In our unpublished data involving 33 depressed adolescents who received ECT (described earlier in this chapter), serious academic impairment was found among 88 %, including inability to attend school, and severe conflict with parents was reported by 65 %.

Evaluation of Past Treatment (Including Adherence and Duration)

Evaluation of an adolescent with TRD must establish whether treatment received thus far has been consistent with empirically based treatment guidelines or recommendations. In addition to obtaining information about previously recommended treatments, the issue of treatment adherence must be taken into consideration. Treatment nonadherence is common among psychiatric patients and possibly higher among adolescents who are known to be highly nonadherent across a variety of disorders. This phenomenon is difficult to predict but should be carefully monitored during the course of treatment and scrutinized before a patient is determined to have TRD. Standard psychiatric interviewing techniques, information from previous treatment providers, and pharmacy records, in some cases, may clarify the extent of adherence to recommended antidepressant treatment.

The most complete and up-to-date guideline for the pharmacological treatment of adolescent depression is described in the Texas Children's Medication Algorithm Project (Hughes et al. 2007). This guideline is a stepwise, empirically based set of pharmacological recommendations for the treatment of adolescent depression (Figure 3–1). The guideline indicates that the first-line (stage 1) antidepressant treatment of moderate to severe depression in an adolescent should be monotherapy with an SSRI (fluoxetine, citalopram, or sertraline). Adults whose depression fails to respond to stage 1 may switch to another drug class. However, among children and adolescents, for whom data are less adequate, failure to respond to the first-stage antidepressant (an SSRI) should be followed by monotherapy with an alternative SSRI in stage 2. Stage 2a includes augmentation with lithium, mirtazapine, or bupropion. In stage 3, monotherapy with an antidepressant from a different class (venlafaxine, bupropion, mirtazapine, or duloxetine) may be used. However, no good evidence is available at this time to recommend these agents (venlafaxine, bupropion, mirtazapine, or duloxetine) as first-line agents. The need for additional assessment, precautions, monitoring, and maintenance treatment is emphasized.

Adequate treatment duration with an antidepressant is necessary for the acute phase of the illness and for maintenance treatment after the patient has achieved remission. It is not unusual for adolescents to discontinue medications once they begin to feel better. Although the exact duration of maintenance antidepressant treatment is not known because virtually no data are available for youths with TRD, adult studies suggest that most adolescents require treatment for 1.5–2 years (Greden 2002) and would recommend considerably longer durations for those with multiple episodes or chronicity and suicide risk.

Tricyclic antidepressants are not recommended, and meta-analyses and controlled trials converge in indicating that this group of antidepressants is not effective or safe for the treatment of adolescent depression (Keller et al. 2001).

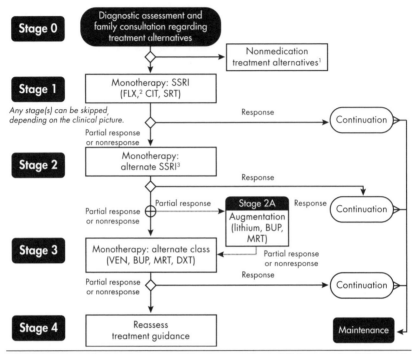

FIGURE 3–1.   Medication algorithm for treating children and adolescents who meet DSM-IV-TR criteria for major depressive disorder.

BUP = bupropion; CIT = citalopram; DXT = duloxetine; FDA = U.S. Food and Drug Administration; FLX = fluoxetine; MRT = mirtazapine; SRT = sertraline; SSRI = selective serotonin reuptake inhibitor; VEN = venlafaxine.

[1]Evidence-based psychotherapy can be used at any stage in the algorithm.
[2]Fluoxetine is the only antidepressant with an FDA-approved indication for depression in youths.
[3]Paroxetine is not recommended for preadolescents.

Source.   Adapted from Hughes et al. 2007. This algorithm is in the public domain and may be used and reprinted without special permission. The authors appreciate proper citation. The authors bear no responsibility for the use of these guidelines by third parties.

Pharmacological augmentation is frequently used, but as noted earlier in this chapter, data on its usefulness among adolescents are limited.

Treatment dose and adherence are also important considerations when evaluating the psychotherapy that has been provided to children and adolescents. In a review and critique of the evidence base for psychotherapy for child and adolescent mental health problems and disorders, Weisz et al. (2005) reported on various treatment characteristics, including dose. It is noteworthy that they identified 18 treatment studies in the depression domain that used random assignment. In more than 80% of these studies, psychotherapy used learning-based approaches that would fit within the broad category of CBT. The mean number of therapy sessions was 12.3 across 9.5 weeks. Clinical findings from the TADS and the TORDIA trial converged to suggest similar parameters for dose. In phase 1 of the TADS trial (March et al. 2004), an initial parent-adolescent session for goal-setting, psychoeducation, and clarification of therapy rationale was followed by 14 hour-long sessions over a 12-week period. The mean number of CBT sessions attended was 11 (median = 12). Similarly, in the TORDIA study (Brent and Birmaher 2006), the mean number of CBT sessions attended during phase 1 (first 12 weeks) was 8.3 (median = 9). In both of these studies, additional sessions were available after this period. With these findings taken together, one can argue that a minimum of 11–12 psychotherapy sessions across a 12- to 15-week period, followed by a second phase of weekly visits for partial responders, could be considered an adequate psychotherapy trial.

Treatment Strategies

Many adolescents and their families feel helpless and desperate by the time they receive a diagnosis of TRD. They may report prolonged absence from school (sometimes years in duration, as described in Vignette 2), loss of peer relationships, and progressive social isolation. Frustration at the possibility of another failed medication trial or additional psychotherapy is common. Therefore, an honest discussion with the patient and family about each available option, the rationale for its use, and the minimum duration necessary for an effective trial is critical. Discussion should include evidence-based information and take patient and family preferences into account.

The following list and Figure 3–2 summarize suggested treatment options for adolescents with TRD:

- ***Empirically supported treatments.*** Clinicians should use one or more empirical treatments suggested in the Texas Children's Medication Algorithm Project (Hughes et al. 2007) guideline if standard treatments have not been used. This option should be preferred for adolescents who did not receive adequate treatment with agents with established efficacy data, such as SSRIs mentioned in stages 1 and 2 (Hughes et al. 2007). Failure to respond to an initial SSRI should be followed by changing to a different SSRI or venlafaxine in combination with CBT (Brent et al. 2008). If the response is still inadequate, augmentation with lithium may be considered, which is also one of the options included in this algorithm; however, it is not well studied in

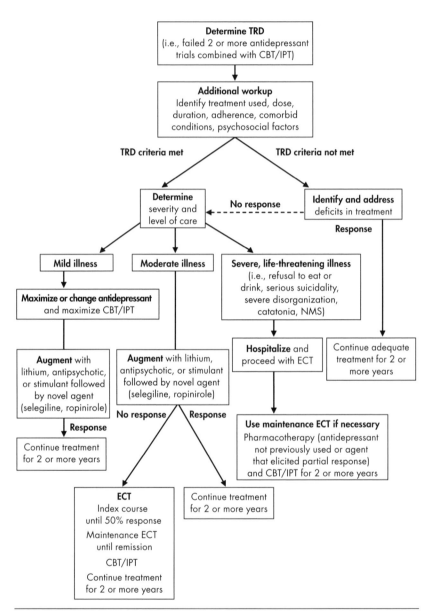

FIGURE 3–2.   Suggested treatment of adolescent Treatment Resistant Depression (TRD).

CBT = cognitive-behavioral therapy; ECT = electroconvulsive therapy; IPT = interpersonal psychotherapy; NMS = neuroleptic malignant syndrome.

any age group with history of multiple failed medication trials. Modest improvement was found, however, in one controlled study involving adults whose depression had not responded to two prior antidepressants (Nierenberg et al. 2006). Specific data involving adolescents consist of a single report of two adolescents who experienced rapid response to the combination of venlafaxine and lithium (Walter et al. 1998). Therefore, lithium augmentation data for adolescents with TRD are at best equivocal. Augmentation with bupropion or mirtazapine is not supported by systematic studies involving adolescents. However, one-third of adults reportedly achieved remission after inadequate response to citalopram alone (Trivedi et al. 2006).

- *A role for CBT or IPT.*   Although relatively few studies have examined the efficacy of CBT or IPT-A for children and adolescents with severe or treatment-refractory depression, several studies indicated that CBT may have a role in this patient group. Benefits noted were an accelerated antidepressant response rate and protection against suicidal thoughts or acts in the major multisite TADS (March et al. 2007). A positive effect of combining CBT with a change in antidepressant was found in comparison with change in medication alone in the TORDIA trial (Brent et al. 2008). Given the increased risk of suicidal behavior and suicide in those with a chronic history of severe depression, and the types of comorbid disorders and symptoms that are common with TRD (recurrent suicidal behaviors, severe conflict, psychosocial failure, anxiety disorders, PDD), safety concerns are a priority with these patients. To obtain the most positive effects—to avoid further affective distress, developmental impairment, risk of suicidality, development of comorbidity, and impaired quality of life—it is recommended that a "strong arm" approach of combination treatment be implemented. Although no trials of IPT for TRD have been published, it may be a reasonable alternative if the primary psychosocial issues are interpersonal in nature, such as conflicts with a new stepparent or a difficult move to a new school.

- *Agents shown effective in other populations.*   Clinicians should consider pharmacological agents shown to be effective in other populations, although class I data may be lacking. These may include changing to a novel class, such as a monoamine oxidase inhibitor, or augmentation with an atypical antipsychotic, stimulant, or ropinirole. Open trials of aripiprazole and a controlled trial of risperidone were found to be effective among adults with TRD (Hellerstein et al. 2008; Simon and Nemeroff 2005). A pilot study in adults found favorable results when ropinirole was added to their antidepressant regimen (Cassano et al. 2005). Selegiline, an irreversible inhibitor of monoamine oxidase type B in humans, may be used in adolescents with TRD because it offers the advantage of a novel class. This agent has been found to be well tolerated and modestly effective for the treatment of ADHD in children (Mohammadi et al. 2004) but has not been studied in the treatment of adolescent mood disorders.

- **Electroconvulsive therapy.**   ECT may be considered for adolescents whose symptoms have not responded to combination treatment and who have a severe and disabling disorder. Controlled trials of ECT in adolescents are lacking, however. Therefore, it is not known how many failed treatment trials are necessary before an adolescent is deemed an appropriate candidate for ECT. We believe that ECT should not be considered as a "treatment of last resort" and that illness severity, rather than the number of failed treatments, should be used as a guide when making a decision between ECT and an additional medication trial. Case reports and case series show an approximate 65% response rate (Cohen et al. 1997; Ghaziuddin et al. 1996; Walter and Rey 1997). Memory disturbance following ECT is a known side effect. However, the available data indicate that short-term impairment and recovery appear to follow adult patterns, with complete recovery within a few months of treatment (Cohen et al. 2000; Ghaziuddin et al. 2000). Adolescents who received ECT and their families are noted to have a favorable view of the treatment (Taieb et al. 2000). Practice guidelines published by the American Academy of Child and Adolescent Psychiatry are a comprehensive resource (Ghaziuddin et al. 2004). Note that the patients in all four case vignettes described earlier in this chapter received ECT because of illness severity and past failure to respond to treatment. Alice and Brian responded with more than 50% reduction in their depressive symptoms, whereas Cindy and David experienced complete remission. All patients continued to receive pharmacotherapy, and two patients continued to receive psychotherapy.

- **Neuromodulation using rTMS.**   Relatively novel treatments include repetitive transcranial magnetic stimulation (rTMS), a neuromodulatory procedure in which a magnetic field is used to alter brain activity. An electromagnetic coil placed on the scalp generates a rapidly alternating magnetic field that passes through the skull to induce small focal electric currents that stimulate nerve cells in the underlying cerebral cortex, inducing neuronal depolarization. The exact mechanism of action for rTMS is not known, but several hypotheses have been proposed, including increase in the regional cerebral blood flow, endogenous dopamine release in the mesolimbic and mesostriatal regions, and increase in serum brain-derived neurotrophic factor.

In contrast to adults, there is a dearth of information on the use of rTMS in children and adolescents. Among the scant data is a review of 49 publications between 1990 and January 2005 that used TMS; however, only seven studies ($n = 34$) used rTMS (the remainder used single-pulse TMS). Only one study ($n = 7$) examined the antidepressant effects of rTMS. In the latter study, two of four subjects (age 16–18 years) with depression or bipolar disorder showed improvement after 10 treatment sessions (Walter et al. 2001). Another publication involving depressed adolescents (Loo et al. 2008) found significant improvement among two adolescents, who were randomly assigned to the active treatment arm of a double-blind, sham-controlled trial of rTMS. Therefore, despite promising preliminary data, this treatment may be used only with caution and only after other better-known treatments are exhausted.

- *Vagus nerve stimulation.* VNS is an established treatment for selected patients with medically refractory seizures and was found to be effective among adults with TRD (Sackeim et al. 2007). It appears that the vagus nerve exerts direct influence on areas of the brain involved in the regulation of mood and increases the level of biogenic amines. Although large studies are lacking for all age ranges, and especially for adolescents, this treatment option may be considered in the future for adolescents with TRD who have exhausted all treatment options, including ECT.

Treatment Follow-Up

The overall goal of follow-up of adolescents with TRD is to maintain treatment response, continue to treat previously missed or treatment-resistant comorbid conditions, maximize treatment adherence, treat secondary complications (academic failure, school refusal, social isolation), and, whenever possible, achieve remission. Wellness is the goal! Careful observation for any increase in suicidal thoughts or acts should be mandatory, and periodic suicide rating scales should be used. Although it is not known what might constitute adequate follow-up, most adolescents are likely to benefit from ongoing treatment and monitoring until they can reach and maintain remission, most likely for 2 or more years.

Future Directions

The following steps are suggested to promote progress in the treatment of children and adolescents with TRD:

- Large-scale studies, such as those that might be conducted in national networks so that they can be combined with long-term follow-up, are necessary to identify prevalence, initial outcomes, and long-term prognosis of adolescent TRD.
- Studies are necessary to identify risk factors that signify later development of TRD.
- TRD should be identified in a timely manner to prevent prolonged suffering and disability.
- Some patients are likely to benefit from treatment with ECT. Therefore, adequate training of child and adolescent psychiatrists in the delivery of ECT is necessary.
- Novel neuromodulation treatments (rTMS, VNS) need to be studied in this population.

Key Clinical Concepts

- ■ TRD often results in severe impairment and distress, with a worsening developmental trajectory over time. "Preventive" strategies are especially needed during childhood and adolescence.

- ■ Clinicians should be trained to identify Treatment Resistant Depression (TRD) among children and adolescents.

- ■ Improved recognition of Axis I and Axis II comorbid disorders is important. Treatment failure can be a result of failure to recognize and treat comorbid conditions.

- ■ Treatment must be comprehensive to prevent or minimize the psychosocial failure and chronicity commonly associated with TRD.

- ■ Sparse but compelling data support adolescent TRD as a valid clinical entity with onset observed during childhood and adolescence.

- ■ Any patient thought to have TRD must receive a careful biopsychosocial evaluation and formulation.

- ■ Careful assessment of treatment history should include extent to which treatments received were empirically based, whether the medication dose was adequate, and whether pharmacotherapy and psychotherapy were of adequate duration.

- ■ Careful follow-up is recommended to maintain remission and to identify relapse rapidly.

References

Botteron KN, Geller B: Refractory depression in children and adolescents. Depress Anxiety 5:212–223, 1997

Brent DA, Birmaher B: Treatment-resistant depression in adolescents: recognition and management. Child Adolesc Psychiatr Clin North Am 15:1015–1034, 2006

Brent DA, Holder D, Kolko D, et al: A clinical psychotherapy trial for adolescent depression comparing cognitive, family, and supportive therapy. Arch Gen Psychiatry 54:877–885, 1997

Brent DA, Emslie G, Clarke G, et al: Switching to another SSRI or to venlafaxine with or without cognitive behavioral therapy for adolescents with SSRI-resistant depression: the TORDIA randomized controlled trial. JAMA 299:901–913, 2008

Bridge JA, Iyengar S, Salary CB, et al: Clinical response and risk for reported suicidal ideation and suicide attempts in pediatric antidepressant treatment: a meta-analysis of randomized controlled trials. JAMA 297:1683–1696, 2007

Brown RT: Journal of Pediatric Psychology (JPP), 2003 2007: Editors Vale Dictum. J Pediatr Psychol 32:1165–1178, 2007

Cassano P, Lattanzi L, Fava M, et al: Ropinirole in treatment-resistant depression: a 16-week pilot study. Can J Psychiatry 50:357–360, 2005

Clarke GN, Rohde P, Lewinsohn PM, et al: Cognitive-behavioral treatment of adolescent depression: efficacy of acute group treatment and booster sessions. J Am Acad Child Adolesc Psychiatry 38:272–279, 1999

Cohen D, Paillere-Martinot ML, Basquin M: Use of electroconvulsive therapy in adolescents. Convuls Ther 13:25, 1997

Cohen D, Taieb O, Flament M, et al: Absence of cognitive impairment at long-term follow-up in adolescents treated with ECT for severe mood disorder. Am J Psychiatry 157:460–462, 2000

Cohen P, Pine DS, Must A, et al: Prospective associations between somatic illness and mental illness from childhood to adulthood. Am J Epidemiol 147:232–239, 1998

Daviss WB, Bentivoglio P, Racusin R, et al: Bupropion sustained release in adolescents with comorbid attention-deficit/hyperactivity disorder and depression. J Am Acad Child Adolesc Psychiatry 40:307–314, 2001

Delgado SV, Saldana SN, Barzman DH, et al: Response to duloxetine in a depressed, treatment-resistant adolescent female. J Child Adolesc Psychopharmacol 17:889–894, 2007

Emslie GJ, Rush AJ, Weinberg WA, et al: A double-blind, randomized, placebo-controlled trial of fluoxetine in children and adolescents with depression. Arch Gen Psychiatry 54:1031–1037, 1997

Emslie GJ, Mayes TL, Laptook RS, et al: Predictors of response to treatment in children and adolescents with mood disorders. Psychiatr Clin North Am 26:435–456, 2003

Emslie GJ, Yeung PP, Kunz NR: Long-term, open-label venlafaxine extended-release treatment in children and adolescents with major depressive disorder. CNS Spectr 12:223–233, 2007

Ghaziuddin N, King CA, Naylor MW, et al: Electroconvulsive treatment in adolescents with pharmacotherapy-refractory depression. J Child Adolesc Psychopharmacol 6:259–271, 1996

Ghaziuddin N, Laughrin D, Giordani B: Cognitive side effects of electroconvulsive therapy in adolescents. J Child Adolesc Psychopharmacol 10:269–276, 2000

Ghaziuddin N, Kutcher SP, Knapp P, et al: Practice parameter for use of electroconvulsive therapy with adolescents. J Am Acad Child Adolesc Psychiatry 43:1521–1539, 2004

Giaconia RM, Reinherz HZ, Paradis AD, et al: Major depression and drug disorders in adolescence: general and specific impairments in early adulthood. J Am Acad Child Adolesc Psychiatry 40:1426–1433, 2001

Greden JF: Unmet need: what justifies the search for a new antidepressant? J Clin Psychiatry 63 (suppl 2):3–7, 2002

Hellerstein DJ, Batchelder S, Hyler S, et al: Aripiprazole as an adjunctive treatment for refractory unipolar depression. Prog Neuropsychopharmacol Biol Psychiatry 32:744–750, 2008

Hughes CW, Emslie GJ, Crismon ML, et al: Texas Children's Medication Algorithm Project: update from Texas Consensus Conference Panel on Medication Treatment of Childhood Major Depressive Disorder. J Am Acad Child Adolesc Psychiatry 46:667–686, 2007

Jastak S, Wilkinson GS, Wilmington DE (eds): Wide Range Achievement Test, Revised. Wilmington, DE, Jastek Associates, 1984

Keller MB, Ryan ND, Strober M, et al: Efficacy of paroxetine in the treatment of adolescent major depression: a randomized, controlled trial. J Am Acad Child Adolesc Psychiatry 40:762–772, 2001

Klerman GL, Weissman M, Rounsaville BJ, et al (eds): Interpersonal Psychotherapy of Depression. New York, Basic Books, 1984

Kovacs M, Obrosky DS, Goldston D, et al: Major depressive disorder in youths with IDDM: a controlled prospective study of course and outcome. Diabetes Care 20:45–51, 1997

Kratochvil CJ, Wagner KD, Emslie G, et al: Pharmacological management of treatment-resistant pediatric depression. J Am Acad Child Adolesc Psychiatry 44:198–200, 2005

Lewinsohn PM, Clarke GN, Hops H, et al: Cognitive-behavioral treatment for depressed adolescents. Behav Ther 21:385–401, 1990

Loo CK, Sachdev P, Mitchell PB, et al: A study using transcranial magnetic stimulation to investigate motor mechanisms in psychomotor retardation in depression. Int J Neuropsychopharmacol 11:935–946, 2008

Lord C, Risi S, Lambrecht L, et al: The Autism Diagnosis Observation Schedule-Generic: a standard measure of social and communication deficits associated with the spectrum of Autism. J Autism Dev Disorder 30:205–223, 2000

Mandoki MW, Tapia MR, Tapia MA, et al: Venlafaxine in the treatment of children and adolescents with major depression. Psychopharmacol Bull 33:149–154, 1997

March JS, Silva S, Petrycki S, et al: Fluoxetine, cognitive-behavioral therapy, and their combination for adolescents with depression: Treatment for Adolescents With Depression Study (TADS) randomized controlled trial. JAMA 292:807–820, 2004

March JS, Silva S, Petrycki S, et al: The Treatment for Adolescents With Depression Study (TADS): long-term effectiveness and safety outcomes. Arch Gen Psychiatry 64:1132–1143, 2007

Masi G, Perugi G, Millepiedi S, et al: Clinical implications of DSM-IV subtyping of bipolar disorders in referred children and adolescents. J Am Acad Child Adolesc Psychiatry 46:1299–1306, 2007

Meighen KG: Duloxetine treatment of pediatric chronic pain and co-morbid major depressive disorder. J Child Adolesc Psychopharmacol 17:121–127, 2007

Mohammadi MR, Ghanizadeh A, Alaghband-Rad J, et al: Selegiline in comparison with methylphenidate in attention deficit hyperactivity disorder children and adolescents in a double-blind, randomized clinical trial. J Child Adolesc Psychopharmacol 14:418–425, 2004

Mufson LH, Moreau D, Weissman M, et al (eds): Interpersonal Psychotherapy for Depressed Adolescents. New York, Guilford, 1993

Mufson LH, Gallagher T, Dorta KP, et al: A group adaptation of interpersonal psychotherapy for depressed adolescents. Am J Psychother 58:220–237, 2004

Nierenberg AA, Fava M, Trivedi MH, et al: A comparison of lithium and T(3) augmentation following two failed medication treatments for depression: a STAR*D report. Am J Psychiatry 163:1519–1530; quiz 1665, 2006

Oreskovic NM, Strother CG, Zibners LM: An unusual case of a central nervous system tumor presenting as a chief complaint of depression. Pediatr Emerg Care 23:486–488, 2007

Patkar AA, Masand PS, Pae CU, et al: A randomized, double-blind, placebo-controlled trial of augmentation with an extended release formulation of methylphenidate in outpatients with treatment-resistant depression. J Clin Psychopharmacol 26:653–656, 2006

Petersen T, Gordon JA, Kant A, et al: Treatment resistant depression and Axis I co-morbidity. Psychol Med 31:1223–1229, 2001

Rao U, Ryan ND, Birmaher B, et al: Unipolar depression in adolescents: clinical outcome in adulthood. J Am Acad Child Adolesc Psychiatry 34:566–578, 1995

Rapaport MH, Gharabawi GM, Canuso CM, et al: Effects of risperidone augmentation in patients with treatment-resistant depression: results of open-label treatment followed by double-blind continuation. Neuropsychopharmacology 31:2505–2513, 2006

Rohde P, Clarke GN, Mace DE, et al: An efficacy/effectiveness study of cognitive-behavioral treatment for adolescents with comorbid major depression and conduct disorder. J Am Acad Child Adolesc Psychiatry 43:660–668, 2004

Rossello J, Bernal G: The efficacy of cognitive-behavioral and interpersonal treatments for depression in Puerto Rican adolescents. J Consult Clin Psychol 67:734–745, 1999

Rutter M, Bailey A, Lord C (eds): Social Communication Questionnaire. Los Angeles, CA, Western Psychiatric Services, 2003

Sackeim HA, Brannan SK, Rush AJ, et al: Durability of antidepressant response to vagus nerve stimulation (VNS). Int J Neuropsychopharmacol 10:817–826, 2007

Semel E, Wiig EH, Wayne A (eds): Clinical Evaluation of Language Fundamentals—4. San Antonio, TX, Harcourt Assessment, 2003

Simon JS, Nemeroff CB: Aripiprazole augmentation of antidepressants for the treatment of partially responding and nonresponding patients with major depressive disorder. J Clin Psychiatry 66:1216–1220, 2005

Solhkhah R, Wilens TE, Daly J, et al: Bupropion SR for the treatment of substance-abusing outpatient adolescents with attention-deficit/hyperactivity disorder and mood disorders. J Child Adolesc Psychopharmacol 15:777–786, 2005

Taieb O, Cohen D, Mazet P, et al: Adolescents' experiences with ECT. J Am Acad Child Adolesc Psychiatry 39:943–944, 2000

Thase ME: The clinical, psychosocial, and pharmacoeconomic ramifications of remission. Am J Manag Care 7 (suppl 11):S377–S385, 2001

Trivedi MH, Fava M, Wisniewski SR, et al: Medication augmentation after the failure of SSRIs for depression. N Engl J Med 354:1243–1252, 2006

Wagner KD, Ambrosini P, Rynn M, et al: Efficacy of sertraline in the treatment of children and adolescents with major depressive disorder: two randomized controlled trials. JAMA 290:1033–1041, 2003

Wagner KD, Robb AS, Findling RL, et al: A randomized, placebo-controlled trial of citalopram for the treatment of major depression in children and adolescents. Am J Psychiatry 161:1079–1083, 2004

Walter G, Rey JM: An epidemiological study of the use of ECT in adolescents. J Am Acad Child Adolesc Psychiatry 36:809–815, 1997

Walter G, Lyndon B, Kubb R: Lithium augmentation of venlafaxine in adolescent major depression. Aust NZ J Psychiatry 32:457–459, 1998

Walter G, Martin J, Kirkby K, et al: Transcranial magnetic stimulation: experience, knowledge and attitudes of recipients. Aust NZ J Psychiatry 35:58–61, 2001

Weisz JR, Doss AJ, Howley KM: Youth psychotherapy outcome research: a review and critique of the evidence base. Annu Rev Psychol 56:337–363, 2005

Wood A, Harrington R, Moore A: Controlled trial of a brief cognitive-behavioural intervention in adolescent patients with depressive disorders. J Child Psychol Psychiatry 37:737–746, 1996

CHAPTER FOUR

Recognizing and Treating Depression and Bipolar Disorder on College Campuses

Early Identification and Intervention

Rachel Lipson Glick, M.D.
Victor Hong, M.D.
Robert Winfield, M.D.
Todd Sevig, Ph.D.

DEPRESSION AND BIPOLAR DISORDER often emerge in patients in their late teens or young adult years. Because nearly 18 million young adults attend colleges and universities in the United States, many patients with mood disorders will first develop symptoms while they are in college. Data on the best treatment approaches in college students are limited, although the evidence base regarding the recognition of mood disorders and suicide prevention in this population is growing. Given the scope of the problem, and the belief that early recognition and intervention can decrease the severity of these chronic disorders, programs to assist college health services, counseling centers, and other student support services may play a key role in both decreasing the overall disease burden of mood disorders across the life span and mitigating the effect on students' academic success. In this chapter, we summarize the epidemiological data on mood disorders in college and university students, discuss some of the current best practices in recognition and early intervention, and suggest future directions for research.

Clinical Vignette 1

Martha is an 18-year-old freshman at a small liberal arts college who comes from a small town where she was valedictorian in her graduating class of 200 students. At college, she completed her first midterm examinations and was disappointed with her grades. She also found adjustment to life in the dormitory difficult and was not getting along with her roommate, who was more interested in meeting boys than in studying. She felt tired all the time but had difficulty sleeping. She cried easily and felt sad, overwhelmed, and unsure that college was the right place for her.

Martha received an e-mail from the counseling services with information about depression and a link to a secure Web site on which she could complete a survey to determine whether she is depressed. The results of her survey prompted the suggestion that she seek an assessment from the student counseling center (Counseling and Psychological Services [CAPS]). Martha was somewhat reluctant to go to CAPS because she did not know anything about counseling and was unsure how it could help. She did make an appointment at the health service, and her physician diagnosed depression, spent some time educating Martha about depression and its treatment, and prescribed citalopram. The physician suggested that Martha consider whether she might benefit from counseling given the issues she is struggling with as she adjusts to college life, and she scheduled an appointment for Martha to return later in the week to check for any side effects or problems with the medication.

When Martha returned for follow-up, she said that she was willing to give CAPS a try. The health service physician, with Martha's permission, called the CAPS office, told the intake staff member about Martha, and obtained specific information for Martha about how most easily to access services there. Martha met with a counselor and began a course of cognitive-behavioral therapy in addition to continuing her citalopram. She has successfully completed her freshman year, feeling that she did pick the right college.

Clinical Vignette 2

Martin is a 21-year-old senior at a state university. He became depressed after a breakup a month earlier with his long-term girlfriend and began taking fluoxetine prescribed by the health service physician. Martin was brought to the local emergency department by the police after he was found trying to steal a car from a used car lot. He was talking incessantly and making little sense to the police officers, as he explained that he had the right to drive the car off the lot because he was the "chosen" test car driver. His roommate was contacted and reported that Martin had not slept in several nights and had been acting "funny." When Martin's parents arrived in the emergency department, they informed the physicians that Martin's maternal grandfather has bipolar disorder.

Martin was admitted to the psychiatric service at the local hospital with a diagnosis of bipolar I disorder, manic episode. He stabilized quickly on a combination of olanzapine and lithium. The social worker on the in-patient unit, with Martin's permission, contacted the dean of students' office to inform the school of Martin's hospitalization. The dean of students arranged for a psychiatric case manager to visit Martin in the hospital and help him contact his professors about making up missed work. When he was discharged from the hospital, the case manager continued to work with Martin, assisting him in continuing college with minimal disruption despite his psychiatric illness. He received follow-up psychiatric care in the community, and the case manager from the dean's office, again with Martin's permission, coordinated care with his outpatient psychiatrist. Martin has completed his senior year and entered graduate school at a nearby university.

Epidemiology

Data suggest a widespread increase in mental health concerns and students seeking mental health services on college campuses. Over a recent 15-year period, rates of depression doubled and suicidal behavior tripled (Kadison and DiGeronimo 2004). More students are asking for help, more students are presenting with acute or serious disturbances, and more students are matriculating with mental disorders (Gallagher 2006).

According to the American College Health Association survey of 20,000 students in 2004 (American College Health Association 2007; Kisch et al. 2005), 59 % of the students reported feeling hopeless at times, 45 % felt depressed to the point that it was difficult to function, 95 % felt overwhelmed at times, and more than 9 % had considered suicide. The 2005 American College Health Association survey also found that depression was the fourth ranked health problem that students experience, and anxiety was the sixth ranked health problem (American College Health Association 2005). A 2007 report from the *Journal of American College*

Health (American College Health Association 2007) reviewed survey data on more than 94,000 students and found that almost 15 % had been given the diagnosis of depression sometime in their lives, and 18 % reported experiencing depression within the last school year. Of those who actually received a diagnosis of depression, only 27 % were receiving therapy, 37 % were taking medication, and 1.3 % had made at least one suicide attempt. Suicide appears to be the second leading cause of death on college campuses (Silverman et al. 1997).

In a 2005 survey, directors of college counseling centers reported a significant increase in the number of students seeking treatment and the number of students taking psychiatric medications. They expressed great concerns in every category on which they were surveyed, including increased reports of self-injury; growing demands for services yet no growth in resources; increased need for crisis intervention services; and the need to find more long-term referral services for students with significant illness (Gallagher 2006). Eisenberg et al. (2007) completed a random survey of almost 3,000 University of Michigan students and found that 15 % of the students sought counseling or took medications, but of these, fewer than 50 % actually received treatment on campus.

In a longitudinal study of counseling center clients, Benton et al. (2003) compared the period 1988–1992 with 1996–2001 and found an increase in suicidal thinking, from 4.8 % to 9.0 %, respectively. Other trends found in this study were increased sexual assault issues and increased stress and anxiety.

A study involving a random sample of undergraduate and graduate or professional students at a large Midwestern university (Soet and Sevig 2006) found that 30 % of the sample reported ever having been in counseling; of those 30 %, approximately 20 % were currently in counseling. Self-reported diagnoses included depression (14.9 %), eating disorders (6.1 %), anxiety (5.9 %), attention-deficit/hyperactivity disorder (4.2 %), and posttraumatic stress disorder (3.4 %).

Graduate students appear to be a population at especially high risk. They have more demanding academic requirements, are in a less structured and less supervised academic environment, and are less likely to be in a supervised residence compared with undergraduates. They are more likely to have financial stress, spouses or partners and children, and a higher risk for suicide. The 2000 Berkeley Graduate and Professional Student Survey (Hyun et al. 2006) found that 45 % of graduate students reported emotional or stress-related problems that interfered with their functioning, 10 % seriously considered suicide, 25 % were unaware of counseling services, and only 27 % of the students used these services. Soet and Sevig (2006) also found that graduate and professional students were almost twice as likely to report depression compared with under-graduates. Cost is a major deterrent to using mental health services be-cause most graduate students are no longer covered on their parents' insurance, although cost is also an issue for undergraduates. Approxi-mately 20% of students were uninsured in 2006 (U.S. Government Ac-countability Office 2008). In addition, many international students in graduate programs face significant additional stress related to accultura-tion and cross-cultural issues.

In a 2009 pilot study from the Center for the Study of Collegiate Men-tal Health involving approximately 28,000 student clients in counseling centers from 66 institutions, 19% of the students reported having coun-seling prior to starting college, with 18% receiving services after starting; 10% had received psychotropic medications prior to college, and 5% had been hospitalized. Further results found that 11% had engaged in nonsui-cidal self-injury, 11% had seriously considered suicide, and 5% had made a suicide attempt, all prior to college.

The reasons for these high and increasing rates of stress and mental health issues have been subject to debate and ultimately are unclear and most likely multifactorial. Students are under tremendous pressure to be admitted into colleges and universities, as well as into professional or graduate programs. Alcohol use is common on campuses (Centers for Dis-ease Control and Prevention 1995; Office of Applied Studies, Substance Abuse and Mental Health Services Administration 2008; Slutske 2005; Wright and Slovis 1996), as is use of stimulants and other drugs to en-hance performance or for recreation (Bronwen et al. 2006; Strote et al. 2002). Anxious or highly pressured parents are often overinvolved in all aspects of high school students' lives, making it more challenging for these students to arrive on campus and take charge of simple things such as sleep and study schedules (Kadison and DiGeronimo 2004). Finally, the availability of evidence-based treatment for depression and other mental illnesses in children and adolescents has increased, allowing them to at-tend competitive colleges and universities. Thus, students who were al-ready being treated for depression must be added to the number who first present with mood disorders in young adulthood.

Case Identification, Interventions, and Treatment

No evidence base is available for specific treatments for college- or univer-sity-age students—or for young adults compared with older adults, for that matter. Treatment of depression and bipolar disorder in these groups of patients should follow the algorithms available in the literature for all patients, such as Sequenced Treatment Alternatives to Relieve Depression (STAR*D) and Systematic Treatment Enhancement Program for Bipolar Disorder (STEP-BD).

Several issues make treatment in college students uniquely challenging. Students represent a captive audience, a group of high-risk individuals who are potentially available for early recognition and intervention trials. They can be educated through public health efforts to recognize early signs and symptoms in themselves or their friends. Residence hall staff, counselors, coaches, professors, and others also can be sensitized to make early referrals. Yet several studies show that most psychiatric illness in college students is not being treated. In fact, Garlow et al. (2008) reported that 85 % of Emory University students with depression were not receiving treatment of any kind. This may be because college students are particularly sensitive to the stigma associated with mental illness. In a study by Van Voorhees et al. (2005), 45.8 % of the young adults reported that they would be embarrassed if their friends knew about their depression. The lack of privacy in residence halls, fraternity or sorority houses, and other communal living situations may lead to denial of symptoms as well as noncompliance with medications or other treatments. Finally, there has been increased awareness and understanding of emerging mental health issues and symptoms and the need for treatment, but it remains difficult for some students to know when to seek treatment, to know the difference between "feeling sad" and being depressed, and to know when professional services are needed.

Research on recognition of suicide risk and prevention of suicide has been conducted on campuses across the United States. These studies can inform how to identify young adults on campus who have psychiatric disorders, including depression and bipolar disorder. In 2002, the American Foundation for Suicide Prevention developed the College Screening Project, which was designed to study the efficacy of online outreach and screening. Students were sent e-mails inviting them to participate in a Web-based screening project, and this Internet screening found similar rates of suicidal ideation, suicidal behavior, depression, and use of mental health services as those cited in previous, more traditional studies (Garlow et al. 2008). In addition, this proved a potentially helpful and novel method of connecting the most at-risk suicidal students with mental health providers because those who engaged in online discussions were three times more likely to eventually enter into treatment (Haas et al. 2008). This project has expanded, with 30 campuses targeted for further research by 2010. The Jed Foundation (2010) and Screening for Mental Health, Inc. (2010), also used online questionnaires to target those most in need of mental health treatment.

The University of Illinois's suicide prevention program is unique and has reduced the rates of suicide by 45% when compared with other Big Ten institutions (Joffe 2008). After a study of coroner's records in Champaign County indicated that most University of Illinois students who committed suicide had previously threatened or attempted suicide, in addition to the fact that many of them were not in treatment, university officials realized that they could not wait for students to ask for help if they wanted to prevent suicides, so they tried a new approach. In 1984, they implemented a suicide prevention program that mandated that any student who threatens or attempts suicide must meet with a mental health professional for four sessions. Those who did not comply faced disciplinary action, including possible removal from the university. These and other methods need to be researched further because it has become clear that the more traditional clinical model of waiting for students to self-refer has fallen short of the ideal.

With the issue of stigma and reluctance to accept diagnosis and treatment in mind, the first case vignette in this chapter underscores the importance of outreach via several different mechanisms, such as online resources, increased advertising on campus, mandatory attendance at seminars during orientation, and increased presence of counseling staff at campus gatherings such as sporting events and Greek Life meetings. Online outreach and access to information are crucial and useful for contacting those individuals who may otherwise not seek out treatment themselves. A study by Haas et al. (2008) indicated that completing an online questionnaire led to 34% of those students designated as high risk (Patient Health Questionnaire score > 5) engaging in an online dialogue with a counselor, 20% attending an in-person session, and 15% entering into treatment.

Other aspects of outreach include student-based groups. One such group is Active Minds (www.activeminds.org), with more than 200 chapters at various colleges and universities. This student-run group emphasizes education, enlightenment, and empowering of college students to ensure their own mental health. Other resources that offer important information include ULifeline.org, presented by The Jed Foundation (2010), and television-based outreach, such as the programs run by mtvU (www.mtvu.com) and Half of Us, which uses public figures to create dialogue about mental illness in an attempt to reduce stigma. These useful resources should be easily accessible through links from CAPS Web sites or online screening tools on all campuses. In addition, given the reluctance of many young adults to take medications, education about all aspects of the treatment of mental illness and maintenance of mental health should be available. Effective, evidence-based therapies; stress reduction techniques; sleep hygiene; responsible use of alcohol; and the importance of physical activity in improving mood (Taliaferro et al. 2008) can all be highlighted in educational materials.

Campus staff, including professors, deans, counselors, and financial aid officers, also can help improve detection of students who are having problems. However, these individuals may not recognize signs of psychological distress in students and may be inadequately prepared to make necessary accommodations with respect to the potentially slowed pace of academic progress.

To address the issue of faculty and staff psychoeducation, several programs have been developed, including the widely used intervention program QPR, or Question, Persuade, and Refer, a gatekeeper behavioral training program that teaches individuals how to recognize warning signs, assess for suicide, listen effectively, and refer for treatment (Quinnett 2006). QPR has been used to educate faculty, resident advisers, coaches, and other staff on how to effectively help students who they are concerned about, particularly those who may be suicidal. Although no studies of the effectiveness of such interventions have been published, studies of QPR and other such programs are currently in development. A growing body of anecdotal and satisfaction data suggests that these types of active programs are helping persuade more students to initiate treatment at counseling centers and be referred to the proper treatment setting. Certainly, more research is needed to determine the effectiveness of such interventions.

If a crisis leads to an inpatient hospitalization or a suicide attempt, postvention becomes critical. Follow-up treatment and basic intermittent contact with clinicians has been shown to be helpful in significantly reducing suicidal risk (Motto and Bostrom 2001). As the second case vignette shows, improved communication among psychiatric emergency services, inpatient units, outpatient providers at CAPS or University Health Services, and the Dean of Students' Office and other student support offices can positively affect outcome. This is critical for continuity of care and the prevention of a student "falling through the cracks." This linking might ideally be done through "case managers" in health care units and staff in the dean of students' office (as we do at the University of Michigan) to provide liaison between students, the academic institution, and clinicians.

Finally, another especially challenging issue is the relationship of college students with their parents. Developmentally, the college years represent an excellent opportunity for students to individuate from parents and develop a strong concept of self. Depression, bipolar disorder, and other mental health issues interfere with this normal progression to independence. The individual student may be worried about academic failure, financial consequences of losing time in school, and parental response to these issues. Students are often dependent on their parents financially and emotionally even though most students are legally adults. Thus, policy makers at colleges and universities struggle with what role parents can and should play when a student receives a diagnosis of a mood disorder (Center for the Study of Collegiate Mental Health 2009).

Understanding the importance of parents in a college student's life, Mowbray (2006) included family involvement in a summary of recommendations for treating mental illness on college campuses. In addition, she concluded that faculty and staff must be knowledgeable about mental illness, universities need to identify people responsible for outreach, universities must offer easy access and a "no wrong door" policy (no matter where students enter treatment, they should reach the appropriate treatment setting), and a well-developed crisis response mechanism should be available.

Conclusion

Although no evidence base exists to guide treatment of Treatment Resistant Depression in college students, we believe that early recognition, diagnosis, and intervention are the keys to decreasing the morbidity and mortality from mood disorders in this population. Evidence suggests that early identification and treatment may diminish the risk of a depressive episode being prolonged, possibly leading to treatment resistance. An emerging data source to lend support to this statement comes from the Center for the Study of Collegiate Mental Health (2009). In this pilot study, 1,500 students of the 28,000 students were selected for examination of pre- and post- data (before and after their treatment). Results from these analyses showed a statistically significant decrease in depressive symptoms after approximately 6 weeks of treatment. Even more important is the finding that students who initially reported higher levels of depressive symptoms compared with the rest of the sample had a greater decrease in symptoms within the same time. Furthermore, in that same treatment period of 6 weeks, data indicated that treatment led to statistically significant reduction in suicidal ideation.

Future Directions

Researchers are just beginning to develop tools for outreach, recognition, and treatment on college and university campuses, but their efforts may be the best approach to decreasing the illness burden of treatment-resistant mood disorders in the years to come. Future efforts might include the following:

- Increased attention to transitioning from home to the university through parental communication, student education of signs and symptoms, and increased attention paid to resources at colleges and universities
- Improved awareness and training of academic, housing, and financial aid staff in recognition and referral through multiple venues of written material, in-person presentations, telephone consultation, and online materials
- Increase in student-friendly interfaces, such as electronic tools and social marketing tools, to encourage contact with mental health resources (At the University of Michigan, for example, two Web sites have been developed. MI Talk [http://mitalk.umich.edu] is a student-developed and student-focused interactive effort that helps students understand mental health issues through short texts and personal stories on video, offers downloadable videos for relaxation, and has a message and tools to help students help themselves and one another. Campus Mind Works [www.campusmindworks.org] supports students who have chronic and long-standing disorders through education, support, and self-management strategies.)
- Increase in student support services in the dean of students' office and other relevant offices or units in an effort to create a web of support
- Improved training of community providers to be familiar with resources available at their local universities to support students in distress
- Investigation of the most beneficial use of family support to improve outcomes
- Creation of electronic tools such as programmable text messaging to help students remember to take medications on time and other self-management strategies to complement treatment services

Sharing of information about all of these efforts is important. The University of Michigan Depression Center's Depression on College Campuses Annual Conference offers college students and personnel from around the United States the opportunity to meet and discuss best practices and emerging trends. The conference is for everyone with an interest in this issue, including health care providers, faculty and staff, administrators, students, and even parents. The goal is to promote a fully engaged campus in which all play a role in supporting student mental health.

Key Clinical Concepts

▪ Depression, distress, and suicidal thinking are increasing on college and university campuses.

▪ Interventions that involve screening and outreach are now being tried and reported. We are just beginning to study the next step— "what to do" when screening is positive.

▪ In the long term, a public health approach that uses outreach and capitalizes on computer and Internet resources may potentially lead to preventive or early intervention strategies that may decrease overall disease burden.

References

American College Health Association: Reference Group Executive Summary Fall 2005. 2005. Available at: http://www.acha-ncha.org/docs/ACHA-NCHA _Reference_Group_ExecutiveSummary_Fall2005.pdf. Accessed January 31, 2011.

American College Health Association: American College Health Association National College Health Assessment Spring 2006 Reference Group data report (abridged). J Am Coll Health 55:195–207, 2007

Benton SA, Robertson JM, Tseng W, et al: Changes in counseling center client problems across 13 years. Prof Psychol Res Pr 34:66–72, 2003

Bronwen CC, McLaughlin TJ, Blake DR: Patterns and knowledge of nonmedical use of stimulants among college students. Arch Pediatr Adolesc Med 160:481–485, 2006

Center for the Study of Collegiate Mental Health (CSCMH): 2009 Pilot Study: Executive Summary. 2009. Available at: http://www.sa.psu.edu/caps/pdf/ 2009-CSCMH-Pilot-Report.pdf. Accessed September 18, 2010.

Centers for Disease Control and Prevention: Youth Risk Behavior Surveillance: National College Health Risk Behavior Survey. Atlanta, GA, National Center for Chronic Disease and Health Promotion, 1995

Eisenberg D, Golberstein E, Gollust SE: Help-seeking and access to mental health care in a university student population. Med Care 45:594–601, 2007

Gallagher RP: National Survey of Counseling Center Directors 2006. Washington, DC, International Association of Community Services, 2006. Available at: http://www.iacsinc.org. Accessed January 31, 2011.

Garlow S, Rosenberg J, Moore JD, et al: Depression, desperation, and suicidal ideation in college students: results from the American Foundation for Suicide Prevention College Screening project at Emory University. Depress Anxiety 25:482–488, 2008

Haas A, Koestner B, Rosenberg J, et al: An interactive web-based method of out-
    reach to college students at risk for suicide. J Am Coll Health 57:15–22, 2008
Hyun JK, Quinn BC, Madon T, et al: Graduate student mental health: needs assess-
    ment and utilization of counseling services. J Coll Stud Dev 47:247–266, 2006
Jed Foundation: ULifeline. 2010. Available at: http://www.ulifeline.org. Accessed
    September 18, 2010.
Joffe P: An empirically supported program to prevent suicide in a college student
    population. Suicide Life Threat Behav 38:87–103, 2008
Kadison R, DiGeronimo TF: College of the Overwhelmed: The Campus Mental
    Health Crisis and What to Do About It. San Francisco, CA, Jossey-Bass, 2004
Kisch J, Leino EV, Silverman MM: Aspects of suicidal behavior, depression, and
    treatment in college students: results from the spring 2000 National College
    Health Assessment Survey. Suicide Life Threat Behav 35:3–13, 2005
Motto JA, Bostrom AG: A randomized controlled trial of post-crisis suicide pre-
    vention. Psychiatr Serv 52:828–833, 2001
Mowbray CT, Megivern D, Mandiberg JM, et al: Campus mental health services:
    recommendations for change. Am J Orthopsychiatry 76:226–237, 2006
Office of Applied Studies, Substance Abuse and Mental Health Services Ad-
    ministration: The NSDUH Report, 2006: Underage alcohol use among full-
    time college students. 2008. Available at: http://www.oas.samhsa.gov/2k6/
    college/collegeunderage.htm. Accessed September 18, 2010.
Quinnett P: The QPR Theory Paper. 2006. Available at: http://www.qprinstitute
    .com. Accessed September 18, 2010.
Screening for Mental Health, Inc: Prevention, early detection and treatment of
    prevalent mental health disorders and alcohol problems. 2010. http://
    www.mentalhealthscreening.org/college/index.aspx. Accessed September
    18, 2010.
Silverman MM, Meyer PM, Sloane F, et al: The Big Ten Student Suicide Study: a
    10-year study of suicides on midwestern university campuses. Suicide Life
    Threat Behav 27:285–303, 1997
Slutske WS: Alcohol use disorders among US college students and their non-
    college-attending peers. Arch Gen Psychiatry 62:321–327, 2005
Soet J, Sevig T: Mental health issues facing a diverse sample of college students:
    results from the College Student Mental Health Survey. NASPA Journal
    43:410–431, 2006
Strote J, Lee JE, Wechsler H: Increasing MDMA use among college students: re-
    sults of national survey. J Adolesc Health 30:64–72, 2002
Taliaferro LA, Rienzo BA, Pigg RM Jr, et al: Associations between physical activ-
    ity and reduced rates of hopelessness, depression, and suicidal behavior
    among college students. J Am Coll Health 57:427–436, 2009
U.S. Government Accountability Office: Health insurance: most college students
    are covered through employer-sponsored plans, and some colleges and states
    are taking steps to increase coverage. March 2008. Available at: http://
    www.gao.gov/new.items/d08389.pdf. Accessed September 19, 2010.
Van Voorhees BW, Fogel J, Houston TK, et al: Beliefs and attitudes associated with
    the intention to not accept the diagnosis of depression among young adults.
    Ann Fam Med 3:38–46, 2005
Wright SW, Slovis CM: Drinking on campus: undergraduate intoxication requir-
    ing emergency care. Arch Pediatr Adolesc Med 150:699–702, 1996

CHAPTER FIVE

Treatment Resistant Depression in Pregnant Women

Maria Muzik, M.D., M.Sc.
Delia Vazquez, M.D.
Sheila M. Marcus, M.D.

DEPRESSIVE SYMPTOMS occur in up to 20 % of women, usually during the childbearing years (Weissman and Olfson 1995). Studies show that 10 % – 16 % of pregnant women fulfill the diagnostic criteria for major depressive disorder (MDD), and greater numbers have subsyndromal illness (O'Hara et al. 1984). However, even when appropriately screened, more than 80 % of women with antenatal depression do not receive treatment during pregnancy (Marcus et al. 2003). The failure to access treatment or the undertreatment of depression may lead to Treatment Resistant Depression (TRD). Frequently cited reasons for undertreatment are concerns about stigma (Roeloffs et al. 2003) and diagnostic uncertainty among professionals confusing depressive symptomatology with normative pregnancy experiences (poor sleep, fatigue, appetite dysregulation). Effective treatment is sometimes also limited by underdosing of otherwise effective medications because many physicians are unsure how to balance maternal medication with risk of exposing the growing fetus to pharmacotherapy. Finally, even if treated aggressively, depression in pregnancy may prove treatment refractory because of secondary maintaining factors. These include the presence of bipolar depression, anxiety disorders, eating disorders, substance abuse, or severe psychosocial stressors. We briefly review clinical features and consequences of antenatal depression, beginning with a clinical vignette followed by an elaboration of factors that may contribute to TRD.

Clinical Vignette 1

Ms. A, a 38-year-old woman with two young children, presented to her primary care physician with a chief complaint of poor-quality sleep and anxious mood during gestational week 25 of her third pregnancy. The primary care physician observed that she had become preoccupied with the notion that the weight of the baby was interfering with her ability to properly digest food. She was referred to gastroenterology for assessment of reflux esophagitis and placed on a histamine blocker. She continued to complain of a myriad of somatic concerns, which were attributed to her pregnancy.

After 2 weeks, Ms. A began to note that her mood was increasingly depressed, and she grew uncharacteristically impatient with her children. Her sleep eroded and she began to ruminate for hours before falling asleep, preoccupied with the notion that she "wanted to be the best mother" to her young children. She again called her physician, who believed that her insomnia was likely secondary to her increased uterine size and suggested diphenhydramine to assist with sleep. Despite this intervention, sleep continued to decline; Ms. A began to pray for hours on end, often repeating her prayers in characteristic fashion, starting over "if I didn't think about them in just the right way" so no harm would befall her fetus.

Ms. A was referred to psychiatric care, and she received pharmacotherapy and interpersonal and cognitive therapy to assist her with role transitions, sleep hygiene, and anxious preoccupation. Citalopram was initiated, titrating to a dose of 40 mg, which significantly improved her mood symptoms. Trazodone, at doses of 50–100 mg, was added for sleep. Ms. A's depressive symptoms significantly improved, but she continued to have residual anxious preoccupation until the time of her delivery at 39 gestational weeks. Following delivery, she found that she continued to ruminate that "something bad" might happen to her infant. She vehemently denied that she would intentionally harm her infant or had any concerns about self-harm. She did feel less anxious when her husband or mother was available and in the home. Citalopram was increased to 60 mg, and Ms. A continued cognitive-behavioral therapy (CBT) to address her anxious ruminations.

By 6 weeks postpartum, her symptoms of anxiety and depression were significantly improved. Issues related to sleep hygiene, ways to garner appropriate support from her extended family, and assertiveness skills were addressed in follow-up treatment. Ms. A did well and contacted the psychiatry clinic for pre-conception planning 2 years later.

Symptomatology and Screening for Antenatal Depression

Vignette 1 highlights the key symptoms of antenatal depression. In general, clinical depression during childbearing presents with the same symptomatology as depressive episodes unrelated to childbearing. According to the DSM-IV-TR (American Psychiatric Association 2000) criteria, a diagnosis of depression must include depressed mood or inability to experience pleasure. Ms. A presented with a depressed and irritable mood and, as with many women who are depressed during the puerperium, noted prominent anxious features. Many women report worrisome cognitions regarding infant health and preoccupations about becoming a competent parent. These preoccupations can take on an obsessional flavor and may deteriorate to psychotic thinking. Many of the classic symptoms of depression (sleep and appetite dysregulation, poor energy) overlap with the physical and mental changes experienced during pregnancy, often resulting in them being misattributed to the physiological changes of gestation.

Practitioners caring for women should be aware of personal and epidemiological factors that place women at greatest risk for antenatal depression. A critical primary risk factor is genetic vulnerability manifesting as previous personal or family history of depression (particularly during pregnancy or postpartum) (O'Hara et al. 1984). Other common risk factors are a woman's perception of limited social support and presence of social conflict, which may be red flags suggesting the need for clinical intervention (Westdahl et al. 2007). Other risk factors include past or present physical, emotional, or sexual abuse; current or past cigarette smoking; alcohol or substance abuse; financial or occupational stressors; medical health concerns; living alone; greater number of children at home; and finally, ambivalence about the pregnancy (Altshuler et al. 1998).

Several user-friendly screening tools for depression can be easily administered during pregnancy. The Edinburgh Postnatal Depression Scale (EPDS) is a 3-minute screening tool initially developed for specific use in postpartum women (Cox et al. 1987) and now the gold standard instrument across the peripartum. Two other commonly used depression screening measures for adults in ambulatory care are the Beck Depression Inventory (Feinman et al. 2000) and the Center for Epidemiologic Studies Depression Scale, Revised (Radloff 1977), both of which are valid for use during pregnancy.

Obstetrics practices may benefit from nursing or care management services to facilitate treatment engagement in women with multiple stressors who screen positive for depression, because these women may be reluctant to access appropriate treatment.

Consequences of Antenatal Depression

Unidentified and untreated depression can lead to detrimental effects in both the mother and her child. Maternal infanticide and suicide are the most catastrophic effects of undertreated depression (Meyer and Oberman 2001). In addition, depressed women are more likely to participate in unhealthy practices during pregnancy, such as smoking and substance use. They may have poor nutrition, in part because of lack of appetite, leading to poor weight gain during pregnancy. Depressed women are less compliant with, and feel less invested in, antenatal care. Women with depression may have increased pain and discomfort during their pregnancies and often complain of myriad somatic concerns, which sometimes lead to medical procedures. Untreated maternal depression in pregnancy has been associated with poor obstetric, fetal, and neonatal outcomes (Alder et al. 2007). Research suggests that maternal depression leads to an alteration in the mother's neuroendocrine axis and uterine blood flow, which may contribute to adverse pregnancy and infant outcomes (Davis et al. 2007).

Clinical Vignette 2

Ms. B, a 21-year-old woman with one child, presented at gestational week 23 of her second pregnancy. Her pregnancy was unplanned and occurred after an evening of heavy alcohol and marijuana abuse at the home of her boyfriend. On discovering the pregnancy, Ms. B's mother "threw her out" of the house because she did not support Ms. B's "choices." Ms. B began living with her boyfriend and his stepmother. Initially, both were accepting of the pregnancy, but as the nutritional and medical demands of the pregnancy began to place a strain on the family's finances, Ms. B's relationship with her boyfriend likewise became conflicted. He began to accuse her of tricking him and wondered whether the infant was biologically his own. He threatened to make her leave his home if she "as much as looked" at another guy. On one occasion when she smiled at one of his friends, he blackened her eye.

Under these stressors, Ms. B grew distressed, tearful, and irritable. She slept fitfully at night with frequent violent nightmares. She tried to sleep throughout the day but found herself increasingly agitated. Her obstetrician noted that her uterine growth was minimally delayed, and when she broke down in his office, he referred her to a social worker to address her psychosocial difficulties. Despite 3 weeks of supportive treatment, Ms. B's symptoms continued to escalate, and the obstetrician prescribed fluoxetine 20 mg to address her depressed and irritable mood.

Over time, Ms. B felt that she was less sad, but approximately 4 weeks later, she grew increasingly dysphoric. She began pacing at night, preoccupied with the notion that her infant would not have a childhood any better than her own. Despite her desire to stay free of substances during her pregnancy, she found herself using marijuana to calm her nerves when she couldn't sleep. She became preoccupied that her infant would be born damaged as a result of her marijuana use. A psychiatrist who was consulted believed that the marijuana use most likely represented a partial attempt to self-treat her depression and increased her fluoxetine dose to 40 mg/day. Her sleep further declined; for a period of 5 nights, she was unable to sleep more than 1–2 hours each night. She became transfixed by the idea that her infant would be malformed if she did not get some sleep.

At 29 gestational weeks, Ms. B took an overdose of diphenhydramine and acetaminophen, stating that she had to put herself to sleep to save her fetus. Her infant son was delivered emergently by cesarean delivery the following day, when Ms. B's hepatic function precipitously declined.

Ms. B remained hospitalized medically, and her hepatic enzyme levels declined over 4 days. Following her delivery, psychiatry was consulted. At that point, quetiapine 100 mg/day was added to her regimen and later increased to 200 mg, and her fluoxetine dose was tapered to 20 mg. She continued to be dysphoric, but her sleep gradually improved. Initially, she perseveratively thought that her infant was damaged and abnormal, but over the course of 7–10 days, this notion dissipated. Ms. B decided to bottle-feed her infant because of concern about the frequency of solo feeding during nocturnal awakenings.

After consultation with social workers, Ms. B's biological mother agreed to accept her and her infant son into her home, albeit reluctantly. Because Ms. B was not dangerous to herself or to her infant, she was discharged at 17 days postpartum. Her infant remained hospitalized until week 8 and had a reasonably favorable neonatal course, with the exception of treatment for sepsis. Ms. B's boyfriend, who visited her briefly in the hospital, gradually withdrew, feeling that the needs of Ms. B and her infant were too overwhelming. Following discharge, Ms. B visited her infant somewhat infrequently, and social work was consulted from the neonatal intensive care unit. A consultation with the perinatal psychiatry team ensued. Ms. B stated that she was feeling better but felt "disconnected" from her infant son. The nurses noted that she seemed poorly attuned to his needs and that the premature infant had significant difficulty with regulation of sleep and feeding. Recommendations of the perinatal team included interpersonal therapy for Ms. B, pharmacotherapy, and attachment-based treatment to support a healthy dyadic relationship during the postpartum phase. Additionally, a substance use treatment team provided concurrent care for Ms. B. Because of difficulty with reliable transportation, a community mental health team was later involved to provide some home-based services to support Ms. B and her infant.

Factors Contributing to Treatment Resistant Depression in Pregnancy

Undiagnosed bipolar depression; other comorbid mental illness, including anxiety disorders, posttraumatic stress disorder (PTSD), and substance abuse; and co-occurring severe psychosocial stress can all contribute to treatment resistance despite adequate treatment with antidepressants. Clinicians who want to prevent TRD in pregnancy need to consider these contributing factors and address them aggressively.

Bipolar Depression

Several features in Ms. B's vignette, such as worsening dysphoria while taking selective serotonin reuptake inhibitors (SSRIs), agitation, extreme insomnia, and emerging psychosis, should alert a clinician to a potential underlying bipolar depression. Bipolar disorder is a severe, recurrent illness, with a lifetime prevalence of 1%–2% (Kessler et al. 1994), without gender specificity. For patients who present for the first time during pregnancy, a differential diagnosis, including infectious, immunological, electrolyte, or endocrine disorders, should be considered. Medications that may contribute to increased mood instability include steroids, bronchodilators, decongestants, antihypertensives, and immunosuppressants; however, "unopposed" antidepressant medication alone also can trigger (hypo)mania and treatment refractoriness (Sharma 2006).

Exacerbation of bipolar illness may be particularly problematic during pregnancy because risk-taking behavior, including sexual promiscuity and excessive use of drugs or alcohol, may place a fetus at risk. Overall, information is limited about the course of bipolar illness in pregnancy (Sharma 2009), whereas exacerbation of bipolar illness in the postpartum period is well documented. Studies suggest that the risk of recurrence of preexisting bipolar illness during pregnancy is greater than 60%, particularly when medication is discontinued (Viguera et al. 2000). Because many of the mood stabilizers may increase the risk for fetal anomalies when used during the first trimester, these medications are often tapered antepartum, leaving women vulnerable to exacerbations during the second and third trimesters.

Key Clinical Message:
- Any woman who experiences significant irritability and a worsening or unstable course of her depressive illness, particularly with psychotic features, during pregnancy or postpartum should be evaluated for bipolarity.
- A history of mood instability and, more specifically, the induction of hypomania, rapid cycling, or mixed episodes following treatment with antidepressants may provide a clue about the underlying bipolar nature of the depression.
- Poor or absent response to antidepressants and severe psychotic features also hint at underlying bipolar illness.

- A personal history of postpartum depression or family history of bipolar illness also may suggest bipolarity.

Anxiety Disorders

Modest levels of anxiety occur in most women during pregnancy; thus, differentiating generalized anxiety disorder (GAD) can be difficult. GAD, characterized by the presence of at least 6 months of excessive worry with additional unique somatic symptoms, occurs at a rate of 8.5 % during the last trimester of pregnancy. This rate exceeds the prevalence rate in non-pregnant samples (~ 3 %), suggesting that the peripartum is a vulnerable period for GAD (Ross et al. 2006).

The prevalence of panic disorder during pregnancy is 1 % –2 %, consistent with the prevalence outside of childbearing. Current studies report conflicting data regarding the course of illness across the peripartum period; several studies suggest that panic symptoms improve during pregnancy and exacerbate postpartum, whereas others note no change in course of illness across the puerperium (Ross et al. 2006).

Co-occurring anxiety and depressive systems are common, with 50 % of women with panic disorder reporting major depression. This comorbidity may complicate treatment regimens and may necessitate the use of both an antidepressant and an anxiolytic (commonly an SSRI and a benzodiazepine).

Obsessive worries centering on pregnancy outcomes are very common in pregnancy. However, the prevalence of obsessive-compulsive disorder (OCD) is lower during pregnancy (0.2 %) relative to both postpartum prevalence (2.7 % –3.9 %) and lifetime prevalence (2.5 %) in the general population (Ross et al. 2006). One of the most common obsessional themes during the peripartum is the fear of intentionally or accidentally harming the fetus or infant. Obsessional thoughts about harming the infant are present in both depressed women (40 %) and healthy community volunteers (30 % –60 %) and thus are not specific to OCD or necessarily pathological. In mild form, they can be viewed as a normative feature of early parenthood. Obsessive thoughts about harming the fetus or infant must be differentiated from psychotic delusions present in psychotic depression or bipolar illness. In general, women with OCD-like thoughts about hurting their child are very distressed and identify these thoughts as unwanted and unreasonable. Such women try to avoid being alone with their child because of concern about their ideations. In contrast, women with psychotic harmful thoughts toward their child lack insight into their delusions and may be at risk to act on them. In such cases, immediate safety measures for the child and treatment for the mother are

warranted. Presence of an OCD spectrum disorder comorbid with antenatal depression complicates treatment and may require higher levels of
medications (SSRIs) or behavior therapy.

Finally, PTSD can be present during pregnancy and postpartum, either as new onset or as exacerbation of preexisting illness (Ross et al.
2006). In general, PTSD is approximately twice as common in women
(12% lifetime prevalence) as in men. Prevalence rates among pregnant
women are as high as 8%. PTSD symptoms also have been described in
women who have experienced prior losses during pregnancy and those
who have had complicated prior deliveries. History of childhood abuse,
particularly sexual abuse, is related to higher rates of perinatal PTSD as
well, with symptoms sometimes precipitated by the intrusive procedures
inherent in the management of pregnancy and delivery. Childhood sexual
abuse survivors are also more likely to have perinatal depression, confirm-
ing the observation that PTSD and depression are commonly comorbid
during the perinatal period, again complicating treatment algorithms and
increasing the likelihood for treatment resistance.

Key Clinical Message:

- Anxiety is common in pregnancy, ranging from increased rates of
  GAD and OCD to possible exacerbation of preexisting panic disorder
  and PTSD.
- Comorbidity with depression is common, and co-occurrence of anxiety and depression complicates treatment, increasing the risk for treatment resistance.

Substance Use Disorders

In Vignette 2, Ms. B presented with preexisting alcohol and marijuana
abuse. Self-medication for mood and anxiety disorders is common (Bolton
et al. 2009; Robinson et al. 2009); and substance use disorders that persist
in pregnancy often co-occur with mood or anxiety disorders. Alcohol and
nicotine are estimated to be the most commonly used substances during
pregnancy. National survey self-report estimates of drug use in pregnancy
indicate that 9%–15% of women consume alcohol, 17% smoke ciga-
rettes, and 3.4% use any illicit drug during pregnancy (Chang et al. 1998).

Substance abuse in pregnancy has significant adverse effects on the
developing fetus. Consuming alcohol while pregnant increases the risk for
first-trimester spontaneous abortion, stillbirth, fetal growth restriction,
and typical fetal anomalies. Alcohol abuse during pregnancy is the most
common preventable risk for child mental retardation (Chudley et al.
2005). Heavy fetal alcohol exposure in late pregnancy or during delivery

can cause a neonatal withdrawal syndrome consisting of tremors, ventricular tachycardia, and seizures. Illicit drug use during pregnancy poses a risk for suboptimal pregnancy outcomes, and dependence on the substance (e.g., amphetamines, opioids) contributes to a higher likelihood of spontaneous abortion or premature delivery, low birth weight, and neonatal withdrawal syndrome (see review by Lester and Twomey 2008).

Key Clinical Message:
- Substance use is frequently comorbid with anxiety and mood disorders and may contribute to treatment resistance if unrecognized and untreated.
- Patients frequently self-medicate with alcohol or other illicit drugs to alleviate anxiety, depression, or insomnia.
- Screening for substance abuse, mainly alcohol consumption, in pregnancy is critical for optimal child outcomes, and several screening tools are available in primary care.

Severe Psychosocial Stress

The presence of psychosocial stressors can trigger the onset of depression in pregnancy or can exacerbate or maintain concurrent depression. Such stressors include exposure to trauma and violence, relationship conflict, and inadequate social support systems. The strain of poverty with resultant food, housing, and financial insecurity may be a further stressor.

Past physical or sexual abuse is common in women with substance use and mental health problems. In general, women in the United States have a 69% chance of being exposed to non-combat-related trauma, including completed rape (13%), other sexual assault (14%), physical assault (10%), and childhood abuse (28%) (Resnick et al. 1993). Additionally, prior trauma and abuse increase the risk for revictimization (Widom et al. 2008), and women may be more likely to enter into abusive relationships.

Domestic violence during pregnancy poses a significant threat to a pregnant woman and the fetus (Parker et al. 1994). Exposure to violence and abuse can lead to adverse physical and mental health consequences for the affected women, including depressive and anxiety disorders. Screening for domestic violence and trauma is essential to begin to address the challenges of these affected women in an empathic and nonjudgmental way and to create a supportive environment for change.

Pregnancy is a time of role transition for all women. The prospect of delivery and a new infant fundamentally alters a woman's role as a self-reliant individual, professional, and partner in various adult relationships, as well as the balance of power within such relationships. Screening for relationship satisfaction and quality of the partner relationship is important because it allows providers to evaluate for relationship conflict, which may underlie the depressive illness and contribute to treatment resistance.

Stress related to lack of social support, as exemplified in Vignette 2 by the ambivalent support for Ms. B from her mother, further confounds depressive illnesses. In addition to such relationship stressors, housing and financial instability can aggravate depressive illness, confound treatment planning, and prevent full remission of antenatal depression. Case management and social work support to help women cope with these issues must be part of a comprehensive treatment package for depression in pregnancy.

Treatment Options

Vignette 2 outlines several of the challenges inherent in treatment planning. Such comorbidities and psychosocial stressors may interfere with rapid treatment response and positive treatment outcomes. To address these multiple and diverse challenges, a comprehensive, multidimensional approach is needed. For patients similar to Ms. B, interpersonal, cognitive, and supportive therapy to assist in role transition, to assert safety and support from a partner, and to address symptoms of mental illness are essential. Additionally, close monitoring of pharmacotherapy is paramount, given the complexity and changing nature of psychiatric symptoms. Provision of social work support to help with housing and income may help minimize psychosocial strain. Involvement of child protective services to provide respite care and to monitor the infant's safety may be needed after the at-risk infants return home with their mothers. Mother-infant therapy supporting the maternal dyad helps to foster a secure attachment relationship. In the next several sections, we provide an overview of current state-of-the art treatment modalities for depression in pregnancy.

Pharmacotherapy

Antidepressants

Few pharmacological standards exist for treatment of depressive disorders during pregnancy, in part because ethical constraints preclude randomized controlled trials in which medication is administered during gestation. In a recent publication (Yonkers et al. 2009), both the American Psychiatric Association and the American College of Obstetricians and Gynecologists suggested that women should consider use of psychotherapy before considering medications but that those with moderate to severe, recurrent depressive symptoms or suicidal thinking should continue taking antidepressants during pregnancy. Many women are reluctant to seek treatment, but for those who do, some physicians are unsure of how to balance maternal medication requirements with risk of exposure to the growing fetus. Because many pregnancies are unplanned or go undetected for some time, all women of childbearing age should have their depression managed as if pregnancy is possible. The primary care provider should engage in pre-conception planning with all women of childbearing age who are at risk for depressive illness. Decisions with regard to the use of pharmacotherapy during conception and the first trimester are among the most critical for a woman and her physician. Women with depression who have been asymptomatic for more than a year may wish to attempt to reduce or discontinue antidepressants prior to conception and throughout the pregnancy (Gonsalves and Schuermeyer 2006). Women should be closely monitored for relapse of symptoms. In one study, 68% of women who discontinued their antidepressants during pregnancy experienced a relapse of symptoms, compared with 26% of women who continued their medication regimens (Cohen et al. 2006). If a woman's depression history contains multiple relapses or severe symptoms such as suicide attempts and multiple inpatient psychiatric admissions, some recommend that she continue antidepressants for her own safety, regardless of pregnancy status (Gonsalves and Schuermeyer 2006).

Although research studies indicate that no major malformations are associated with antidepressant use during pregnancy, they have not shown that any specific antidepressant is completely safe. All psychotropic medications cross the placenta and enter the amniotic fluid. General guidelines include some straightforward principles: 1) keep the medication regimen simple by using monotherapy when possible, 2) discuss risks and consequences of both pharmacotherapy and untreated depression, and 3) choose agents with demonstrated fetal safety. Use of multiple medications in sequence and medication augmentation strategies increases the exposure of the fetus (ACOG Practice Bulletin 2008). The woman's history of response to pharmacotherapy should be considered when choosing a medication (ACOG Practice Bulletin 2008). Although many factors influence pharmacotherapy during pregnancy, drugs with fewer metabolites and drug-drug interactions, more protein binding (preventing placental passage), and lesser teratogenic risk (if known) should be used when possible (ACOG Practice Bulletin 2008).

Spontaneous abortion and preterm birth. Research results for the rates of antidepressant use and the relation of use to spontaneous

abortion are mixed and may be confounded by the effect of the illness itself (Hemels et al. 2005). One study suggested that women taking antidepressants during pregnancy have a statistically significantly higher rate of
spontaneous abortion (3.9%) regardless of the type of antidepressant
(Hemels et al. 2005), whereas other studies showed that spontaneous
abortion rates are elevated for exposure to several different antidepressant
classes, but only exposure to bupropion is statistically significant (Chun-
Fai-Chan et al. 2005; Einarson et al. 2009). A recent study showed that
rates of preterm birth are greater than 20% for both women with untreated gestational depression and women with continuous SSRI exposure during pregnancy (Wisner et al. 2009).

Teratogenicity.   Research on antidepressant teratogenicity is growing,
and there is considerable scientific debate about the safety of antidepressants during pregnancy. Although the mainstream media have reported
controversy about the safety of the SSRIs, most research to date does not
confirm major congenital malformations greater than the 2%–4% baseline rate cited for the general population (Wichman et al. 2009). A recent
meta-analysis confirmed no increased risk of major congenital malformations with in utero exposure to SSRIs (Einarson 2009). In 2005, Glaxo-
SmithKline published a report based on a claims database study of 815
infants that showed that infants born to mothers who were taking paroxetine during their first trimester had a 1.5- to 2-fold increased risk of congenital heart defects, particularly atrial and ventricular septal defects
(GlaxoSmithKline 2005). A more recent study negated these findings by
determining that the rate of cardiac defects for infants exposed to paroxetine in the first trimester and nonexposed infants was the same (0.7%)
and within the expected cardiac malformation risk range for all pregnancies (Einarson et al. 2008). At the time of this writing, perinatal psychiatrists continue to debate the use of paroxetine. Most practitioners choose
other agents, except for those women who have had a preferential past
positive response to paroxetine. When paroxetine is used, monitoring the
fetus with fetal echocardiography is recommended (ACOG Practice Bulletin 2008).

A 2007 study found no significant relation between SSRIs and congenital cardiovascular malformations; however, the authors suggested an
association between maternal use of SSRIs (especially paroxetine during
the first trimester) and infants with anencephaly, craniosynostosis, and
omphalocele (Alwan et al. 2007). These findings were refuted by another
study published in 2007 that found no increased risk of these anomalies
with SSRI use by pregnant women (Louik et al. 2007). However, Louik
and colleagues reported significant relations between sertraline and

omphalocele and between paroxetine and right ventricular outflow tract obstruction defects. Although these findings indicated some increased risk of specific rare birth defects with specific drug exposures, the overall absolute risk of birth defects with the use of SSRIs is small (Alwan et al. 2007; Louik et al. 2007).

Poor neonatal adaptation.   Studies show that up to 30% of infants exposed to SSRIs in the third trimester are likely to have symptoms of poor neonatal adaptation (Koren et al. 2005). These symptoms include short-term self-limited cardiorespiratory symptoms, hypothermia, hypoglycemia, irritability, hyper- and hypotonia, feeding disturbances, and seizures (Koren et al. 2005). These infants may have increased neonatal intensive care unit admissions, in part because of vigilance of staff. Studies assessing neonatal outcomes and complications do not correct for commonly co-occurring risk factors such as substance and tobacco use (Ross et al. 2006). One author who corrected for these confounding variables found no increased rate of premature labor or intensive care monitoring for infants exposed to SSRIs or venlafaxine in utero. As in other studies, some infants did show symptoms of neonatal adaptation syndrome (Ferreira et al. 2007). In a 2006 case-control study, infants exposed to SSRIs after 20 weeks' gestation had a 1% increased risk of persistent pulmonary hypertension of the newborn (Chambers et al. 2006); however, another recent study refuted this increased risk (Andrade et al. 2009). Although some international literature suggests tapering of SSRIs to avoid the late-gestation exposure, most practitioners in the United States avoid this because it predisposes women to a substantially heightened risk of late pregnancy and postpartum morbidity secondary to depression (Einarson et al. 2001) and predisposes the infant to medication withdrawal symptoms in utero.

The bulk of the literature to date does not indicate increased risk of congenital malformations associated with tricyclic antidepressant (TCAs) use by pregnant women (Einarson 2009). Doses of TCAs may need to be increased as much as 1.6 times the prepregnancy dose in the second half of pregnancy to establish therapeutic levels as a result of increased plasma volumes and metabolism (Sharma 2006). Case reports have described infants with TCA exposure experiencing temporary withdrawal symptoms within the first 12 hours of life, including jitteriness, irritability, urinary retention, bowel obstruction, and occasionally seizures (Einarson 2009). Nulman et al. (1997) found no associations between mothers' use of TCAs or fluoxetine during pregnancy and long-term effects on global IQ, language, or behavioral development in preschool children. Further research is needed to examine long-term outcomes for these children. Much more limited information is available for exposure to atypical antidepressants such as bupropion, mirtazapine, nefazodone, trazodone, duloxetine, and venlafaxine in utero; however, data so far indicate a satisfactory safety profile (Einarson 2009). Like SSRIs and TCAs, venlafaxine has been implicated in cases of neonatal withdrawal (Einarson 2009). For an overview, see Table 5–1.

Mood Stabilizers

The challenges in managing bipolar disorder in women center around the potential risk of teratogenicity associated with the major mood stabilizers (Sharma 2009). See Table 5–2 for a summary.

Lithium.   Lithium originally had been associated with a substantially increased risk of Ebstein's anomaly, prompted in part by reporting of the 1970s International Register of Lithium Babies. Original estimates of Ebstein's anomaly, reported at a rate 400-fold higher than in the general population, were called into question as a result of selective overreporting of anomalies within these retrospective registries. More recent pooled analyses of all scientific data estimated the risk of Ebstein's anomaly following first-trimester lithium exposure at 0.05 %–0.1 %. This represents a relative risk 10- to 20-fold higher than in the general population. Use of lithium in later pregnancy has, however, been associated with neonatal withdrawal symptoms (Gentile 2006).

Anticonvulsants.   Compared with lithium, the anticonvulsant medications may pose a somewhat greater risk of teratogenicity (Cohen 2007). It is important to recognize, however, that the bulk of information about congenital anomalies with anticonvulsants derives from epilepsy literature, and it is well known that infants born to women with unmedicated epilepsy are at an increased risk for major malformations; thus, the relative risk of the anticonvulsants themselves is unknown (Holmes et al. 2001).

Carbamazepine.   The overall rate of carbamazepine-related teratogenicity is approximately 6 %, with specific increases in rates of spina bifida ranging from 0.5 % to 1 % (Cohen 2007). There have also been sporadic case reports of coagulopathies, microcephaly, craniofacial anomalies, and growth retardation.

Valproic acid.   Valproic acid may be an even more serious teratogen than carbamazepine, conferring an approximately fivefold increased risk (11 %) of major malformations when used within the first trimester. The

TABLE 5–1. Use of antidepressants in pregnancy

Medication class	Use in pregnancy/ teratogenicity	Spontaneous abortion/ preterm birth	Neonatal adaptation and monitoring at birth
Selective serotonin reuptake inhibitors (SSRIs)	No increased risk of teratogenicity above baseline rate (Einarson 2009; Wichman et al. 2009); small risk of septal defects and other anomalies; paroxetine controversial (Alwan et al. 2007; Einarson et al. 2008; Louik et al. 2007)	Mixed findings (Chun-Fai-Chan et al. 2005) suggesting increased rates of spontaneous abortion regardless of antidepressant type; findings may be confounded by effect of illness; preterm birth rates >20% for SSRIs (Wisner et al. 2009) but equal to rates in untreated illness	Of exposed infants, 30% have transient difficulty in first days of life (Koren et al. 2005); risk for pulmonary hypertension suggested in some (Chambers et al. 2006) but not all (Andrade et al. 2009) studies
Tricyclic antidepressants	No increased risk of teratogenicity above baseline rate (Einarson 2009)	Mixed findings (Chun-Fai-Chan et al. 2005) suggesting increased rates of spontaneous abortion regardless of antidepressant type; findings may be confounded by effect of illness	Difficulties with neonatal adaptation and withdrawal symptoms well established (Einarson 2009)
Serotonin-norepinephrine reuptake inhibitors and other anti-depressants	No increased risk of teratogenicity above baseline rate (Einarson 2009)	Bupropion exposure in pregnancy linked with significant risk for spontaneous abortion (Einarson et al. 2009)	Difficulties with neonatal adaptation and withdrawal symptoms well established with venlafaxine (Boucher et al. 2009)

TABLE 5–2.   Use of mood stabilizers in pregnancy

Medication	Use in pregnancy/teratogenicity	Neonatal adaptation	Monitoring at birth
Lithium	First trimester: increased risk of cardiovascular anomalies but lower than initially stated (Gentile 2006)	Neonatal withdrawal symptoms, including respiratory symptoms, hypotonia; poor neonatal adaptation (Gentile 2006)	May be reinstituted in second trimester to prevent relapse of bipolar illness Lithium dosage should be increased in third trimester to control for increased plasma volumes Following delivery, dosage should be decreased to prepregnancy levels. Fetal survey should be obtained at 18 weeks. Infants should be monitored following delivery for respiratory symptoms and tone (Cohen 2007).
Valproic acid	First-trimester use contraindicated Associated with high rates (up to 11%) of congenital anomalies, including neural tube defects (Cohen 2007; Gentile 2006)	Poor neonatal adaptation reported in some infants, with cognitive delays seen longer term (Gentile 2006)	When used in second and third trimester, plasma levels should be monitored because of increased plasma volumes. Fetal survey at 18 weeks is essential; folate supplementation is recommended. Compatible with breastfeeding (Cohen 2007)

TABLE 5–2.	Use of mood stabilizers in pregnancy *(continued)*		
Medication	Use in pregnancy/teratogenicity	Neonatal adaptation	Monitoring at birth
Lamotrigine	Data are limited but to date are relatively favorable. One study suggested risk of major anomalies similar to that of population at large (Dolk et al. 2008; Holmes et al. 2001).	Limited data	As in nonpregnant state; careful monitoring for rash Monitor maternal liver function tests.
Antipsychotic agents	The high-potency first-generation antipsychotics (e.g., haloperidol) are best studied, with no clear evidence of increased risk of teratogenicity (Einarson 2009). Case reports and small studies are emerging for the atypical agents; no clear evidence of teratogenic risk at this time, but all studies are insufficiently powered to be conclusive (McKenna et al. 2005).	No data	Continued monitoring for extrapyramidal side effects, complete blood count, liver function tests, and electrocardiogram necessary in women taking antipsychotics in pregnancy (Cohen 2007).

relative risk of neural tube defects is 50-fold greater than the spontaneous rate, and these defects occur in 1%–2% of all pregnancies in which valproate is used within the first trimester. Prenatal use of folate is essential in this population. Fetal exposure to valproate also has been associated with craniofacial anomalies and cognitive delays (Cohen 2007).

Lamotrigine. The estimated risk of congenital anomalies with lamotrigine monotherapy (2.7%) is similar to the base rate in the general population, according to data from the Lamotrigine Pregnancy Registry (Cunnington et al. 2007). Data from the U.K. Prospective Pregnancy Registry suggests a similar risk (Morrow et al. 2001). A recent article from Europe refutes a previous report on increased risk for orofacial clefts (Dolk et al. 2008; Einarson 2009).

Antipsychotics. Until recently, literature on the use of antipsychotics during pregnancy was limited to studies and case reports involving the conventional neuroleptics. Studies of newer atypical antipsychotics are ongoing but are insufficiently powered to definitively determine rates of teratogenicity beyond the baseline rate; however, one study on use of atypical antipsychotic medications during pregnancy did not show increased teratogenicity (McKenna et al. 2005). The same study also reported increased rates of spontaneous abortions in the group taking atypical antipsychotics compared with women not taking atypical antipsychotics (McKenna et al. 2005). For an overview, see Table 5–2.

Benzodiazepines

Early studies reported increased risk for major malformations and oral cleft malformations, especially during first-trimester exposure; however, recent studies have not confirmed these previous reports (Einarson 2009). High-dose use late in pregnancy may predispose the infant to neonatal withdrawal symptoms, including hypotonia, neonatal apnea, and temperature instability (Fisher et al. 1985). Some investigators had concluded that third-trimester discontinuation was indicated to avoid these sequelae, but most had concluded that such discontinuation would unnecessarily predispose women to relapse of anxiety disorders.

Electroconvulsive Therapy

Electroconvulsive therapy (ECT) use in pregnancy is considered effective for TRD and relatively safe without risk of teratogenicity and with only a moderate rate of adverse complications. Standard practice should include an obstetric consultation to assess potential preexisting risk prior to the ECT procedure. When receiving ECT, women in the second and third trimester of pregnancy should be positioned slightly toward their left side with support under the right hip to prevent a vena caval compression syndrome (Rabheru 2001).

Psychotherapy

Psychotherapy has been studied extensively in the treatment of depression and is empirically validated for treatment of mood disorders. Psychotherapy is recommended as the treatment of choice for mild to moderate depression (Yonkers et al. 2009) and should be included in the treatment of all treatment-resistant symptoms in women because of the severity of illness and psychosocial issues seen in complicated TRD. Both interpersonal psychotherapy (IPT) and CBT are evidence-based approaches for treatment of depression outside of pregnancy (Bhatia and Bhatia 1999). Data are very limited, however, on CBT with specific timing during pregnancy. CBT has been investigated as a modality for postpartum depressed women and found effective. IPT, which focuses on role transitions or role conflicts that may surface in the context of depression, may be particularly relevant for childbearing women because this may be a time of significant role transitions and role disputes with significant others. Studies have reported effectiveness of IPT in pregnant and postpartum women. For a review of CBT and IPT as treatments for depression in pregnancy, see Misri and Kendrick (2007).

Informed Consent

A careful process of informed consent and its documentation is essential when prescribing pharmacotherapy and considering psychotherapy during pregnancy. Review of maternal symptom severity, course of illness, prior treatment response, and relapse risk without medication, as well as consideration of fetal safety when prescribing specific medications, is crucial to decision making. Women should be informed about and understand the potential risks of pharmacotherapy and the documented risks of undertreated illness. Patients and their families should be informed about the latest recommendations by the American Psychiatric Association and the American College of Obstetricians and Gynecologists (Yonkers et al. 2009) that psychotherapy is the first choice in treating mild to moderate illness prior to the institution of pharmacotherapy. Psychotherapy should be used as relapse prevention when mood stabilizers or antidepressants are discontinued at conception. Documentation of the informed consent process, distribution of relevant educational materials (REPROTOX is one reputable source; see www.reprotox.org), and written medication consents are suggested for all women during pregnancy.

Alternative Treatments

Data on bright-light therapy during the peripartum period are limited yet promising. Light therapy has been studied in both pregnancy and postpartum. Although application during pregnancy has resulted in clear reduction of depressive symptoms, beneficial use postpartum has not yet been demonstrated (Misri and Kendrick 2007).

Epidemiological studies have found that consumption of two to three seafood meals per week is associated with a decreased risk for depression and other mood disorders. Fish is the premier dietary source of the omega-3 fatty acids EPA (eicosapentaenoic acid) and DHA (docosahexaenoic acid), neither of which is synthesized by the human body. During pregnancy and postpartum, maternal omega-3 fatty acid stores are progressively depleted because women in the United States fall short in the recommended dietary intake, mainly owing to fear of mercury-contaminated fish. However, omega-3 fatty acids are essential for healthy fetal brain development. Several studies to date have confirmed that intake of EPA and DHA is safe and beneficial as an adjunctive treatment for depression and bipolar depression (with effective doses ranging from 1 to 9 g/day across studies); however, only limited data are available regarding their intake during pregnancy and postpartum. Continued research on fish oil supplementation during peripartum is needed. Current guidelines recommend EPA and DHA supplementation of at least 1g/day in capsule form, during or outside of childbearing, to support mood stabilization, or at least two fish meals per week outside of pregnancy, with concern about mercury contamination affecting guidelines for fish consumption during pregnancy. For a meta-analysis of current studies, dosing recommendations, and safety considerations, see the review by Freeman and colleagues (2006).

More recently, there has been interest in research on mind-body modalities, some of which have been practiced over thousands of years, such as progressive muscle relaxation, yoga, and awareness-enhancing meditation (Beddoe and Lee 2008). Although much of this research has methodological limitations (e.g., lack of randomized controlled trials), there appears to be converging evidence for the efficacy of mind-body modalities used during pregnancy in conjunction with prenatal care.

Summary

Primary care providers should be aware that depression in pregnancy is common ($\sim 15\%$). Routine depression screening during prenatal visits, coupled with the use of physician collaborators to assist in connecting women with care, is critical to facilitate treatment engagement with appropriate providers. Providers should be aware of risk factors for depression, including history of depression, life events, and interpersonal conflict, and should appropriately screen for such conditions. Links have been made between depression during pregnancy and poor pregnancy outcomes such as preeclampsia, insufficient weight gain, decreased compliance with prenatal care, and premature labor. Current literature suggests that overall the risks of antidepressant treatment in pregnancy (SSRIs, serotonin-norepinephrine reuptake inhibitors, bupropion) may be favorable relative to the risk of untreated depression for mother and child. Poor neonatal adaptation or withdrawal symptoms in the neonate may occur with fetal exposure in late pregnancy, but the symptoms are mild to moderate and transient. Among mothers who decide to stop taking their antidepressants during pregnancy, most experience relapsing symptoms. If depression continues postpartum, the risk increases for poor mother-infant attachment, delayed cognitive and linguistic skills in the infant, impaired emotional development, and behavior problems in later life. Bipolar depression, comorbid Axis I disorders (anxiety and substance use disorders), and severe psychosocial stress can cause treatment resistance. Modified and more complex treatment algorithms are then warranted. Psychiatric medications and IPT or CBT, as well as social work support, are often-needed modalities to address all issues surrounding the illness comprehensively.

Future Directions

Treatment of depression during pregnancy is complex and almost always involves multimodal treatments and many providers, including those in obstetrics, pediatrics, psychiatry, and child psychiatry. Coordination of care among such providers and the relative merit of psychotherapeutic, supportive, and psychopharmacological modalities require further investigation. Moreover, because ethics constrain the study of medication in pregnancy and preclude randomized controlled trials, the specific contribution of pharmacotherapy, compared with that of illness, to maternal and fetal risk has been difficult to quantify to date, yet preliminary data show similar neonatal risks (Wisner et al. 2009). Novel treatment strategies such as vagus nerve stimulation and transcranial magnetic stimulation are also untested in pregnancy.

Researchers are beginning to explore the epigenetic influences on infants during gestation and the neonatal period, and the effect of maternal illness on the infant's developing stress axis and predisposition to later psychiatric illness also merits further research. Moreover, the effects of maternal depressive illnesses and treatments on the infant's capacity for self-regulation, temperament, subsequent attachment, cognitive development, and predisposition to psychiatric illness all are areas for further exploration.

Key Clinical Concepts

■ Depression during pregnancy is common yet often unrecognized and undertreated.

■ Antenatal depression frequently can be comorbid with other psychiatric conditions, which complicates treatment.

■ Not treating maternal mental illness during pregnancy has negative consequences, not only for the mother but also for the developing fetus, the infant, and the child.

■ Psychotherapy should be considered the treatment of first choice for less severe antenatal mood and anxiety disorders.

■ Pharmacological treatment of maternal mental illness needs careful risk-benefit analysis, weighing fetal exposure to the medicine against the effects of maternal illness itself.

■ Alternative and complementary treatments such as light therapy, omega-3 fatty acids, and mind-body techniques show promising preliminary results, yet more rigorous and well-powered studies are needed.

References

ACOG Practice Bulletin: Clinical management guidelines for obstetrician-gynecologists no 92, April 2008 (replaces practice bulletin no 87, November 2007). Use of psychiatric medications during pregnancy and lactation. ACOG Committee on Practice Bulletins—Obstetrics. Obstet Gynecol 111:1001–1020, 2008

Alder J, Fink N, Bitzer J, et al: Depression and anxiety during pregnancy: a risk factor for obstetric, fetal and neonatal outcome? A critical review of the literature. J Matern Fetal Neonatal Med 20:189–209, 2007

Altshuler LL, Hendrick V, Cohen LS: Course of mood and anxiety disorders during pregnancy and the postpartum period. J Clin Psychiatry 59 (suppl 2):29–33, 1998

Alwan S, Reefhuis J, Rasmussen SA, et al: Use of selective serotonin-reuptake inhibitors in pregnancy and the risk of birth defects. N Engl J Med 356:2684–2692, 2007

American Psychiatric Association: Diagnostic and Statistical Manual of Mental Disorders, 4th Edition, Text Revision. Washington, DC, American Psychiatric Association, 2000

Andrade S, McPhillips H, Loren D, et al: Antidepressant medication use and risk of persistent pulmonary hypertension of the newborn. Pharmacoepidemiol Drug Saf 18:246–252, 2009

Beddoe AE, Lee KA: Mind-body interventions during pregnancy. J Obstet Gynecol Neonatal Nurs 37:165–175, 2008

Bhatia SC, Bhatia SK: Depression in women: diagnostic and treatment considerations. Am Fam Physician 60:225–234, 239–240, 1999

Bolton JM, Robinson J, Sareen J: Self-medication of mood disorders with alcohol and drugs in the National Epidemiologic Survey on Alcohol and Related Conditions. J Affect Disord 115:367–375, 2009

Boucher N, Koren G, Beaulac-Baillargeon L: Maternal use of venlafaxine near term: correlation between neonatal effects and plasma concentrations. Ther Drug Monit 31:404–409, 2009

Chambers CD, Hernandez-Diaz S, Van Marter LJ, et al: Selective serotonin-reuptake inhibitors and risk of persistent pulmonary hypertension of the newborn. N Engl J Med 354:579–587, 2006

Chang G, Wilkins-Haug L, Berman S, et al: Alcohol use and pregnancy: improving identification. Obstet Gynecol 91:892–898, 1998

Chudley AE, Conry J, Cook JL, et al: Fetal alcohol spectrum disorder: Canadian guidelines for diagnosis. CMAJ 172 (suppl 5):S1–S21, 2005

Chun-Fai-Chan B, Koren G, Fayez I, et al: Pregnancy outcome of women exposed to bupropion during pregnancy: a prospective comparative study. Am J Obstet Gynecol 192:932–936, 2005

Cohen LS: Treatment of bipolar disorder during pregnancy. J Clin Psychiatry 68 (suppl 9):4–9, 2007

Cohen LS, Altshuler LL, Harlow BL, et al: Relapse of major depression during pregnancy in women who maintain or discontinue antidepressant treatment. JAMA 295:499–507, 2006

Cox JL, Holden JM, Sagovsky R: Detection of postnatal depression: development of the 10-item Edinburgh Postnatal Depression Scale. Br J Psychiatry 150:782–786, 1987

Cunnington M, Ferber S, Quartey G; International Lamotrigine Pregnancy Registry Scientific Advisory Committee: Effect of dose on the frequency of major birth defects following fetal exposure to lamotrigine monotherapy in an international observational study. Epilepsia 48:1207–1210, 2007

Davis E, Glynn L, Schetter C, et al: Prenatal exposure to maternal depression and cortisol influences infant temperament. J Am Acad Child Adolesc Psychiatry 46:737–746, 2007

Dolk H, Jentink J, Loane L, et al: Does lamotrigine use in pregnancy increase orofacial cleft risk relative to other malformations? Neurology 71:714–722, 2008

Einarson A: Risks/safety of psychotropic medication use during pregnancy—
Motherisk Update 2008. Can J Clin Pharmacol 16:58–65, 2009

Einarson A, Selby P, Koren G: Abrupt discontinuation of psychotropic drugs during pregnancy: fear of teratogenic risk and impact of counselling. J Psychiatry
Neurosci 26:44–48, 2001

Einarson A, Pistelli A, DeSantis M, et al: Evaluation of the risk of congenital cardiovascular defects associated with use of paroxetine during pregnancy. Am
J Psychiatry 165:749–752, 2008

Einarson A, Choi J, Einarson T, et al: Rates of spontaneous and therapeutic abortions following use of antidepressants in pregnancy: results from a large prospective database. J Obstet Gynaecol Can 31:452–456, 2009

Feinman JA, Cardillo D, Palmer J, et al: Development of a model for the detection
and treatment of depression in primary care. Psychiatr Q 71:59–78, 2000

Ferreira E, Carceller AM, Agogue C, et al: Effects of selective serotonin reuptake
inhibitors and venlafaxine during pregnancy in term and preterm neonates.
Pediatrics 119:52–59, 2007

Fisher JB, Edgren BE, Mammel MC, et al: Neonatal apnea associated with maternal clonazepam therapy: a case report. Obstet Gynecol 66 (suppl 3):34S–35S,
1985

Freeman MP, Hibbeln JR, Wisner KL, et al: Omega-3 fatty acids: evidence basis
for treatment and future research in psychiatry. J Clin Psychiatry 67:1954–
1967, 2006

Gentile S: Prophylactic treatment of bipolar disorder in pregnancy and breastfeed-
ing: focus on emerging mood stabilizers. Bipolar Disord 8:207–220, 2006

GlaxoSmithKline: Important prescribing information. December 2005. Available
at: http://www.gsk.com/media/paroxetine/pregnancy_hcp_letter.pdf. Accessed September 20, 2010.

Gonsalves L, Schuermeyer I: Treating depression in pregnancy: practical suggestions. Cleve Clin J Med 73:1098–1104, 2006

Hemels ME, Einarson A, Koren G, et al: Antidepressant use during pregnancy
and the rates of spontaneous abortions: a meta-analysis. Ann Pharmacother
39:803–809, 2005

Holmes LB, Harvey EA, Coull BA, et al: The teratogenicity of anticonvulsant
drugs. N Engl J Med 344:1132–1138, 2001

Kessler RC, McGonagle KA, Zhao S, et al: Lifetime and 12-month prevalence of
DSM-III-R psychiatric disorders in the United States: results from the National Comorbidity Survey. Arch Gen Psychiatry 51:8–19, 1994

Koren G, Matsui D, Einarson A, et al: Is maternal use of selective serotonin reuptake inhibitors in the third trimester of pregnancy harmful to neonates?
CMAJ 172:1457–1459, 2005

Lester BM, Twomey JE: Treatment of substance abuse during pregnancy. Womens Health (Lond Engl) 4:67–77, 2008

Louik C, Lin AE, Werler MM, et al: First-trimester use of selective serotonin-
reuptake inhibitors and the risk of birth defects. N Engl J Med 356:2675–
2683, 2007

Marcus SM, Flynn HA, Blow FC, et al: Depressive symptoms among pregnant
women screened in obstetrics settings. J Womens Health (Larchmt) 12:373–
380, 2003

McKenna K, Koren G, Tetelbaum M, et al: Pregnancy outcome of women using atypical antipsychotic drugs: a prospective comparative study. J Clin Psychiatry 66:444–449; quiz 546, 2005

Meyer C, Oberman M: Mothers Who Kill Their Children: Inside the Minds of Moms From Susan Smith to the "Prom Mom." New York, New York University Press, 2001

Misri S, Kendrick K: Treatment of perinatal mood and anxiety disorders: a review. Can J Psychiatry 52:489–498, 2007

Morrow JI, Craig JJ, Russell AJ: Epilepsy and pregnancy: a prospective register in the United Kingdom. J Neurol Sci 187 (suppl 1):S299, 2001

Nulman I, Rovet J, Stewart DE, et al: Neurodevelopment of children exposed in utero to antidepressant drugs. N Engl J Med 336:258–262, 1997

O'Hara MW, Neunaber DJ, Zekoski EM: Prospective study of postpartum depression: prevalence, course, and predictive factors. J Abnorm Psychol 93:158–171, 1984

Parker B, McFarlane J, Soeken K: Abuse during pregnancy: effects on maternal complications and birth weight in adult and teenage women. Obstet Gynecol 84:323–328, 1994

Rabheru K: The use of electroconvulsive therapy in special patient populations. Can J Psychiatry 46:710–719, 2001

Radloff L: The CES-D scale: a self-report depression scale for research in the general population. Appl Psychol Meas 1:385–401, 1977

Resnick HS, Kilpatrick DG, Dansky BS, et al: Prevalence of civilian trauma and posttraumatic stress disorder in a representative national sample of women. J Consult Clin Psychol 61:984–991, 1993

Robinson J, Sareen J, Cox BJ, et al: Self-medication of anxiety disorders with alcohol and drugs: results from a nationally representative sample. J Anxiety Disord 23:38–45, 2009

Roeloffs C, Sherbourne C, Unützer J, et al: Stigma and depression among primary care patients. Gen Hosp Psychiatry 25:311–315, 2003

Ross AS, Hall RW, Frost K, et al: Antenatal and neonatal guidelines, education and learning system. J Ark Med Soc 102:328–330, 2006

Sharma V: A cautionary note on the use of antidepressants in postpartum depression. Bipolar Disord 8:411–414, 2006

Sharma V: Management of bipolar II disorder during pregnancy and the postpartum period—Motherisk Update 2008. Can J Clin Pharmacol 16:E33–E41, 2009

Viguera AC, Nonacs R, Cohen LS, et al: Risk of recurrence of bipolar disorder in pregnant and nonpregnant women after discontinuing lithium maintenance. Am J Psychiatry 157:179–184, 2000

Weissman MM, Olfson M: Depression in women: implications for health care research. Science 269:799–801, 1995

Westdahl C, Milan S, Magriples U, et al: Social support and social conflict as predictors of prenatal depression. Obstet Gynecol 110:134–140, 2007

Wichman C, Moore K, Lang T, et al: Congenital heart disease associated with selective serotonin reuptake inhibitor use during pregnancy. Mayo Clin Proc 84:23–27, 2009

Widom CS, Czaja SJ, Dutton MA: Childhood victimization and lifetime revictimization. Child Abuse Neglect 32:785–796, 2008

Wisner KL, Sit DK, Hanusa BH, et al: Major depression and antidepressant treatment: impact on pregnancy and neonatal outcomes. Am J Psychiatry 166:557–56, 2009

Yonkers KA, Wisner KL, Stewart DE, et al: The management of depression during pregnancy: a report from the American Psychiatric Association and the American College of Obstetricians and Gynecologists. Gen Hosp Psychiatry 31:403–413, 2009

CHAPTER SIX

Treatment Resistant Depression in Later Life

Erin Miller, M.S.
Lisa S. Seyfried, M.D.
Susan Maixner, M.D.
Kara Zivin, Ph.D.
Helen C. Kales, M.D.

Clinical Vignette

Mrs. V, a 78-year-old woman, had a remote history of postpartum depression 50 years earlier that had resulted in a lengthy inpatient hospitalization with "some kind" of medication treatment. According to the patient, she "resumed her life" following that episode; although she had "down periods over the years," she had no further severe depression until approximately 6 months before the present evaluation. Starting 4 months prior to the evaluation, Mrs. V was seen by an outside psychiatrist who prescribed a trial of unclear duration of fluoxetine up to 60 mg/day. At some point, the fluoxetine was augmented with aripiprazole 4 mg. At the time of the evaluation, Mrs. V was taking duloxetine 60 mg twice per day and alprazolam 0.5 mg twice per day, but her symptoms had not responded to this treatment, even after an adequate trial. Mrs. V stated that despite the medications, her symptoms were worsening over time, and she wondered whether she would ever get back to her baseline and "be a functional person."

On examination, Mrs. V stated that she had been severely depressed over the last few months. Mornings were the worst, she said; she had extreme difficulty getting out of bed but felt somewhat better toward the evening hours. She made herself "do chores" but said that she was nearly housebound in terms of not wanting to go out. She did not want to see her grandchildren "in her condition." She had stopped coloring her hair, which was unusual for her. Mrs. V had psychomotor retardation, and her affect was generally downcast. She had the appearance of an almost constant frown. She stated that her concentration was very poor and that she could not sustain the attention to read anything. Her appetite had been very low, and she had lost about 15 pounds. Mrs. V described a feeling of her body "involuting on itself" and of near-constant anxiety. Although she stated that she would never commit suicide given what it would do to her family, she noted that it was "hard to think about going on this way." She was sleeping about 8 hours per night and napping throughout the day, noting that sleep was her "only respite." She worried about being a burden on her family and felt that she was "scaring my husband." She wanted to cry almost constantly, but she stated that the alprazolam helped to "numb" some of these feelings. She brought out a notebook in which she had been journaling some of her thoughts and feelings and drawing some depictions of herself with depression. These drawings were quite poignant and showed her sitting under her "happy light" (a Verilux) and inscriptions such as "not the start of another day, please; I can't take another day; please come evening, please."

Mrs. V's medical history was significant for hypertension, elevated cholesterol levels, and hypothyroidism. The patient admitted that she often forgot to take the thyroid replacement medication but was taking her psychotropic regimen adherently. In terms of cognition, Mrs. V scored 22 out of 30 on cognitive screening (Montreal Cognitive Assessment), missing items for the mini-trails test as well as correct placement of the hands on the clock. She had difficulty sustaining her attention in terms of sequencing digits. On delayed recall, she missed two words. She appeared to be giving good effort during the test, but she was noted to be quite anxious throughout the screening process.

Later-life depression is a heterogeneous syndrome. Although depression in elderly patients is highly treatable, several factors make overall management challenging and contribute to treatment resistance in later-life depression. The case of Mrs. V illustrates many of the themes that will be discussed in this chapter as contributors to Treatment Resistant Depression (TRD): 1) medical comorbidity; 2) neuropsychiatric comorbidity, including vascular depression, executive dysfunction, dementia, and co-occurring psychiatric illness (e.g., anxiety, substance use, personality disorders); 3) nonadherence to prescribed treatments; and 4) psychosocial factors (e.g., social support, caregiving issues, relationship changes). The chapter concludes with a discussion of potential treatments for TRD in late life.

Prevalence, Scope, and Estimates of Treatment Resistant Depression in Later Life

Later-life depression is a significant public health concern in the United States and worldwide. Depression is the most common psychiatric disorder in the geriatric population, with prevalence estimates of up to 3 % in the general population and 12 % among those in medical settings (Shanmugham et al. 2005). By 2030, depressive disorders are projected to be the leading cause of disability and disease burden among developed countries worldwide and the second leading cause among all countries, outranked only by HIV/AIDS (Mathers and Loncar 2006). As the population ages, the burden of geriatric depression will continue to grow. Depression is associated with increased rates of morbidity and mortality, medical burden, health service use, longer hospital stays, and disability. However, treatments for depression among the elderly do exist, and approximately 60 % of depressed older adults recover within 6 months, which is comparable to recovery in younger patients (Alexopoulos et al. 1996).

In younger or mixed-age samples, depression that does not remit despite adequate treatment (e.g., trials of antidepressant medication at adequate dosage and duration) is considered TRD (Bonner and Howard 1995). Among the geriatric population, it has been estimated that up to 40 % of patients have depression that does not adequately respond to initial treatment (Flint 1995). However, determining accurate estimates of TRD in this population is difficult because of a lack of definitive diagnostic criteria and scientific research in this area. In addition, many factors can contribute to and complicate the presentation, diagnosis, and treatment of geriatric TRD. These factors include several psychological and medical comorbidities, dementia and cognitive impairment, treatment nonadherence, and other psychosocial components such as interpersonal and familial relationship changes and social support insufficiency. Because of the heterogeneity of later-life depression, as well as the paucity of definitive criteria and research regarding later-life TRD, for the purposes of this chapter, TRD is considered to be depression that does not remit despite the provision of adequate treatment by a provider to an elderly patient.

Contributors to Treatment Resistance

Medical Comorbidity

Medical illness is common in elderly patients who have late-life depression; 88 % of such patients have at least one significant medical disorder, and 48 % have three or more significant medical disorders (Lacro and Jeste 1994). The prevalence of major depression increases in clinical settings that are marked by high levels of medical illness and physical disability, with rates of major depression lower than 3 % among community elderly, at least 10 % –12 % in inpatient medical settings (Shanmugham et al. 2005), and 20 % –25 % among cognitively intact patients in nursing homes (Katz et al. 1993). In many cases, specific medical illnesses may be less important as contributors to depression severity and treatment resistance than are overall medical burden and degree of functional disability. However, some illness-specific cohorts, including patients with stroke, myocardial infarction, and coronary artery disease, appear to have higher-than-expected rates of depression (Alexopoulos 2001a). Depression also has been cited as a possible risk factor for several medical and psychiatric illnesses.

Medical illness has been documented as the most powerful predictor of poor outcomes in patients with late-life depression, but depression itself is associated with poor outcomes of medical illness. Depression in older adults with medical illness may delay recovery by decreasing motivation and compliance and interfering with rehabilitation and thus prolonging hospitalizations. In medical inpatients, depression has been associated with longer hospital stays, prolonged recovery periods, and increased use of medical services (Koenig et al. 1989).

In the few studies of TRD in the elderly to date, the effect of physical illness on depression treatment response has been mixed. In one study (Small et al. 1996), more than 80 % of geriatric patients with depression also reported physical illnesses; however, the number of comorbid physical illnesses did not influence their treatment response. In another study of 205 consecutively admitted elderly inpatients (Zubenko et al. 1994), the number of medical problems and length of hospital stay independently contributed to significantly poorer response to pharmacotherapy for depression. The mixed results from these studies may, in part, reflect the fact that treatment response is less related to the number of medical conditions and more related to the degree of disability caused by those illnesses.

In the case of Mrs. V, hypothyroidism was a comorbid medical condition. Hypothyroidism is very common in older adults, its prevalence increases with older age, and it affects women more commonly than men (Shanmugham et al. 2005). As noted in the history, Mrs. V admitted being nonadherent to her thyroid supplementation, which was reflected in an elevated thyrotropin level on evaluation laboratory testing. Hypothyroidism in an older adult can mimic depression, causing a slowed, apathetic appearance and cognitive difficulties.

Vascular Depression and Executive Dysfunction

Although it has been recognized for some time that depression may occur in association with acute cerebrovascular events, more recent attention has been given to depression associated with chronic ischemic changes in the brain. With the availability of magnetic resonance imaging (MRI) and other imaging techniques, identification of subtle in vivo structural brain change became possible, and late-onset depression was linked to brain changes on MRI (white matter hyperintensities [WMH]) beginning in the late 1980s (Krishnan et al. 1988). Fujikawa et al. (1994) described finding "silent stroke" in most patients with late-onset major depression, particularly in the absence of a family history of depressive illness or psychosocial stressors. This mounting evidence led to the proposal of the "vascular depression" hypothesis in 1997 (Alexopoulos et al. 1997).

The vascular depression hypothesis, as proposed by Alexopoulos et al. (1997), describes depression with the following characteristics: 1) late onset (after age 65) or change in course after early onset, 2) persistent symptoms, and 3) the association of depression with vascular disease or vascular risk factors and diffuse or multifocal cerebrovascular lesions. Alexopoulos et al. (1997) also noted the large amount of existing indirect support for the vascular depression hypothesis, including the high rates of depression in patients with hypertension, hyperlipidemia, and coronary artery disease; the high rate of poststroke depression; the frequency of silent stroke and WMH in late-onset depression (Fujikawa et al. 1994; Krishnan et al. 1988); and the rarity of a family history of depression in those with depression and silent stroke (Fujikawa et al. 1994).

One placebo-controlled study did not find a significant difference in response to sertraline between groups of depressed older patients with either low or high levels of subcortical hyperintensities (Salloway et al. 2002). The authors noted that the lack of difference may have been related to the small sample size, the lack of consistent drug effect overall, the small number of patients with high subcortical hyperintensity severity, and the use of a visual rating scale to measure hyperintensities. In Simpson et al.'s (1997) study, total WMH load was not associated with poor treatment outcomes; however, patients with lesions in the pontine reticular formation, basal ganglia, and deep white matter had an especially poor response to pharmacotherapy. The latter findings suggest that the association between subcortical hyperintensities and treatment response may be related to lesion location. A subsequent study (Taylor et al. 2003) found that greater progression of WMH volume was associated with poor outcomes of geriatric depression. In the study, a 1% increase in WMH volume was associated with a 7% increased risk of poor outcome. Although this study appeared to validate the vascular depression hypothesis, the measure of comorbidity used did not capture subtler distinctions (mean blood pressure over time, cigarette use) that may have affected WMH progression.

Executive dysfunction involving compromised integrity of frontal structures and subcortical connections ("striatofrontal dysfunction"; Tranel et al. 1994) manifests as impairments in planning, organization, and abstraction, as often seen in late-life depression. Although it is not the only cause of executive dysfunction, ischemic brain damage is thought to be a major potential contributor to such pathology (Alexopoulos 2001b). Other causes of executive dysfunction include disorders affecting subcortical structures, such as Parkinson's disease, and those involving degeneration of the basal ganglia. Studies of patients with executive dysfunction (Alexopoulos 2001b) or vascular depression (Simpson et al. 1997) indicate that these patients have a poorer and delayed response to antidepressants, decreased long-term recovery, increased relapse risk, and more adverse events and disability.

In the case of Mrs. V, she had only one cerebrovascular risk factor (hypertension), but an MRI following the evaluation detected multiple areas of focal white matter signal change in both cerebral hemispheres that were thought likely to represent chronic microvascular ischemic disease changes. Mrs. V also had evidence of some executive dysfunction (poor performance on the mini-trails portion of the Montreal Cognitive Assessment) when she was seen for evaluation. On the basis of the research findings for vascular depression and executive dysfunction and poorer treatment outcomes, it is not surprising that Mrs. V's response to antidepressant trials had been suboptimal.

Dementia

The overall prevalence rate for major depression in dementia patients is estimated to be approximately 20%, with even more patients experiencing symptoms (Ballard et al. 1996). A study examining the prevalence of depression among dementia patients and control subjects without dementia in chronic care facilities in the last 6 months of life found that major depression was highly prevalent regardless of cognitive status (Evers et al. 2002).

The diagnosis of depression in dementia is complicated by several factors: overlapping symptoms, symptom persistence, cohort effects, ageist myths (e.g., senility and depression are "normal" outgrowths of aging), communication difficulties in later stages of dementia, anosognosia, and uncertain reliability of caregiver reports (Thorpe and Groulx 2001). The possibility of a superimposed depression in dementia should be considered when chronic symptoms associated with dementia progression, such as weight loss, sleep changes due to loss of diurnal rhythms, and amotivation, become more severe over the course of a few weeks (Thorpe and Groulx 2001). Depressed patients with dementia (especially those with mild dementia) can have symptom profiles similar to those of patients without dementia.

In 2002, a group of investigators with extensive research and clinical experience related to late-life depression and Alzheimer's disease (AD) proposed provisional diagnostic criteria for depression in AD for the purpose of facilitating hypothesis-driven research in this area and providing a consistent target for treatment research (Olin et al. 2002). These investigators noted the widely varying prevalence estimates for depression in AD as part of the background and rationale for the new criteria. The investigators also acknowledged that the proposed criteria are broad, rely on clinical judgment, and reflect both the overlap between the two syndromes and the current evidence base. Unlike the DSM-IV-TR (American Psychiatric Association 2000) diagnostic criteria for a major depressive episode, the provisional diagnostic criteria for depression in AD require the presence of only three or more symptoms within the same 2-week period (vs. five or more for major depressive episode); incorporate criteria for irritability and social isolation; and revise the criteria for loss of interest so that they reflect decreased positive affect in response to social contact or activities.

It is difficult to compare among the treatment studies of depression in dementia patients, given the varying diagnostic categories used (symptoms vs. depressive syndromes) and types of studies performed (case reports, case series, chart reviews, open trials). There have been few placebo-controlled outcome trials of antidepressants in patients with AD who met criteria for major depression. Only one placebo-controlled trial examined the use of a selective serotonin reuptake inhibitor (SSRI) in dementia patients with major depression; this trial found a significantly greater antidepressant effect for sertraline (Lyketsos et al. 2000). Magai et al. (2000) studied late-stage AD nursing home patients with depressive symptoms in a double-blind trial of sertraline and found no significant benefits of sertraline over placebo (although they hypothesized that a trend effect on a "knit brow" facial measure might be more sensitive to signs of depression in their population). The significant placebo response indicated that such response may be frequent in dementia patients, who may show wide fluctuations in depressive symptomatology (Alexopoulos 1996); thus, early improvement of depression in dementia should be viewed with caution. Alexopoulos (1996) pointed out that such patients are prone to early relapse and should receive careful follow-up.

Psychiatric Comorbidity

In addition to medical and neurological comorbidities, psychiatric comorbidities such as anxiety, substance use, and personality disorders may play a role in treatment resistance in later-life depression.

Anxiety

One risk factor for poor outcomes of treatment for late-life depression, including treatment resistance, is anxiety. Depression associated with clinically significant anxiety, primarily generalized anxiety disorder or subsyndromal anxiety characterized by generalized anxiety or panic symptoms, is found in approximately half of older outpatients with depression (Lenze et al. 2005). Steffens and McQuoid (2005) found that older depressed patients with anxiety were less likely to have remitted depression than were nonanxious depressed patients; anxiety influenced depression outcomes, even after the investigators controlled for use of benzodiazepines, which itself was an independent predictor of poor depression outcomes. In the Prevention of Suicide in Primary Care Elderly: Collaborative Trial (PROSPECT) study, which used care management strategies to treat late-life depression, the intervention was more effective than usual care in patients with low anxiety severity, but it added little benefit for patients with higher anxiety severity (Alexopoulos et al. 2005). Thus, poor adherence and poor outcomes in later-life depression may be most likely among those with comorbid anxiety, and care management may be insufficient treatment for such anxious depressed elderly primary care patients.

Somatic symptoms are a core feature of anxiety disorders in older patients. Anxious individuals may be hypervigilant about their bodily sensations and may overestimate the dangerousness of medications or the severity of side effects (Lenze et al. 2005). Older patients with anxious depression frequently misattribute somatic symptoms of anxiety to adverse medication effects, contributing to both dropout and poor response in antidepressant treatment trials (Lenze et al. 2003). Additionally, older adults with anxiety symptoms and a somatic focus may tend to discount psychological explanations for psychiatric symptoms and to refuse treatment (Lenze et al. 2005). The potential negative effect of anxious somatization on adherence is of particular concern because anxious depression is associated with higher rates of suicidality in older patients (Lenze et al. 2003). However, comorbid anxiety is also modifiable; in one study, Nelson et al. (2005) found that symptoms of psychic and somatic anxiety were among the symptoms showing the greatest change during adequate antidepressant treatment of late-life depression.

Mrs. V. described nearly constant generalized anxiety symptoms. These symptoms created an increased reliance on the use of benzodiazepines "to get through the day." In addition, it was thought that the benzodiazepines were contributing to cognitive difficulties and to a potential fall risk.

Substance Use

Many depressed patients have comorbid substance use disorders, but data on addictive behaviors in older adults are scarce, and studies of TRD and comorbid alcoholism or substance use are virtually nonexistent for elderly patients. The limited existing data are inconclusive. Some data suggest that depression treatment can be effective in elderly patients who also use alcohol (Oslin et al. 2000). However, other studies suggest a negative relation between problem drug or alcohol use and depression treatment outcomes. This may be attributable, in part, to depression treatment nonadherence. One study of nearly 4,000 older adults in 11 countries (Cooper et al. 2005) found that nonadherence was associated with problem drinking. More studies need to be conducted to determine the relation between addictive disorders and TRD in older adults.

Personality Disorders

Personality traits and disorders are important comorbid factors that may complicate the course and treatment of depression. Many clinicians believe that personality disorders interfere with depression treatment and lead to worse outcomes. Despite their potential importance, personality disorders in the elderly have received little attention. Most existing data suggest that the prevalence of personality disorders in older adults is slightly lower than in younger adults. Yet a meta-analysis of 30 studies published between 1980 and 1997 found that the prevalence and distribution of personality disorders are similar in adults younger and older than 50 years (Abrams and Horowitz 1999), suggesting that personality issues remain a significant problem in later life. However, few studies have focused on the relation between personality disorders and depression in the elderly.

Personality disorders appear to be more common in depressed individuals than in nondepressed individuals. It has been estimated that 30%–70% of depressed patients have personality disorders (Thase 1996). In later life, personality disorder comorbidity has been associated with an earlier age at depression onset, interpersonal difficulties, and high rates of Axis I comorbidities. Some personality disorders are associated with increased risk of rehospitalization following a psychiatric admission. Personality traits also may predict negative outcomes through medication nonadherence (Thase 1996). Therefore, it is important to conduct future research on the relation between personality disorders and depression (particularly TRD) in older adult populations.

Nonadherence

Another large contributor to treatment resistance in elderly patients with depression is nonadherence to depression treatment regimens. A recent review by Zivin and Kales (2008) examined the problem of treatment nonadherence in later-life depression in detail; a summary of this information is presented here.

Although rates of antidepressant treatment among the elderly have increased with the availability of newer antidepressants such as SSRIs, among those who begin treatment, nonadherence ranges from 40 % to 75 %. Thus, even though evidence indicates that providers are increasingly diagnosing depression and recommending treatment for older patients (addressing a "first-generation problem"), greater effort is needed to ensure that patients actually initiate and continue appropriate care throughout the course of their depressive illness (a "second-generation problem") (Zivin and Kales 2008). In this way, patients may maximize improvement in both emotional and physical quality of life domains.

Poor adherence to depression treatment is an important source of drug exposure variability, but adherence is often poorly measured in both research trials and clinical practice: TRD may, in fact, represent undertreatment because of poor adherence (Mulsant and Pollock 1998). Thus, even with successful screening and diagnosis of late-life depression in health care settings, a large treatment gap remains. Poor adherence to depression treatment may limit the extent to which older patients with depression realize the benefits of efficacious treatment options, and this problem can be viewed as the next frontier in the treatment of late-life depression.

Adherence to antidepressant regimens has been studied somewhat more extensively in mixed-age primary care samples, in which patients' enhanced attitudes about depression or antidepressants and confidence in managing side effects have been found to be predictors of adherence (Lin et al. 2003). However, these findings cannot be directly extrapolated to older adults and therefore cannot adequately inform late-life intervention development because mean ages in primary care samples are typically in the 40s (Lin et al. 2003) and ages within a sample can have a wide range. Sample age is a critical issue given that 1) medical and neurological comorbidities increase with age and may affect adherence behaviors to a greater degree in older-age samples than in mixed-age samples, and 2) beliefs and attitudes also may differ in older populations (Wetherell et al. 2004).

Information is very limited about the effect of patient-level beliefs and attitudes toward depression treatment in older adults. Preliminary data from the Primary Care Research in Substance Abuse and Mental Health for Elderly (PRISMe) study suggested that most older adults surveyed from a random primary care sample believe that depression is a medical illness (Oslin et al. 2001). However, only 50% were willing to take an antidepressant. Thus, it appears that barriers exist that may outweigh older patients' perceptions of depression as a serious illness. One such barrier to antidepressant adherence may be stigma or the belief that most people will devalue or discriminate against individuals who have a mental health diagnosis. One prior study (Sirey et al. 2001) examined the effects of stigma, age, and treatment discontinuation. In this study of younger ($n = 63$) and older ($n = 29$) patients with depression, stigma was higher in younger patients but affected treatment discontinuation only in older patients. We are not aware of any studies examining the effect of past treatment on adherence, but this factor, as well as other beliefs and attitudes, may affect late-life antidepressant adherence.

Medication adherence problems also increase with the total number of drugs prescribed, and 25% of elderly patients take three or more drugs. Complexity of medication regimens resulting from medical comorbidity also may be associated with decreased medication adherence in the elderly. Other illness factors that may affect late-life depression medication adherence include depression severity, comorbid substance abuse, and cognitive impairment (Zivin and Kales 2008).

Experts have suggested that inadequate education and support from providers, complexity of dosing regimens, medication cost, inadequate insurance coverage, concern for side effects, and caregiver agreement with treatment recommendations also may be contributors (Bogardus et al. 2004). Although studies such as PROSPECT (Alexopoulos et al. 2005) and Improving Mood—Promoting Access to Collaborative Treatment (IMPACT; Unützer et al. 2002) have shown that collaborative care models do improve the recognition, treatment, and outcomes of depressive illness in older primary care patients, geriatric-specific patient factors likely affect how and whether such interventions will succeed in real-world settings.

In Mrs. V's case, she admitted being nonadherent to her thyroid medication. Although she stated that she was compliant with her psychotropics, this remained a question, particularly given the presence of some executive dysfunction. Adherence is predicated on taking the correct amount of medication at the correct times, for which intact memory and executive function are needed. Nonadherence because of cognitive issues can be improved by the use of pill boxes, caregiver support, and newer technologies such as medication alarm reminder systems.

Psychosocial Components

Many psychosocial changes occur in later life; these include losses (e.g., the death of loved ones or increasing disability) and role transitions (e.g., retirement or moves to be closer to family caregivers). Although most of these changes are met with resilience, some are associated with an increased risk of depression in later life. The research literature on the effect of many of these psychosocial changes is limited. However, ample clinical evidence shows that these factors may be contributors to poor depression outcomes, including treatment resistance.

One of these late-life transitions is widowhood. Although in this age group widowhood is frequent and is considered an "in-phase" life transition, a significant risk of bereavement-related depression remains. In the first month after being widowed, about 33 % of people are depressed according to DSM criteria (Zisook and Shuchter 1991). Six months after the death of a spouse, about 25 % of the survivors still meet depression criteria, with about 15 % of survivors still having depression at 13 months (Zisook and Shuchter 1991). In addition to the loss of a life partner, the surviving spouse often must take on responsibilities that were previously the domain of the spouse. In some cases, performing such responsibilities might be difficult for the widow or widower because of medical or cognitive issues, and thus, dependency may increase. This dependency may evolve into role reversal of lifetime patterns with adult children. Such dependency also may alter the person's ability to take medications adherently.

Caregivers are at an increased risk for depression, often neglecting their own medical, dental, and mental health needs. Additionally, the caregiving responsibilities may lead to inadequate sleep and nutrition. Social contacts can be reduced as well because of the intensity of the workload.

In one meta-analysis, caregivers' rates of major depressive disorder were approximately 22 % (Cuijpers 2005). Spousal caregivers are thought to be at higher risk for depression because of their older age and medical comorbidities. A study by Martire et al. (2008) noted the importance of "the dyad" in depressed caregivers—in other words, the relationship between the caregiver and the dependent person. In this study, a significant association was found between reduced response to depression treatment in the dependent person and the presence of significant depressive symptoms in the caregiver. Similarly, depression may be treatment resistant in the caregiver if the dependent person remains depressed.

Social contacts and support networks change with age and infirmity. Retirement, moves, illness or death of friends, transportation, mobility, and cognitive or sensory impairments all may cause the disruption or constriction of social networks. Primary contacts with friends may be replaced by increased contacts with family or formal caregivers. Relocations may be required for medical or cognitive reasons; moves may take place within communities, within facilities, or at a long distance. It may be difficult to create new social networks. Research, both cross-sectional and longitudinal, indicates that social support protects older adults from depressive disorders; thus, any factor that decreases social support may make an elderly person vulnerable to depression (Oxman and Hull 2001). The latter was confirmed in a study of community-dwelling older adults, in which smaller social networks increased the risk of depression (Oxman and Hull 2001). Decreased social support has been convincingly linked with the *development* of depression in later life, but is the level of social support related to depression *outcomes?* Bosworth et al. (2008) determined that lower perceived social support and less interaction with non-family members were predictive of poorer outcomes in depression treatment over 1-year follow-up.

Financial issues also may affect the course and treatment of depression. A patient may choose not to fill a medication prescription because of cost. He or she may not be able to afford an increased copayment for mental health treatment. The latter issue eventually may be addressed by parity legislation, but it remains a current reality for many patients.

For Mrs. V, psychosocial issues were a definite component of her TRD. After several visits, it was revealed that when Mrs. V had the episode of postpartum depression that resulted in a lengthy inpatient hospitalization, her husband had made a "promise" to her that he would never again allow her to be hospitalized. This promise led him to be wary of any psychiatric treatments in general. In addition, the children of Mr. and Mrs. V noted that Mr. V had begun to have some cognitive issues himself and would become anxious if his wife left the house for any length of time.

Clinical Management of Treatment Resistant Depression in Later Life

In this section of this chapter, we cover clinical management of TRD in the older adult, taking into account the comorbidity and psychosocial factors that were discussed in earlier sections. In many cases, the older adult with TRD comes in for a geriatric psychiatry evaluation after several recent unsuccessful SSRI trials. In addition, augmentation strategies might have been attempted. This was true in the case of Mrs. V: she had undergone recent trials of fluoxetine and duloxetine; in addition, she had received augmentation with an antipsychotic and a benzodiazepine. None of these strategies had resolved her symptoms. We then use Mrs. V's case as a starting point, assuming that the typical treatments for depression already would have been attempted.

General Treatment Considerations

In the case of Mrs. V, the first choice of antidepressant may have been problematic. As noted earlier in the section on comorbid anxiety, such patients are often prone to attribute somatic symptoms of anxiety to adverse medication effects, contributing to both dropout and poor response in antidepressant treatment trials (Lenze et al. 2003). Thus, the choice of fluoxetine was not optimal in an elderly patient with anxiety symptoms. Given that all SSRIs have similar mechanisms of action, the choice should be made on the basis of side-effect and pharmacokinetic profiles. Citalopram and sertraline were the top antidepressant choices for later-life depression in expert consensus guidelines because of their more benign side-effect profiles and lower risk of drug interactions compared with fluoxetine, which may be associated with increased symptoms of anxiety (Alexopoulos et al. 2001b).

Other important considerations are to ensure that the patient had a trial of adequate dose and duration (e.g., 6 weeks or longer); many antidepressant trials lack this and result in poorer response (Mulsant et al. 2001). The axiom of treatment of later-life depression is "start low, go slow, but don't stop." The latter phrase is added because many older patients may receive suboptimal doses over a long time, whereas older patients with depression may require doses similar to those given to younger patients but simply require a longer period of titration (Mulsant et al. 2001).

Following initial treatment of adequate dose and duration and very limited response, one could switch to another antidepressant. This could include a different SSRI, a serotonin-norepinephrine reuptake inhibitor (SNRI; e.g., venlafaxine), or bupropion (Alexopoulos et al. 2001a). Switching may be preferable to augmentation because the patient has to take only one antidepressant, resulting in better compliance and fewer drug interactions and side effects (Papakostas et al. 2008). Note that a switch to bupropion would not likely be helpful in a case of anxious depression such as that in Mrs. V, and she had a trial of an SNRI (duloxetine).

If the patient has had a partial response to the initial antidepressant, an augmentation or combination therapy strategy could be used (Alexopoulos et al. 2001b). The advantage of this strategy is that the improvements gained by the current antidepressant will be maintained; it also prevents a delay from having to stop one antidepressant and then start another and allows for a longer overall antidepressant trial. Despite the limited evidence base for combining multiple antidepressants for TRD in the elderly, it is now a common clinical practice. We discuss three such strategies here: 1) lithium augmentation, 2) the addition of bupropion to an SSRI, and 3) the use of antipsychotic medication.

Lithium augmentation at levels lower than 0.5 mEq/L has been shown to be useful in improving antidepressant response in older adults (Flint and Rifat 1994). However, problematic side effects in the elderly may occur even at lower doses and include tremor, polyuria, and cognitive impairment (Flint and Rifat 1994). In addition, older adults are more prone to lithium toxicity than are young adults because of comorbidity and polypharmacy. Particularly close monitoring of renal function and lithium levels is needed in most cases, as well as caution with medications such as nonsteroidal antiinflammatory drugs, thiazide diuretics, and angiotensin-converting enzyme inhibitors, which can increase lithium levels.

The addition of bupropion to SSRIs is a frequently used strategy in older adults (Alexopoulos et al. 2001b), and response rates have been greater than 50% (Dodd et al. 2005). This combination has been used safely and effectively in mixed-age populations, but side effects including delirium and seizures can occur and result in discontinuation.

The use of antipsychotics for augmentation is somewhat controversial. One open trial of older adults whose symptoms did not respond to a trial of SSRIs found that nearly all of them experienced a reduction in their depression symptoms and 50% met remission criteria following augmentation with antipsychotics. However, almost half also experienced side effects, some of which were severe (Rutherford et al. 2007). Although antipsychotics may have some sedating properties for patients with anxious depression, their use in patients without psychotic depression is not recommended in light of their side-effect profiles and recent evidence that they may be associated with a significant risk of increased mortality in the elderly. In 2005, the U.S. Food and Drug Administration issued a "black box" warning that the "treatment of behavioral disorders in elderly patients with dementia with atypical (second-generation) antipsychotic medications is associated with increased mortality" (Weintraub and Katz 2005, p. 974). A similar warning for conventional antipsychotics followed in June 2008. Thus, the risk-benefit profile for antipsychotics as an augmentation strategy for later-life depression would appear very heavily weighted toward the risks.

Electroconvulsive Therapy

Because electroconvulsive therapy (ECT) is the subject of another chapter in this text (see Chapter 11 by Taylor and colleagues), we do not discuss it in detail here except to describe its use in the elderly. ECT remains the most highly effective treatment for later-life depression; ECT can cause retrograde and anterograde amnesia but is often quite effective in the cognitively impaired patient (Kamholz and Mellow 1996). Recovery rates from amnesia have been shown to be high in elderly patients.

In the case of Mrs. V, the clinicians decided to admit her as an inpatient for ECT because of the severity of her symptoms and poor functioning. Not surprisingly, her husband was resistant to the admission given the "pact" he had made with her previously. However, Mrs. V herself was in favor of the admission, and this, as well as social work efforts with him, eventually won her husband over. On admission, Mrs. V had a head computed tomographic scan, which indicated no acute abnormality but small areas of white matter changes. Her duloxetine was tapered off, but she continued taking lorazepam 0.5 mg twice a day. Mrs. V received six bilateral ECT treatments. However, she developed increased cognitive impairment following the sixth ECT treatment (overall confusion and decline in Montreal Cognitive Assessment score to 18). ECT was held for several days, and Mrs. V showed clearing of the confusion as well as resolution of depressive symptoms. She then started taking nortriptyline for maintenance therapy as an inpatient, and this was titrated up to 50 mg. By the time Mrs. V was discharged, her memory had improved and her Montreal Cognitive Assessment score was up to 26. An MRI performed before discharge showed multiple areas of focal white matter T2 signal change noted in both cerebral hemispheres as likely representing chronic microvascular ischemic disease changes. Mrs. V's dose of nortriptyline was eventually titrated up to 75 mg as an outpatient to a therapeutic level. She remains stable and doing well.

Other Specific Treatment Issues

Vascular Depression

The treatments needed for vascular depression and striatofrontal dysfunction in older adults may be different from current standard antidepressant treatments. Alexopoulos et al. (2001) noted that such treatments might include drugs that modify neurotransmitters involved in striatofrontal pathways (e.g., dopamine, acetylcholine, opiates) such as dopamine D_3 receptor agonists, cholinesterase inhibitors, and opiate receptor agonists and antagonists, as well as medications that may improve executive dysfunction (modafinil). Considering the evidence that vascular disease is one of the strongest potential contributors to striatofrontal dysfunction, the future treatment of vascular depression also may involve primary prevention of vascular disease (Alexopoulos et al. 2001). The latter would entail the continued emphasis on advising the discontinuation of smoking and excessive drinking, given their effects on the vascular system, as well as modification of treatable vascular risk factors (e.g., blood pressure, cholesterol level).

Other strategies for the treatment of vascular depression may include nonpharmacological approaches to address executive dysfunction. Problem-solving therapy may be particularly useful for those with late-life depression and executive dysfunction. Specifically, Alexopoulos et al. (2003) proposed that problem-solving therapy with components of behavioral activation, increased exposure to positive events, and remediation of communication deficits might potentially target symptoms, including lack of interest in activities, diminished insight, and substantial disability. These investigators then compared problem-solving therapy with supportive therapy in elderly patients with major depression and executive dysfunction. Problem-solving therapy was more effective than supportive therapy in leading to remission of depression and decreasing disability (Alexopoulos et al. 2003).

Depression in Dementia

Current expert recommendations describe SSRIs as first-line agents for depression in dementia (Katz 1998). Given the limited data available, this recommendation is largely based more on benign side-effect profiles than on an evidence base. Katz (1998) noted that the pronounced improvement of depressive symptoms in placebo groups in those trials suggests that interpersonal or behavioral approaches might be effective in the treatment of depression in dementia. Teri et al. (1997) studied two types of behavioral interventions—the use of pleasant events for patients living in the community and teaching caregiver problem solving for caregivers—compared with a wait-list control condition in depressed patients with AD. Both approaches were associated with significant improvement in depressive symptoms in patients and caregivers, and the improvements were maintained for 6 months. These results suggest that caregiver treatment may be an important factor in the treatment of the patient or that some type of supportive intervention is needed for the patient-caregiver dyad.

Depression and Comorbid Anxiety

If appropriately identified, anxious depression may be effectively managed via 1) pretreatment accounting of physical symptoms of anxiety for comparison with later adverse effects, which may allow the patient to compare more objectively those physical symptoms that are new and may be drug related with those that predated the medication and may be caused by the underlying illness; 2) altered antidepressant titration schedules (start low, go slow, aim high, treat long); 3) psychoeducation; 4) early supportive contact (Lenze et al. 2005); and 5) cognitive-behavioral treatment strategies. Such structured support of older patients with anxious depression may achieve outcomes similar to those achieved in patients without anxiety (Lenze et al. 2003).

Summary

Treatment Resistant Depression remains an important barrier to the effective management of later-life depression, which is often complicated by medical, neuropsychiatric, and psychiatric comorbidities, as well as nonadherence and psychosocial barriers. Future research is needed to examine ways to best manage the challenge of TRD in older adults to improve quality of life and well-being among this growing population subgroup.

Key Clinical Concepts

- Depression in later life is very prevalent but treatable; numerous factors such as medical and psychiatric comorbidities, dementia, treatment nonadherence, and psychosocial components make management more complex and contribute to higher rates of Treatment Resistant Depression in this population.

- Chronic ischemic changes in the brain are also associated with depression in later life and contribute to vascular depression and executive dysfunction.

- Patients with vascular depression and executive dysfunction have been found to have reduced response to antidepressants, increased risk of relapse and disability, and worse outcomes.

- It is important in the treatment of depression in later life to "start low, go slow, but don't stop" to obtain an adequate dose and duration of treatment to achieve a response.

■ If the patient's symptoms still have not sufficiently responded after an adequate medication trial, switching to a different antidepressant is preferable to augmenting, in the interest of reducing the total number of medications taken by the older patient.

■ Other treatment options include augmentation with lithium or antipsychotics (although antipsychotics should be used with caution), adding bupropion to a selective serotonin reuptake inhibitor, and electroconvulsive therapy.

References

Abrams R, Horowitz S: Personality disorders after age 50: a meta-analytic review of the literature, in Personality Disorders in Older Adults: Emerging Issues in Diagnosis and Treatment. Edited by Rosowsky E, Abrams R, Zweig R. Mahwah, NJ, Erlbaum, 1999, pp 55–68

Alexopoulos GS: The treatment of depressed demented patients. J Clin Psychiatry 57 (suppl 14):14–20, 1996

Alexopoulos GS: Interventions for depressed elderly primary care patients. Int J Geriatr Psychiatry 16:553–559, 2001a

Alexopoulos GS: New concepts for prevention and treatment of late-life depression. Am J Psychiatry 158:835–838, 2001b

Alexopoulos GS, Meyers BS, Young RC, et al: Recovery in geriatric depression. Arch Gen Psychiatry 53:305–312, 1996

Alexopoulos GS, Meyers BS, Young RC, et al: "Vascular depression" hypothesis. Arch Gen Psychiatry 54:915–922, 1997

Alexopoulos GS, Katz IR, Reynolds CF III, et al: Pharmacotherapy of depression in older patients: a summary of the expert consensus guidelines. J Psychiatr Pract 7:361–376, 2001

Alexopoulos GS, Raue P, Arean P: Problem-solving therapy versus supportive therapy in geriatric major depression with executive dysfunction. Am J Geriatr Psychiatry 11:46–52, 2003

Alexopoulos GS, Katz IR, Bruce ML, et al: Remission in depressed geriatric primary care patients: a report from the PROSPECT study. Am J Psychiatry 162:718–724, 2005

American Psychiatric Association: Diagnostic and Statistical Manual of Mental Disorders, 4th Edition, Text Revision. Washington, DC, American Psychiatric Association, 2000

Ballard C, Bannister C, Solis M, et al: The prevalence, associations and symptoms of depression amongst dementia sufferers. J Affect Disord 36:135–144, 1996

Bogardus ST Jr, Bradley EH, Williams CS, et al: Achieving goals in geriatric assessment: role of caregiver agreement and adherence to recommendations. J Am Geriatr Soc 52:99–105, 2004

Bonner D, Howard R: Clinical characteristics of resistant depression in the elderly. Int J Geriatr Psychiatry 10:1023–1027, 1995

Bosworth HB, Voils CI, Potter GG, et al: The effects of antidepressant medication adherence as well as psychosocial and clinical factors on depression outcome among older adults. Int J Geriatr Psychiatry 23:129–134, 2008

Cooper C, Carpenter I, Katona C, et al: The AdHOC Study of older adults' adherence to medication in 11 countries. Am J Geriatr Psychiatry 13:1067–1076, 2005

Cuijpers P: Depressive disorders in caregivers of dementia patients: a systematic review. Aging Ment Health 9:325–330, 2005

Dodd S, Horgan D, Malhi GS, et al: To combine or not to combine? A literature review of antidepressant combination therapy. J Affect Disord 89:1–11, 2005

Evers MM, Samuels SC, Lantz M, et al: The prevalence, diagnosis and treatment of depression in dementia patients in chronic care facilities in the last six months of life. Int J Geriatr Psychiatry 17:464–472, 2002

Flint AJ: Augmentation strategies in geriatric depression. Int J Geriatr Psychiatry 10:137–146, 1995

Flint AJ, Rifat SL: A prospective study of lithium augmentation in antidepressant-resistant geriatric depression. J Clin Psychopharmacol 14:353–356, 1994

Fujikawa T, Yamawaki S, Touhouda Y: Background factors and clinical symptoms of major depression with silent cerebral infarction. Stroke 25:798–801, 1994

Kamholz BA, Mellow AM: Management of treatment resistance in the depressed geriatric patient. Psychiatr Clin North Am 19:269–286, 1996

Katz IR: Diagnosis and treatment of depression in patients with Alzheimer's disease and other dementias. J Clin Psychiatry 59 (suppl 9):38–44, 1998

Katz IR, Beaston-Wimmer P, Parmelee P, et al: Failure to thrive in the elderly: exploration of the concept and delineation of psychiatric components. J Geriatr Psychiatry Neurol 6:161–169, 1993

Koenig HG, Shelp F, Goli V, et al: Survival and health care utilization in elderly medical inpatients with major depression. J Am Geriatr Soc 37:599–606, 1989

Krishnan KR, Goli V, Ellinwood EH, et al: Leukoencephalopathy in patients diagnosed as major depressive. Biol Psychiatry 23:519–522, 1988

Lacro JP, Jeste DV: Physical comorbidity and polypharmacy in older psychiatric patients. Biol Psychiatry 36:146–152, 1994

Lenze EJ, Mulsant BH, Dew MA, et al: Good treatment outcomes in late-life depression with comorbid anxiety. J Affect Disord 77:247–254, 2003

Lenze EJ, Karp JF, Mulsant BH, et al: Somatic symptoms in late-life anxiety: treatment issues. J Geriatr Psychiatry Neurol 18:89–96, 2005

Lin EH, Von Korff M, Ludman EJ, et al: Enhancing adherence to prevent depression relapse in primary care. Gen Hosp Psychiatry 25:303–310, 2003

Lyketsos CG, Sheppard JM, Steele CD, et al: Randomized, placebo-controlled, double-blind clinical trial of sertraline in the treatment of depression complicating Alzheimer's disease: initial results from the Depression in Alzheimer's Disease study. Am J Psychiatry 157:1686–1689, 2000

Magai C, Kennedy G, Cohen CI, et al: A controlled clinical trial of sertraline in the treatment of depression in nursing home patients with late-stage Alzheimer's disease. Am J Geriatr Psychiatry 8:66–74, 2000

Martire LM, Schulz R, Reynolds CF, et al: Impact of close family members on older adults' early response to depression treatment. Psychol Aging 23:447–452, 2008

Mathers CD, Loncar D: Projections of global mortality and burden of disease from 2002 to 2030. PLoS Med 3:2011–2030, 2006

Mulsant BH, Pollock BG: Treatment-resistant depression in late life. J Geriatr Psychiatry Neurol 11:186–193, 1998

Mulsant BH, Alexopoulos GS, Reynolds CF, et al: Pharmacological treatment of depression in older primary care patients: the PROSPECT algorithm. Int J Geriatr Psychiatry 16:585–592, 2001

Nelson JC, Clary CM, Leon AC, et al: Symptoms of late-life depression: frequency and change during treatment. Am J Geriatr Psychiatry 13:520–526, 2005

Olin JT, Schneider LS, Katz IR, et al: Provisional diagnostic criteria for depression of Alzheimer disease. Am J Geriatr Psychiatry 10:125–128, 2002

Oslin DW, Katz IR, Edell WS, et al: Effects of alcohol consumption on the treatment of depression among elderly patients. Am J Geriatr Psychiatry 8:215–220, 2000

Oslin D, Zubritsky C, Katz I, et al: The impact of beliefs about depression among elderly primary care patients. Presented at the annual meeting of the American Association for Geriatric Psychiatry, San Francisco, CA, 2001

Oxman TE, Hull JG: Social support and treatment response in older depressed primary care patients. J Gerontol B Psychol Sci Soc Sci 56:P35–P45, 2001

Papakostas GI, Fava M, Thase ME: Treatment of SSRI-resistant depression: a meta-analysis comparing within- versus across-class switches. Biol Psychiatry 63:699–704, 2008

Rutherford B, Sneed J, Miyazaki M, et al: An open trial of aripiprazole augmentation for SSRI non-remitters with late-life depression. Int J Geriatr Psychiatry 22:986–991, 2007

Salloway S, Boyle PA, Correia S, et al: The relationship of MRI subcortical hyperintensities to treatment response in a trial of sertraline in geriatric depressed outpatients. Am J Geriatr Psychiatry 10:107–111, 2002

Shanmugham B, Karp J, Drayer R, et al: Evidence-based pharmacologic interventions for geriatric depression. Psychiatr Clin North Am 28:821–835, 2005

Simpson SW, Jackson A, Baldwin RC, et al: 1997 IPA/Bayer Research Awards in Psychogeriatrics: subcortical hyperintensities in late-life depression: acute response to treatment and neuropsychological impairment. Int Psychogeriatr 9:257–275, 1997

Sirey JA, Bruce ML, Alexopoulos GS, et al: Perceived stigma as a predictor of treatment discontinuation in young and older outpatients with depression. Am J Psychiatry 158:479–481, 2001

Small GW, Birkett M, Meyers BS, et al: Impact of physical illness on quality of life and antidepressant response in geriatric major depression. J Am Geriatr Soc 44:1220–1225, 1996

Steffens DC, McQuoid DR: Impact of symptoms of generalized anxiety disorder on the course of late-life depression. Am J Geriatr Psychiatry 13:40–47, 2005

Taylor WD, Steffens DC, MacFall JR, et al: White matter hyperintensity progression and late-life depression outcomes. Arch Gen Psychiatry 60:1090–1096, 2003

Teri L, Logsdon RG, Uomoto J, et al: Behavioral treatment of depression in dementia patients: a controlled clinical trial. J Gerontol B Psychol Sci Soc Sci 52:P159–P166, 1997

Thase ME: The role of Axis II comorbidity in the management of patients with treatment-resistant depression. Psychiatr Clin North Am 19:287–309, 1996

Thorpe L, Groulx B: Depressive syndromes in dementia. Can J Neurol Sci 28 (suppl 1):S83–S95, 2001

Tranel D, Andersen SW, Benton A: Development of the concept of "executive function" and its relationship to frontal lobes, in Handbook of Neuropsychology, Vol 9. Edited by Boller F, Spinnler J, Hendler JA. Amsterdam, Netherlands, Elsevier, 1994, pp 125–148

Unützer J, Katon W, Callahan CM, et al: Collaborative care management of late-life depression in the primary care setting: a randomized controlled trial. JAMA 288:2836–2845, 2002

Weintraub D, Katz IR: Pharmacologic interventions for psychosis and agitation in neurodegenerative diseases: evidence about efficacy and safety. Psychiatr Clin North Am 28:941–983, 2005

Wetherell JL, Kaplan RM, Kallenberg G, et al: Mental health treatment preferences of older and younger primary care patients. Int J Geriatr Psychiatry 34:219–233, 2004

Zisook S, Shuchter SR: Depression through the first year after the death of a spouse. Am J Psychiatry 148:1346–1352, 1991

Zivin K, Kales HC: Adherence to depression treatment in older adults: a narrative review. Drugs Aging 25:559–571, 2008

Zubenko GS, Mulsant BH, Rifai AH, et al: Impact of acute psychiatric inpatient treatment on major depression in late-life and prediction of response. Am J Psychiatry 151:987–994, 1994

CHAPTER SEVEN

Treatment Resistant Depression and Comorbid Medical Problems

Cardiovascular Disease and Cancer

Kevin Kerber, M.D.
Kiran Taylor, M.D.
Michelle B. Riba, M.D., M.S.

A FAILURE to respond to initial efforts to treat depression can occur for many different reasons, but the presence of comorbid medical problems is surely a common one (Rush et al. 2008). Treatment resistance can arise in association with many medical illnesses and can involve a large number of potential pathways. In this chapter we will focus on two major groups of such illnesses: first, on cardiovascular disease, and second, on cancer. Potential mechanisms and specific treatment considerations will be reviewed.

Cardiovascular Disease and Treatment Resistant Depression

Although there has been a great deal of interest in recent years in the relation between depression and cardiovascular disease (CVD), little research has specifically addressed Treatment Resistant Depression (TRD). In this section of the chapter, we therefore have two broad goals: 1) to discuss areas of intersection, identifying factors that may either increase the co-occurrence of depression and CVD or reduce treatment response for both illnesses; and 2) to describe some treatment considerations relevant to patients with CVD whose symptoms do not respond to initial treatments for depression.

These areas of intersection between cardiovascular and depressive illnesses most likely reflect shared etiologies and interacting behavioral, psychological, and biological processes. The suggestion of a causal interaction arises from data showing that depression is associated with a threefold increase in morbidity and mortality from cardiovascular causes (Glassman and Bigger 2007). Because CVD and depressive disorders are the first and second leading causes of overall disability worldwide, the dynamics of their interaction is of great interest (Murray et al. 1997). Despite some methodological limitations, the preponderance of the evidence supports depression as a risk factor for cardiac disease (Frasure-Smith and Lesperance 2005). Even mild depressive symptoms seem to increase the risk of mortality 4 months after an acute myocardial infarction, with severe depression having a still greater effect (Bush et al. 2001). In patients who had undergone coronary artery bypass surgery, depressive symptoms were a stronger predictor of poor functional benefits than were previous myocardial infarction, heart failure, diabetes, or ejection fraction (Mallik et al. 2005).

Note that the significance of the basic temporal relation between the onset of cardiovascular and depressive disorders is not at all clear. Several investigators have found that the increased risk of cardiovascular morbidity and mortality results not from depression in general but rather from first episodes of depression that occur after hospitalization for an acute coronary syndrome (i.e., from incident episodes of depression). Patients with prior (or recurrent) episodes of depression do not appear, at least in certain studies, to have the increased risk of poor cardiovascular outcomes (de Jonge et al. 2006). Other investigators have reported data to the contrary—that cardiac risks are greater for those with recurrent depression (Lesperance et al. 1996). One study suggested that dysthymia has a particularly strong association with CVD (Baune et al. 2006). A more recent study suggested that it is the timing of depressive episodes that is crucial—that the occurrence of *any* depressive episode, whether incident or recurrent, after hospitalization for an acute coronary syndrome raises the risk for poor cardiac outcomes (Parker et al. 2008).

When depression develops after an acute myocardial infarction, some evidence indicates that recurrent depression, compared with incident depression, responds better to antidepressant treatment, suggesting some heterogeneity of depression subtypes and etiology (Lesperance et al. 2007). This is one area of many of ongoing uncertainty in the relation between CVD and depressive illness. The question of diagnostic and etiological heterogeneity is a major issue in the study of depressive illness generally.

Possible Shared Mechanisms Leading to Depression and Poor Cardiovascular Outcomes

A wide range of possible mechanisms connects poor cardiovascular outcomes with depressive disorders. These mechanisms are of interest in raising the risk of TRD and contributing to worse cardiac outcomes, especially when a patient has several of these risk factors or some are present in a severe form.

In the most immediate behavioral way, depressed mood and poor motivation appear to worsen medication adherence in treatment of CVD (Gehi et al. 2005; Rieckmann et al. 2006). This could certainly contribute to depression, resulting in worse cardiac outcomes. However, determining which way the causal arrows run can be difficult. For example, depression is associated with greater risks of obesity, diabetes, poor diet, smoking, and physical inactivity (Bonnet et al. 2005; Whooley et al. 2008). But do smoking, poor diet, and physical inactivity come first and then lead to weight gain, diabetes, and CVD? Can depressive illness develop at either end of that causal chain—that is, can it be either a cause or a consequence of these behaviors? A recent study suggested a bidirectional association between depression and diabetes (Golden et al. 2008). Evidence indicates that severity of acute myocardial infarctions is predictive of occurrence of incident depressive symptoms (Spijkerman et al. 2005). Thus, can the causal effect also run from cardiac events to shaping or effecting depressive outcomes? For those who experience new or incident episodes of depression after a myocardial infarction, the cardiac event certainly does appear to have such effects. It is plausible too that the causality can run in the other direction, from low mood, anhedonia, and poor motivation to physical inactivity, poor diet, obesity, diabetes, and heart disease. Perhaps the apparent heterogeneity of depressive illnesses arises in this way, from patients taking different causal pathways—out of many possible different pathways—through this interlinked net of relations between behavior and biology.

Hypercholesterolemia is another possible mediator of a relation between CVD and depression. It may not only worsen CVD but also reduce responses to antidepressant medication (Papakostas et al. 2003). More broadly, increasing numbers of cardiovascular risk factors are associated with diminished response to antidepressant medication (Iosifescu et al. 2005). These factors that increase the risk of CVD also may increase the risk of TRD.

Another potential mediator is psychosocial disadvantage and its many consequences. Psychosocial disadvantage is associated with greater risk for CVD. In fact, the risk of cardiac disease increases with each additional source of psychosocial disadvantage (such as unemployment, less than high school education, poverty, divorced or widowed status), such that individuals with four or more such risks had a relative risk of 2.63 for incident CVD (Thurston et al. 2007). Job loss and financial stress also have been shown to be associated with TRD (Amital et al. 2008). This role for psychosocial disadvantage is further supported by data regarding predictors of poor treatment response in the Sequenced Treatment Alternatives to Relieve Depression (STAR*D) study (Trivedi et al. 2006). This study, the largest of its kind, found that a wide range of patient characteristics were associated with reduced likelihood of remission in depression treatment. A wide range of anxiety disorders, somatoform disorder, and the total number of psychiatric comorbidities were all associated with decreased likelihood of remission after treatment with citalopram. Other characteristics, such as unemployment, low educational attainment, and having public insurance, also were very strongly associated with poor treatment response. Individuals who are unfortunate enough to have several of these characteristics seem to be at increased risk for both CVD and TRD.

Adverse childhood environments, including a history of abuse, neglect, or household dysfunction, appear to be related to increased risk for both CVD and depression. In fact, a dose-response relation was seen between adverse childhood experiences and ischemic heart disease as well as an adjusted prevalence of depression and anger that was two to three times higher in those individuals with four or more adverse experiences (Dong et al. 2004). These effects may well be mediated through chronic stress and hypothalamic-pituitary-adrenal (HPA) axis dysregulation. A major risk for developing TRD may be found in those individuals with adverse childhood environments. These patients are familiar and frustrating to many clinicians, presenting with a distressing litany of common comorbidities, including depression, anxiety, substance use disorders, chronic fatigue syndrome, fibromyalgia or other chronic pain syndromes, functional gastrointestinal disorders, and CVD (Heim et al. 2008). Psychotherapies that address the chronic mood disorders that often accompany this pathway seem to have a better chance of success than antidepressant medication alone, although the combination of both may be better still (Nemeroff 2003). Many such patients present to psychiatrists already having tried and failed to respond to numerous antidepressants, atypical antipsychotics, and mood stabilizers, in various combinations. Many experienced clinicians believe that these types of patients are disproportionately represented among the TRD population.

Other possible pathways may mediate a relation between TRD and poor cardiac outcomes. Atherosclerosis may cause both heart disease and cerebrovascular disease, leading to a "vascular depression" that may be more difficult to treat with antidepressant medication (Iosifescu et al. 2005). In general, there is reason to believe that comorbid medical illnesses reduce the likelihood of satisfactory response to treatment for depression (Rush et al. 2008). Common genetic mechanisms also may predispose to both depression and CVD (McCaffery et al. 2006).

Given the richness and variety of these intersections between CVD and poor depression treatment response, and the fact that CVD and depressive disorders are the first and second leading causes, respectively, of worldwide disability, it is reasonable to hypothesize that these factors may interact in a destructive positive-feedback cycle, creating a *cumulative disadvantage* that, with each additional factor, leads increasingly to poor cardiac and mood outcomes. These types of cumulative, mutually reinforcing, and multifactorial processes may lead to outcomes that have a power law distribution common in complex systems rather than a normal distribution and that therefore resist simple reductive explanations and interventions. This has treatment implications that are explored in the next section.

Treatment Considerations in Patients With Cardiovascular Disease and TRD

Because of the wide range of possible mechanisms linking CVD and depression and the complexity of the relations between genes, environment, stress, and behavior, no one intervention may be sufficient for patients with TRD and CVD. Multiple avenues of intervention should be considered.

The real difficulty in successfully treating TRD and CVD seems to be the result of many interacting and mutually reinforcing biological, behavioral, and environmental processes. The final result of TRD and CVD may occur after a long interaction between psychosocial disadvantage, adverse childhoods, HPA dysregulation, weight gain, diabetes, cardiovascular risk factors, and the poor self-regard that leads to unhealthy behaviors, poor relationships, and interpersonal stress and loss. Each individual may take a particular path through these related processes, with depression sometimes coming near the beginning and other times as a later result, but, for many, it may be a story of cumulative disadvantage. Treatment must begin, then, by trying to unwrap the collective contributions of each of these factors.

Clinicians should begin with the most immediate potential problem and ask the patient about medication adherence and, if possible, confirm this information with a family member. Clinicians can determine whether refills are being sought or obtained at the proper frequency. It will also be worthwhile to establish whether other medications are being used that may be decreasing antidepressant blood levels. Checking for cytochrome P450 (CYP) interactions may suggest the presence of such a problem. Sometimes it may simply be that previous clinicians have been too cautious about using higher antidepressant doses in medically ill patients who are taking several other medications.

To try to remedy some of the possible pathways mentioned earlier, the clinician should work with the patient to ensure that a healthy diet is followed and that excessive alcohol use and smoking are avoided. In conjunction with the patient's primary care physician or cardiologist, the clinician should try to improve diabetic control, the lipid profile, and exercise frequency. Given the poor motivation that often accompanies depression, a focus on behavioral activation may be especially important. The co-occurrence of CVD and TRD may come about after years of inactivity and unhealthy behaviors, and yet such patients may take a very passive stance regarding what will be needed for them to improve their mood and health. They may wish that antidepressants alone would be sufficient to address their problems, but for patients with several social, environmental, and behavioral risk factors, engaging the patient in an active role to take responsibility for behavior change may be essential. Motivational interviewing is a technique that can be helpful in encouraging a patient to attempt healthy eating and exercising. Additionally, use of omega-3 fatty acids should be considered, as these may be helpful for depression and perhaps even more helpful for cardiac disease (Logan 2004).

In this population, tricyclic antidepressants should, in general, be avoided because they may cause conduction block and orthostatic hypotension. Venlafaxine should not be used because it has some risk of causing elevated blood pressure. Atypical antipsychotics also are inadvisable because they can contribute to a metabolic syndrome with increased body weight and increased levels of blood glucose, triglycerides, and cholesterol.

By contrast, both sertraline and citalopram appear safe in patients with CVD and have a lower frequency of drug-drug interactions (Glassman et al. 2002; Lesperance et al. 2007). This is quite important in patients with CVD, who may be taking numerous medications for various medical problems. Mirtazapine also has been shown to be safe and tolerable in this population (Honig et al. 2007). These findings provide an alternative drug mechanism and a possible strategy of combining a selective serotonin reuptake inhibitor (SSRI) with mirtazapine for patients with TRD. Weight gain must be monitored when mirtazapine is used. Augmentation strategies mentioned in other chapters, such as use of lithium or thyroid supplementation, may be used for patients with CVD and TRD, provided no other contraindications exist.

Electroconvulsive therapy can be safe and effective for treatment of TRD even in patients with CVD. Other newer methods of neuromodulation, such as repetitive transcranial magnetic stimulation (rTMS) or deep brain stimulation, also may have some promise, but much more experience and data are needed for them to be recommended in this population.

Antidepressants and their combination and augmentation may work well for many patients with CVD and TRD, but many others will need a broad behavioral approach that targets the possible mechanisms that connect CVD and TRD. Some patient groups, such as those who experience their first depression after a major cardiac event, may not respond as well to antidepressants and, in addition to the behavioral focus, may benefit from psychotherapy to address the demoralization and pessimism that can result from these reminders of our mortality.

Clinical Vignette

Ms. C, a 61-year-old woman with established CVD, was referred to the psychiatry department for her apparent TRD. She presented a familiar and complex picture of comorbidities and risk factors, including a history of socioeconomic disadvantage, a history of childhood abuse, poor and exploitative relationships in adulthood, poor self-care, unhealthy diet, obesity, type 2 diabetes, hypertension, elevated cholesterol level, and physical inactivity. All of these factors placed her at greater risk for both CVD and poor response to treatment of her depression. In addition, her history of abuse and her general difficulty with trust and relationships complicated the development of an effective therapeutic alliance with her physicians. Prior trials of two different antidepressants lasted only a couple of months and were characterized by only moderate doses (at best), variable adherence, and a lack of any attention to concomitant behavior change.

A more effective intervention for Ms. C's depression began with directly addressing her sense of self-blame, passivity, and pessimism about her ability to be effective on her own behalf. It was our view that Ms. C should not feel that her medical care is simply something that is done to her without her own effort and responsibility. The relation between her difficult history and her depression could be explained to her but should be balanced by a discussion of her ability and responsibility for improving her self-care, largely through having a better diet, beginning a very modest exercise program, and ensuring good medication adherence. She did have some strengths, such as her ability to work hard and take good care of others, even though she saw self-care as somehow "selfish." It was explained to her that depression had an amplifying effect on her other difficulties and that it may be improved by consistent medication use and some initial behavioral activation.

Given Ms. C's stated sensitivity to side effects, sertraline was started at 25 mg/day for several days, until she could clearly tolerate that dose, and then increased to 50 mg. The daily dose was slowly increased to 200 mg; however, although this did help somewhat with her mood and anxiety, it did not yield sufficient improvement. Bupropion was added not only for additional mood benefits but also because it is least likely to cause weight gain and sedation, both very undesirable in Ms. C, for whom behavioral activation was a major goal. Although initially unsuccessful, efforts to begin a modest exercise program finally began to progress when Ms. C found a friend who was willing to walk with her on a regular basis.

Four months after the consultation, Ms. C was improved but not entirely asymptomatic; however, she had a significantly better level of physical activity, better medication adherence, and at least some sense of hope and shared goals in the treatment alliance with the physician.

Cancer and Treatment Resistant Depression

Depression is a common complication of cancer, occurring in about 10 % – 38 % of all patients, a rate approximately fourfold higher than in the general population (Ell et al. 2007; Onitilo et al. 2006). Approximately 50 % of patients with advanced cancer meet criteria for a psychiatric disorder. The most common are adjustment disorders (11 % –35 %) and major depression (5 % –26 %) (Miovic and Block 2007). Prevalence of depressive symptoms in cancer patients varies from 0 % to 58 % (Jones and Doebbeling 2007). Rates appear to increase as the severity of the illness increases (Ciaramella and Poli 2001).

The prevalence of depression appears to vary by the site of the cancer: 50 % prevalence in pancreatic cancer, 22 % –40 % prevalence in oropharyngeal cancers, 10 % –26 % prevalence in breast cancer, 13 % –32 % prevalence in colon cancer, 23 % –25 % prevalence in gynecological cancers, 17 % prevalence in lymphomas, and 11 % prevalence in gastric cancer (Onitilo et al. 2006). The mechanism by which cancer may lead to depression remains controversial. Metabolic and endocrine alterations, treatment with immune response modifiers, chemotherapy regimens, chronic pain, and extensive surgical interventions have been posited as possible reasons for the increased susceptibility to depression in patients with cancer. Patients with premorbid depression, particularly TRD, or poorly controlled depression may be even more vulnerable to such mechanisms, which can lead to an exacerbation of preexisting depressive symptoms (McDaniel et al. 1995; Spiegel and Giese-Davis 2003).

Overall cancer mortality is decreasing as a result of progress in cancer prevention, screening, and treatment programs. Several factors have been suggested to explain the observed variations in cancer mortality, including unequal access to cancer screening and treatment, lifestyle factors (i.e., diet, exercise, alcohol use, and smoking), socioeconomic status, tumor biology, and depression (Onitilo et al. 2006). The observation of a possible relation between cancer and depression dates back to the time of Galen, who observed that cancer was more frequent in "melancholic" women than in "sanguine" women (Kowal 1955).

Depression is a serious, costly, debilitating, and deadly condition in cancer patients. Depressive disorders often worsen over the course of cancer treatment; persist long after cancer therapy; recur when cancer returns; and significantly affect health outcomes such as mortality, quality of life, and treatment adherence (Onitilo et al. 2006). Rates of depression appear to be higher among patients who have greater disability, more pain, and more advanced disease (Gibson et al. 2006).

Depression in patients with cancer also has been shown to have adverse effects on health outcomes other than mortality. Depressed patients with cancer experience a poorer quality of life, are less compliant with medical care, and have longer hospital stays. Depression is also associated with higher pain levels and greater functional limitations. Depression in cancer patients has been found to influence significantly the severity and number of side effects of cancer treatment and to increase the burden of fatigue, cognitive dysfunction, and anxiety (Mossey and Gallagher 2004; Newport and Nemeroff 1998).

Patient depression and caregiver burden and distress are significant problems in families of cancer patients. As a result of a spouse's cancer, 20%–30% of partners experience psychological impairment and mood disturbance (Blanchard et al. 1997; Pitceathly and Maguire 2003). Psychological distress in cancer patients is a major predictor of distress and decreased quality of life in their spouses, parents, or other caregivers (Osborn 2007; Valdimarsdottir et al. 2002). Evidence also indicates that untreated depression in cancer patients may cause higher rates of depression in their family members (Valdimarsdottir et al. 2002). Evidence from depressed cancer patients and other patient populations has shown that depression leads to caregiver burden and stress at levels similar to or greater than those that accompany care of patients with cognitive or behavioral impairment (Andrews 2001; Chen et al. 2004). Children of depressed mothers with cancer are at increased risk for developing adjustment problems (Osborn 2007). Therefore, TRD affects the quality of life of not only the cancer patient but also the patient's caregivers and close family members.

Because depressive symptoms can be similar to symptoms of several illness-related organic syndromes, it is important that practitioners carefully rule out alternative causes, such as chemotherapeutic agents, corticosteroids, central nervous system complications, and whole-brain radiation (Gibson et al. 2006). To diagnose major depressive disorder among the terminally ill (or monitor symptoms), the clinician must place a greater emphasis on psychological or cognitive mood symptoms (worthlessness, excessive guilt, and suicidal ideation) than on the neurovegetative or somatic symptoms (Gibson et al. 2006). Pain and fatigue often coexist with depression, and consequently, it can be difficult to discern whether the etiology of these symptoms is related to cancer or mood. Of those cancer patients who received a psychiatric diagnosis, 39% reported significant pain, whereas only 19% of the individuals without a psychiatric diagnosis had significant pain (Gibson et al. 2006; Onitilo et al. 2006). Fatigue is associated with sleep problems (Bower et al. 2000), which are further exacerbated by depression (Spiegel and Giese-Davis 2003). Despite studies assessing treatment for fatigue, pain, and depression individually, almost no studies have examined a combined treatment modality for the symptom cluster of pain, fatigue, and depression. However, research has found that cognitive-behavioral therapy (CBT) decreased fatigue and depression as well as increased sleep efficiency in breast cancer patients (Fleishman 2004).

As early detection and treatment have improved, survival rates have increased to the extent that 89% of breast cancer patients now survive 5 years beyond diagnosis (Fann et al. 2008). Thus, focus has turned toward maximizing quality of life among survivors, who often experience persisting aversive symptoms such as fatigue, pain, and cognitive problems. Depression, and likewise TRD, may be an important determinant of health behavior for cancer survivors. In a Norwegian study of 1,260 long-term survivors of testicular cancer, participants who identified themselves as physically active were 44% less likely to be depressed compared with physically inactive participants (Shinn et al. 2007). Studies of other cancer survivors have shown an inverse relation between depression and various health behaviors, such as diet and physical activity (Ell et al. 2007).

Psychosocial problems tend to fluctuate with the clinical course of cancer. Patients who have a history of psychiatric illness or have trouble coping are at increased risk for renewed difficulties at the end of life. Sadness, grief, and anticipatory feelings of loss are all appropriate responses to dying. However, feelings of hopelessness, helplessness, guilt, anhedonia, and suicidal ideation are among the best indicators of clinical depression in these patients (Gibson et al. 2006). Depressive symptoms can impair cancer patients' capacity for pleasure, meaning, connection, and doing the emotional work of separating and saying good-bye. Terminally ill cancer patients who have depression are also at high risk for suicide and suicidal ideation, and they have an increased desire for a hastened death (Breitbart et al. 2000). As many as 59 % of all terminally ill patients requesting assisted suicide are depressed (Emanuel et al. 2000). The clinical diagnosis of depression, the severity of depressive symptoms, and a sense of hopelessness are all strong and independent predictors of a desire for a hastened death in the terminally ill (Breitbart et al. 2000). In a review of psychiatric consultation data from Memorial Sloan-Kettering Cancer Center, one-third of suicidal cancer patients had major depression (Breitbart 1987). Another study concluded that suicidal ideation was relatively infrequent in cancer and limited to those who were significantly depressed (Chochinov et al. 1995). Hence patients with TRD are at increased risk for desiring a hastened death when in palliative care.

Treatment Considerations

Extensive reviews of published studies of pharmacological and psychotherapy interventions in depressed patients who had cancer have concluded that antidepressants seem to be effective in reducing depression or depressive symptoms in these patients. In placebo-controlled trials, mianserin, fluoxetine, paroxetine, and sertraline were all superior to placebo in the treatment of major depressive disorder in patients who had cancer (Williams and Dale 2006). No significant difference was detected between fluoxetine and desipramine or between paroxetine and amitriptyline; all treatments were equally useful for depression in patients who had cancer (Penninx et al. 1998). Data on the efficacy of psychotherapeutic interventions in treating depression or depressive symptoms in patients who have cancer are more limited, but CBT seems to be effective in reducing depressive symptoms in this population (Williams and Dale 2006). Some evidence suggests that combining antidepressant therapy with cognitive therapy may enhance long-term recovery from depression compared with cognitive therapy or supportive therapy alone or pharmacological management (Williams and Dale 2006).

With efficacy of most antidepressants being equal, it is important to consider coexisting medical problems when choosing an antidepressant regimen. For example, tricyclic antidepressants have analgesic properties and the ability to potentiate the effects of opioid analgesics. Secondary amines (desipramine and nortriptyline) are less sedating and less anticholinergic than the tertiary amines. Thus, many patients can tolerate secondary amines in higher doses, allowing for greater therapeutic benefit. Cancer patients with comorbid CVD and older patients should take medications that cause the least orthostatic hypotension (e.g., fluoxetine, sertraline). Patients with reduced intestinal motility, urinary retention, stomatitis secondary to chemotherapy, or radiotherapy should receive medications with the fewest anticholinergic effects (e.g., SSRIs) (Stoudemire et al. 1991). One open-label pilot study of mirtazapine (15 or 30 mg at bedtime) suggested that patients with advanced cancer may derive benefit from this medication with regard to mood, appetite, and sleep (Theobald et al. 2002). Treatment was well tolerated at either starting dose (Fernandez et al. 1987; Valdimarsdottir et al. 2002). Liquid formulations are available for some antidepressants (fluoxetine, sertraline, paroxetine, citalopram, escitalopram, doxepin, and nortriptyline), which may be better options for patients who have trouble swallowing pills. SSRIs are still considered first-line treatment, but care should be taken to determine whether drug-drug interactions with chemotherapy agents or other medications are relevant given that SSRIs can increase blood levels of other medications by dislodging them from blood proteins. Various SSRIs also inhibit the CYP isoenzymes to different degrees, allowing drug-drug interactions to occur (Stoudemire et al. 1991).

Psychostimulants such as methylphenidate, dextroamphetamine, and modafinil can be an alternative for depressed patients with cancer, particularly when more urgent relief from neurovegetative symptoms is needed than traditional antidepressants often provide (Fernandez et al. 1987). Mood, appetite, and a sense of well-being can be improved in patients while the medication is decreasing feelings of weakness and fatigue. An additional benefit of methylphenidate and dextroamphetamine is reduction of the sedation caused by opioid analgesics; these stimulants also provide adjuvant analgesia in patients with cancer (Bruera et al. 1987). Additionally, psychostimulants may play a useful role in helping cancer patients feel energetic enough to engage in rehabilitation efforts until their energy level ultimately improves from the direct effects of such efforts. Tolerance can develop, and these medications can exacerbate anxiety, high blood pressure, headache, tremors, and insomnia. Therefore, caution must be used in deciding which cancer patients are prescribed psychostimulants. Modafinil has not been directly compared with amphetamines in the cancer population, but early indications are that it is better tolerated and has less abuse potential.

In a meta-analysis of the potential benefits of psychotherapy in patients with advanced, incurable cancer, psychotherapy was associated with a significant decrease in depression when compared with treatment as usual. However, no randomized trials have focused on psychotherapy in cancer patients with clinically diagnosed depression (Akechi et al. 2008). Types of psychotherapy most commonly used in the cancer population include crisis intervention or supportive psychotherapy, CBT, dignity therapy, and support groups. Crisis intervention or supportive psychotherapy involves helping to alleviate the immediate effect of the stressful triggers. Normalizing feelings and adjustment reactions to a myriad of cancer-related issues and answering questions about the illness or treatment help to improve the patient's morale and sense of control. CBT tries to elicit the patient's irrational or rigid thoughts that lead to feelings of helplessness. Therapists help to provide new coping skills such as relaxation strategies (e.g., guided imagery, progressive muscle relaxation, biofeedback, breathing exercises, meditation). Both group and individual CBT are effective in reducing depressive symptoms and distress and improving quality of life (Spiegel et al. 1989). Dignity therapy is often used to help patients with end-of-life issues by addressing existential concerns of patients and exploring issues that matter the most to them. Additionally, it helps the patients to reflect on the legacy they would like to leave behind for others.

Depression is often perceived as an expected and reasonable reaction to cancer; thus, depression is frequently underrecognized and undertreated in oncology practice (Fallowfield et al. 2001). Oncologist-patient agreement in rating patient depression is high only when the patient reports no significant level of depression. Agreement was only 33 % for mild to moderate depression and 13 % for severe depression, showing that there is a marked tendency to underestimate the level of depressive symptoms in patients who are more severely depressed (Passik et al. 1998).

Patient, provider, and health system barriers to care contribute to the failure to manage depression symptoms effectively. Patients may be reluctant to report symptoms or to see a mental health professional and may not adhere to prescribed treatment, citing concerns about side effects, drug interactions, and preoccupation with cancer treatments. Perceived stigma, family perceptions, and practical barriers such as cost and transportation to therapy also may impede receipt of mental health care, particularly among low-income populations (Ell et al. 2005). Providers may be reluctant to raise the issue and may be less aware of effective treatments, whereas organizational barriers reduce timely and integrated access to mental health professionals. Implementation of routine depression screening and application of evidence-based practice guidelines and algorithms, such as those delineated in the National Comprehensive Cancer Network guidelines for distress, can help minimize some of these barriers to mental health care by creating a more integrated care environment. Efforts have been made in the primary care setting to enhance treatment of depression by implementing routine screening. However, oncology patients often decrease visits to their primary care providers, particularly during active cancer treatments, thus making it all the more important for such screening to occur in the oncology clinics (Reuben 2002).

Special Issues in Patients With Cancer and TRD

With vagus nerve stimulation (VNS) becoming a more accepted treatment option for TRD, potential concerns arise about VNS in patients being evaluated for breast cancer. These issues have been identified previously in patients with cardiac pacemakers (Roelke et al. 1999). The placement of the pulse generator in the left pectoral region may interfere with manual breast examination and mammography (Cascino et al. 2007). The diagnostic yield of mammography in patients with pacemakers has been evaluated in 74 patients. The pacemaker interfered with the mammograms in 7 patients (9%) (Cascino et al. 2007). Hence the treatment of breast cancer also may be affected by VNS when the pulse generator is placed in the left pectoral region. Therapeutic irradiation has been shown to significantly alter the functioning of a cardiac pacemaker (Sundar et al. 2005). The safety of radiation therapy has not been evaluated in patients undergoing VNS. The generator may need to be explanted in a patient requiring this treatment modality. Finally, the follow-up studies performed after definitive treatment may not permit satisfactory evaluation of residual or recurrent tumor in the presence of VNS. Changes related to the placement of the pulse generator, even if the device is explanted, may alter the diagnostic yield of these studies (Cascino et al. 2007).

There are case reports of breast cancer developing at the site of the cardiac pacemaker generators (Cascino et al. 2007). Whether this is coincidental or related to oncogenesis is unknown. To date, breast cancer in association with VNS has not been reported. The most common location for breast cancer is the outer upper quadrant because of the predominance of breast tissue in this region. It may be appropriate, as with a cardiac pacemaker, for women to be screened with mammography and clinical breast examination before implantation of the VNS device (Roelke et al. 1999). Patients at higher risk for developing breast cancer (e.g., those with a positive family history) should have the generator implanted in a location that minimizes disruption of the screening techniques (Roelke et al. 1999). After initiation of VNS, women should have appropriate techniques recommended for breast cancer screening, including mammography with special positioning (Cascino et al. 2007).

Some overlap exists between alternative treatments for cancer and depression. An extract of the herbal medicinal product St. John's wort— hypericin—has been noted to have a cytotoxic effect on tumor cells after photoactivation (Delaey et al. 2000). In vitro studies and in vivo investigations in mice have found that intralesional hypericin has the potential for use in several tumors, including bladder, squamous cell, pancreatic, and prostate cancer (Chen and de Witte 2000). The only human study has involved intralesional injection of hypericin into basal cell and squamous cell carcinomas of the skin. Selective tumor targeting and generation of new epithelium at the surface of the malignancy were noticed. Clinical remissions were observed after 6–8 weeks (Alecu et al. 1998). These preliminary results require replication in a randomized trial. Some scientific evidence shows that St. John's wort is useful for treating mild to moderate depression. However, concerns have been raised about potential interactions of St. John's wort with other treatments. St. John's wort induces CYP3A4, which can lead to subtherapeutic levels of chemotherapeutic agents metabolized by the CYP3A4 system (e.g., taxanes, irinotecan, imatinib), as well as suboptimal levels of several psychotropic agents (Budzinski et al. 2000). When combined with certain antidepressants, St. John's wort may increase side effects such as nausea, anxiety, headache, and confusion.

Fish oil is often used as part of a pharmacological regimen for TRD. Studies in adults have suggested a beneficial effect of omega-3 fatty acids in the treatment of depression (Conklin et al. 2007; Hallahan et al. 2007; Nemets et al. 2002). Fish oil also has been studied as a treatment for cancer-related anorexia or cachexia. At least one trial has examined the benefit of fish oil for control of cancer-related symptoms in addition to anorexia. However, such symptoms were not noted to be significantly influenced by the fish oil (Bruera et al. 2003).

Need for Early Intervention

Depression negatively pervades all aspects of cancer—from diagnosis to death. Untreated depression, particularly TRD that is premorbid to the cancer experience, exacerbates the negative influences of depression on cancer. This influence can negatively affect the quality of life and hasten mortality, whether by the patient's intention or unintentionally. Increased screening for depression and integrated care among oncology, surgery, and psychiatry can lead to earlier interventions and maximized control of the illness. Patients with TRD are already at higher risk for the negative effect of depression on cancer. Therefore, multidisciplinary collaboration is needed beginning with the very first oncology visit.

Key Clinical Concepts

■ Depression is common among patients with either cardiovascular disease or cancer, especially those with histories of depression.

■ Depression reduces quality of life and adherence to treatment in both patients with cardiovascular disease and patients with cancer.

■ Shared risks for cardiovascular disease and depression include behavioral factors (such as physical inactivity, obesity, poor diet, and poor medication adherence), psychosocial factors (such as adverse childhood environments and socioeconomic disadvantages), and biological factors (such as diabetes, metabolic syndrome, hypercholesterolemia, hypothalamic-pituitary-adrenal axis dysregulation, and common genetics).

■ For patients with depression and cardiovascular disease or cancer, the suggested first-line agents are selective serotonin reuptake inhibitors—particularly sertraline and citalopram, which appear less likely to cause drug-drug interactions.

References

Akechi T, Okuyama T, Onishi J, et al: Psychotherapy for depression among incurable cancer patients. Cochrane Database of Systematic Reviews 2008, Issue 2. Art. No.: CD005537. DOI: 10.1002/14651858.CD005537.pub2.

Alecu M, Ursaciuc C, Halalau F, et al: Photodynamic treatment of basal cell carcinoma and squamous cell carcinoma with hypericin. Anticancer Res 18:4651–4654, 1998

Amital D, Fostick L, Silberman A, et al: Serious life events among resistant and non-resistant MDD patients. J Affect Disord 110:260–264, 2008

Andrews SC: Caregiver burden and symptom distress in people with cancer receiving hospice care. Oncol Nurs Forum 28:1469–1474, 2001

Baune BT, Adrian I, Arolt V, et al: Associations between major depression, bipolar disorders, dysthymia and cardiovascular diseases in the general adult population. Psychother Psychosom 75:319–326, 2006

Blanchard CG, Albrecht TL, Ruckdeschel JC: The crisis of cancer: psychological impact on family caregivers. Oncology (Williston Park) 11:189–194; discussion 196, 201–202, 1997

Bonnet F, Irving K, Terra JL, et al: Anxiety and depression are associated with unhealthy lifestyle in patients at risk of cardiovascular disease. Atherosclerosis 178:339–344, 2005

Bower JE, Ganz PA, Desmond KA, et al: Fatigue in breast cancer survivors: occurrence, correlates, and impact on quality of life. J Clin Oncol 18:743–753, 2000

Breitbart W: Suicide in cancer patients. Oncology (Williston Park) 1:49–55, 1987

Breitbart W, Rosenfeld B, Pessin H, et al: Depression, hopelessness, and desire for hastened death in terminally ill patients with cancer. JAMA 284:2907–2911, 2000

Bruera E, Chadwick S, Brenneis C, et al: Methylphenidate associated with narcotics for the treatment of cancer pain. Cancer Treat Rep 71:67–70, 1987

Bruera E, Strasser F, Palmer JL, et al: Effect of fish oil on appetite and other symptoms in patients with advanced cancer and anorexia/cachexia: a double-blind, placebo-controlled study. J Clin Oncol 21:129–134, 2003

Budzinski JW, Foster BC, Vandenhoek S, et al: An in vitro evaluation of human cytochrome P450 3A4 inhibition by selected commercial herbal extracts and tinctures. Phytomedicine 7:273–282, 2000

Bush DE, Ziegelstein RC, Tayback M, et al: Even minimal symptoms of depression increase mortality risk after acute myocardial infarction. Am J Cardiol 88:337–341, 2001

Cascino GD, Eversman CL, Hamre MK, et al: Breast cancer at site of implanted vagus nerve stimulator. Neurology 68:703, 2007

Chen B, de Witte PA: Photodynamic therapy efficacy and tissue distribution of hypericin in a mouse P388 lymphoma tumor model. Cancer Lett 150:111–117, 2000

Chen ML, Chu L, Chen HC: Impact of cancer patients' quality of life on that of spouse caregivers. Support Care Cancer 12:469–475, 2004

Chochinov HM, Wilson KG, Enns M, et al: Desire for death in the terminally ill. Am J Psychiatry 152:1185–1191, 1995

Ciaramella A, Poli P: Assessment of depression among cancer patients: the role of pain, cancer type and treatment. Psychooncology 10:156–165, 2001

Conklin SM, Harris JI, Manuck SB, et al: Serum omega-3 fatty acids are associated with variation in mood, personality and behavior in hypercholesterolemic community volunteers. Psychiatry Res 152:1–10, 2007

de Jonge P, van den Brink RHS, Spijkerman TA, et al: Only incident depressive episodes after myocardial infarction are associated with new cardiovascular events. J Am Coll Cardiol 48:2204–2208, 2006

Delaey E, Vandenbogaerde A, Merlevede W, et al: Photocytotoxicity of hypericin in normoxic and hypoxic conditions. J Photochem Photobiol B 56:19–24, 2000

Dong M, Giles WH, Felitti VJ, et al: Insights into causal pathways for ischemic heart disease: adverse childhood experiences study. Circulation 110:1761–1766, 2004

Ell K, Sanchez K, Vourlekis B, et al: Depression, correlates of depression, and receipt of depression care among low-income women with breast or gynecologic cancer. J Clin Oncol 23:3052–3060, 2005

Ell K, Quon B, Quinn DI, et al: Improving treatment of depression among low-income patients with cancer: the design of the ADAPt-C study. Gen Hosp Psychiatry 29:223–231, 2007

Emanuel EJ, Fairclough DL, Emanuel LL: Attitudes and desires related to euthanasia and physician-assisted suicide among terminally ill patients and their caregivers. JAMA 284:2460–2468, 2000

Fallowfield L, Ratcliffe D, Jenkins V, et al: Psychiatric morbidity and its recognition by doctors in patients with cancer. Br J Cancer 84:1011–1015, 2001

Fann JR, Thomas-Rich AM, Katon WJ, et al: Major depression after breast cancer: a review of epidemiology and treatment. Gen Hosp Psychiatry 30:112–126, 2008

Fernandez F, Adams F, Holmes VF, et al: Methylphenidate for depressive disorders in cancer patients: an alternative to standard antidepressants. Psychosomatics 28:455–461, 1987

Fleishman SB: Treatment of symptom clusters: pain, depression, and fatigue. J Natl Cancer Inst Monogr (32):119–123, 2004

Frasure-Smith N, Lesperance F: Reflections of depression as a cardiac risk factor. Psychosom Med 67 (suppl 1):519–525, 2005

Gehi A, Haas D, Pipkin S, et al: Depression and medication adherence in outpatients with coronary heart disease. Arch Intern Med 165:2508–2513, 2005

Gibson CA, Lichtenthal W, Berg A, et al: Psychologic issues in palliative care. Anesthesiol Clin 24:61–80, 2006

Glassman AH, Bigger JT Jr: Antidepressants in coronary heart disease: SSRIs reduce depression, but do they save lives? JAMA 297:411–412, 2007

Glassman AH, O'Conner CM, Califf RM, et al: Sertraline Antidepressant Heart Attack Randomized Trial (SADHEART) Group: sertraline treatment of major depression in patients with acute MI or unstable angina. JAMA 288:701–709, 2002

Golden SH, Lazo M, Carnethon M, et al: Examining a bidirectional association between depressive symptoms and diabetes. JAMA 299:2751–2759, 2008

Hallahan B, Hibbeln JR, Davis JM, et al: Omega-3 fatty acid supplementation in patients with recurrent self-harm: single-centre double-blind randomised controlled trial. Br J Psychiatry 190:118–122, 2007

Heim C, Newport DJ, Mletzko T, et al: The link between childhood trauma and depression: insights from HPA axis studies in humans. Psychoneuroendocrinology 33:693–710, 2008

Honig A, Kuyper AM, Schene AH, et al: Treatment of post-myocardial infarction depressive disorder: a randomized, placebo-controlled trial with mirtazapine. Psychosom Med 69:606–613, 2007

Iosifescu DV, Clementi-Craven N, Fraguas R, et al: Cardiovascular risk factors may moderate pharmacological treatment effects in major depressive disorder. Psychosom Med 67:703–706, 2005

Jones LE, Doebbeling CC: Suboptimal depression screening following cancer diagnosis. Gen Hosp Psychiatry 29:547–554, 2007

Kowal SJ: Emotions as a cause of cancer; 18th and 19th century contributions. Psychoanal Rev 42:217–227, 1955

Lesperance F, Frasure-Smith N, Talajic M: Major depression before and after myocardial infarction: its nature and consequences. Psychosom Med 58:99–110, 1996

Lesperance F, Frasure-Smith N, Koszycki D, et al: Effects of citalopram and inter-personal psychotherapy on depression in patients with coronary artery dis-ease. JAMA 297:367–379, 2007

Logan AC: Omega-3 fatty acids and major depression: a primer for the mental health professional. Lipids Health Dis 3:25, 2004

Mallik S, Krumholz HM, Lin ZQ, et al: Patients with depressive symptoms have lower health status benefits after coronary artery bypass surgery. Circulation 111:271–277, 2005

McCaffery JM, Frasure-Smith N, Dube MP, et al: Common genetic vulnerability to depressive symptoms and coronary artery disease: a review and develop-ment of candidate genes related to inflammation and serotonin. Psychosom Med 68:187–200, 2006

McDaniel JS, Musselman DL, Porter MR, et al: Depression in patients with can-cer: diagnosis, biology, and treatment. Arch Gen Psychiatry 52:89–99, 1995

Miovic M, Block S: Psychiatric disorders in advanced cancer. Cancer 110:1665–1676, 2007

Mossey JM, Gallagher RM: The longitudinal occurrence and impact of comorbid chronic pain and chronic depression over two years in continuing care retire-ment community residents. Pain Med 5:335–348, 2004

Murray CJ, Lopez AD: Alternative projections of mortality and disability by cause 1990–2020: Global Burden of Disease Study. Lancet 349:1498–1504, 1997

Nemeroff CB: Advancing the treatment of mood and anxiety disorders: the first 10 years' experience with paroxetine. Psychopharmacol Bull 37 (suppl 1):6–7, 2003

Nemets B, Stahl Z, Belmaker RH: Addition of omega-3 fatty acid to maintenance medication treatment for recurrent unipolar depressive disorder. Am J Psy-chiatry 159:477–479, 2002

Newport DJ, Nemeroff CB: Assessment and treatment of depression in the cancer patient. J Psychosom Res 45:215–237, 1998

Onitilo AA, Nietert PJ, Egede LE: Effect of depression on all-cause mortality in adults with cancer and differential effects by cancer site. Gen Hosp Psychia-try 28:396–402, 2006

Osborn T: The psychosocial impact of parental cancer on children and adoles-cents: a systematic review. Psychooncology 16:101–126, 2007

Papakostas GI, Petersen T, Sonawalla SB, et al: Serum cholesterol in treatment-resistant depression. Neuropsychobiology 47:146–151, 2003

Parker GB, Hilton TM, Walsh WF, et al: Timing is everything: the onset of depres-sion and acute coronary syndrome. Biol Psychiatry 64:660–666, 2008

Passik SD, Dugan W, McDonald MV, et al: Oncologists' recognition of depression in their patients with cancer. J Clin Oncol 16:1594–1600, 1998

Penninx BW, Guralnik JM, Pahor M, et al: Chronically depressed mood and cancer risk in older persons. J Natl Cancer Inst 90:1888–1893, 1998

Pitceathly C, Maguire P: The psychological impact of cancer on patients' partners and other key relatives: a review. Eur J Cancer 39:1517–1524, 2003

Reuben DB: Organizational interventions to improve health outcomes of older persons. Med Care 40:416–428, 2002

Rieckmann N, Kronish IM, Haas D, et al: Persistent depressive symptoms lower aspirin adherence after acute coronary syndromes. Am Heart J 152:922–927, 2006

Roelke M, Rubinstein VJ, Kamath S, et al: Pacemaker interference with screening mammography. Pacing Clin Electrophysiol 22:1106–1107, 1999

Rush AJ, Wisniewski SR, Warden D, et al: Selecting among second-step antidepressant medication monotherapies. Arch Gen Psychiatry 65:870–881, 2008

Shinn EH, Basen-Engquist K, Thornton B, et al: Health behaviors and depressive symptoms in testicular cancer survivors. Urology 69:748–753, 2007

Spiegel D, Giese-Davis J: Depression and cancer: mechanisms and disease progression. Biol Psychiatry 54:269–282, 2003

Spiegel D, Bloom JR, Kraemer HC, et al: Effect of psychosocial treatment on survival of patients with metastatic breast cancer. Lancet 2:888–891, 1989

Spijkerman T, de Jonge P, van den Brink RH, et al: Depression following myocardial infarction: first-ever versus ongoing and recurrent episodes. Gen Hosp Psychiatry 27:411–417, 2005

Stoudemire A, Fogel B, Gulley L: Psychopharmacology in the medically ill, in Medical Psychiatric Practice. Edited by Stoudemire GA, Fogel BS. Washington, DC, American Psychiatric Press, 1991, pp 31–57

Sundar S, Symonds RP, Deehan C: Radiotherapy to patients with artificial cardiac pacemakers. Cancer Treat Rev 31:474–486, 2005

Theobald DE, Kirsh KL, Holtsclaw E, et al: An open-label, crossover trial of mirtazapine (15 and 30 mg) in cancer patients with pain and other distressing symptoms. J Pain Symptom Manage 23:442–447, 2002

Thurston RC, Kubzansky LD: Multiple sources of psychosocial disadvantage and risk of coronary heart disease. Psychosom Med 69:748–755, 2007

Trivedi MH, Rush AJ, Wisniewski SR, et al: Evaluation of outcomes with citalopram for depression using measurement-based care in STAR*D: implications for clinical practice. Am J Psychiatry 163:28–40, 2006

Valdimarsdottir U, Helgason AR, Furst CJ, et al: The unrecognised cost of cancer patients' unrelieved symptoms: a nationwide follow-up of their surviving partners. Br J Cancer 86:1540–1545, 2002

Whooley M, de Jonge P, Vittinghoff E, et al: Depressive symptoms, health behaviors, and risk of cardiovascular events in patients with cardiovascular disease. JAMA 300:2379–2388, 2008

Williams S, Dale J: The effectiveness of treatment for depression/depressive symptoms in adults with cancer: a systematic review. Br J Cancer 94:372–390, 2006

CHAPTER EIGHT

Alcohol and Drug Use

Contributions to Treatment Resistance in Patients With Depression

Kirk J. Brower, M.D.
Iyad Alkhouri, M.D.

Epidemiology

Mood disorders and substance use disorders (SUDs) are highly comorbid. In the general population, data from the National Epidemiologic Survey on Alcohol and Related Conditions (NESARC) indicated that people with a current diagnosis of major depressive disorder were nearly four times as likely to have alcohol dependence and nine times as likely to have other drug dependence compared with those without major depression (Grant et al. 2004). These numbers are higher in clinical samples. For example, up to one-third of psychiatric patients receiving treatment for depression have co-occurring SUDs (Davis et al. 2008), and estimates for co-occurrence of bipolar I disorder and SUD exceed 60%. Overall, comorbidity is high enough to justify screening all patients with major depression for SUDs, not just patients with Treatment Resistant Depression (TRD). Doing so may enable the clinician to develop treatment strategies that actually prevent the development of some resistant mood disorders.

Classification of Major Depression in the Context of Substance Use Disorders

Major depressive episodes (MDEs) in individuals with SUDs generally have been categorized as either substance induced or substance independent. By DSM-IV-TR (American Psychiatric Association 2000) definition, a substance-induced disorder is one that has its onset during either the course of intoxication with or the course of withdrawal from a substance. DSM-IV-TR recognizes that the following substances can be associated with mood disorders during intoxication, withdrawal, or both: alcohol (intoxication, withdrawal), amphetamines (intoxication, withdrawal), cocaine (intoxication, withdrawal), hallucinogens (intoxication), inhalants (intoxication), opioids (intoxication), phencyclidine (intoxication), and sedative-hypnotics (intoxication, withdrawal). This classification does not recognize cannabis- or nicotine-induced mood disorders, nor does it recognize opioid-induced depression during withdrawal; however, both the epidemiological and the clinical literature support comorbidity between these substances and MDE (Catley et al. 2005; Havard et al. 2006; Wiesbeck et al. 2008). Moreover, smoking tobacco appears to increase the risk for suicidality (Breslau et al. 2005), and successful quitting may be associated with remission of depressive symptoms (Blalock et al. 2008; Kinnunen et al. 2008). In clinical practice, therefore, all substances require an assessment for their effects on the development and course of TRD.

The notion that all substances associated with dependence can influence the development and course of TRD is also consistent with one of the leading theories of addiction. Specifically, the hedonic dysregulation model postulates that all dependence-producing substances impair, if not damage, those parts of the limbic system that mediate the experience of pleasure (Kalivas and O'Brien 2008; Koob and Kreek 2007). Moreover, what starts as substance-induced euphoria, which positively reinforces repeated drug-taking in the early stages of addiction, culminates in withdrawal states dominated by negative affect, which negatively reinforce repeated drug-taking (Koob and Kreek 2007). In other words, in the later stages of addiction, users take drugs to avoid experiencing negative affect and other withdrawal symptoms.

The clinical implications of the distinction between substance-induced and substance-independent MDEs are not clear. Originally, clinicians tended to assume that substance-induced depression would remit after an appropriate period of abstinence such as 3–4 weeks, even without depression-specific treatment. Given the high rates of suicide and suicide attempts in depressed substance users, however, the course of illness is not necessarily more benign with one etiology than with the other. For example, rates of suicide attempts in 2,945 alcoholic patients were significantly higher among those with substance-independent major depression (30.3%) than among those with substance-induced depression (24.8%), but both rates are high and challenge the assumption that substance-induced depression has a benign course (Schuckit et al. 1997). Similarly, in a sample of 371 alcohol-dependent individuals, patients with independent major depression made nearly twice the number of suicide attempts (mean = 4.6) compared with those with substance-induced major depression (mean = 2.4), but the two groups did not differ in terms of their intention to die or likelihood of hospitalization after their most serious attempt (Preuss et al. 2002).

In addition, patients often have episodes of both types of depression. One lifetime episode of substance-induced depression, for example, does not exclude the possibility of a substance-independent depressive episode occurring at another time. Moreover, substance-induced MDEs and substance-independent MDEs appear to be similarly responsive to antidepressants (Nunes and Levin 2004). Therefore, although classifying depressive episodes as either substance induced or substance independent may have some utility, especially for research purposes, such classification should not necessarily be the primary concern of the treatment professional. Far more important is seeking to resolve both the substance use and the depressive disorders that are contributing synergistically to the individual's burdens and disabilities.

Course of Comorbid Depression and Substance Use Disorders

Among clinical populations, alcohol use disorders predict greater severity of, and poorer outcomes for, mood disorders. Among psychiatric inpatients and outpatients with major depression, for example, having an alcohol use disorder increased the odds for suicidal ideation and attempts by factors of 2.2 and 6.3, respectively (Sokero et al. 2003). Pages et al. (1997) reported that suicidal ideation was more severe among hospitalized inpatients with major depressive disorder when the depression was accompanied by SUDs. Sullivan et al. (2005) reviewed four other studies that showed an increase in suicidal symptoms or acts in depressed patients with a current or lifetime history of an alcohol problem, including two studies with statistically significant increases.

This team (Sullivan et al. 2005) also reviewed six studies investigating the effects of alcohol problems on the course of depression, two of which found that alcohol problems significantly worsened the course of depression. One of these studies followed 588 patients with major depression for 10 years and found that remissions from depression were less likely among patients with current alcohol dependence than among patients with either no history or a past history of alcohol dependence (Mueller et al. 1994). Depressed patients with and without a past history of alcohol dependence did not differ significantly in their course, whereas those with a current history had the worst course. These results suggest that successfully treating alcohol dependence should improve the prognosis for major depression.

Theoretically, substance use may help precipitate, contribute to, or perpetuate depression in several ways. First, substances may cause dysregulation of the limbic system through direct neurotransmitter effects, because all known substances of abuse are capable of influencing, if not impairing, this system of emotional processing (Kalivas and O'Brien 2008; Koob and Kreek 2007). Second, patients with an SUD are likely to feel ashamed and guilty about things they have done because of substances. Third, patients may have endured significant losses, including marriages, friendships, and jobs, as a consequence of using substances. Fourth, substance use may interfere with adherence to treatment for depression. A substance-related chaotic lifestyle also may interfere with adherence. Finally, alcohol may affect sleep patterns, general medical health, and metabolism of antidepressant medications.

Assessment and Differential Diagnosis

How one asks about substance use may affect a patient's willingness to answer truthfully. As mentioned earlier, shame and guilt are among the adverse emotional consequences of substance abuse and dependence, as are anxiety, depression, and irritability. These painful emotions may contribute to secretiveness during the clinical interview. Legal problems associated with drunk driving, domestic violence, or possession of illicit drugs may contribute as well. Not unexpectedly, therefore, some patients may quicken to anger and defensiveness when questioned about their use of substances to avoid feeling painful emotions. Other defenses may include denial, minimization, and rationalization. Such reactions are best viewed as symptoms rather than character traits, but either way, they can present obstacles to making a diagnosis from a single clinical interview.

Several good screening instruments are available for SUDs. Among the most frequently used for alcohol are the Michigan Alcoholism Screening Test (MAST), the CAGE questionnaire, and the Alcohol Use Disorders Identification Test (Connors and Volk 2003). Specialized instruments for older adults (MAST–Geriatric Version) (Beullens and Aertgeerts 2004), adolescents (CRAFFT Screening Test; Knight et al. 2003), and pregnant women (T-ACE test and TWEAK alcohol screening test; Connors and Volk 2003) are also available. The Drug Abuse Screening Test is commonly used for drugs other than alcohol. A composite of these screening tools has been developed for general use: the 16-item self-administered Simple Screening Instrument for Substance Abuse Interview Form (Center for Substance Abuse Treatment 2005). It is surprising, however, that few of these screening tools have been tested specifically in psychiatric populations as opposed to primary care and medically hospitalized patients.

Moreover, these questionnaires have obvious face validity, which means that patients will know what is being asked of them. Consequently, they neither eliminate defensiveness nor guarantee truthfulness. Nevertheless, they do provide a structure for identification and evaluation. Ultimately, however, there is no substitute for a trusting and nonjudgmental therapeutic relationship to facilitate honest dialogue with a patient. Such a relationship may require many sessions to evolve, so the extent of substance-related problems may not immediately be known. Meanwhile, TRD may be the only manifest indicator of an SUD. Therefore, SUDs are always part of the differential diagnosis for TRD.

The diagnostic criteria for substance abuse and dependence are provided in DSM-IV-TR. A few key points are mentioned here. First, substance abuse and dependence are mutually exclusive diagnoses in DSM-IV-TR. Once an individual meets criteria for dependence, he or she no longer qualifies for a diagnosis of abuse for that substance. Instead, dependence may be either active or in remission to some degree (i.e., partial or full remission). Second, DSM-IV-TR substance dependence should not be confused with pharmacological concepts of physical or physiological dependence, which are characterized by tolerance and withdrawal symptoms. Although physical tolerance and withdrawal may occur with, and are among the criteria for, substance dependence, they are not required for the diagnosis. Third, abuse and dependence are differentiated primarily on the basis of impaired control over substance use, which occurs with dependence but not with abuse. Impaired control is specifically operationalized in DSM-IV-TR by two criteria: 1) inability to stop or cut down use despite a persistent desire or multiple attempts and 2) using a substance more than intended in terms of frequency, amount, or both.

Impaired control is crucial to understanding the disorder and the patient who has it. In general, people like to feel in control, so any awareness that one is not in control may contribute to feelings of shame and defensive behaviors, as discussed earlier. Impaired control is also sometimes baffling to patients. Patients may know all the reasons they need to stop, and have good intentions to stop, yet feel hopeless about changing because of many failed attempts.

Tolerance and withdrawal are manifestations of *neuroadaptation.* The brain counters the neurochemical actions of the abused substance to maintain its state of homeostasis. Eventually, it can no longer maintain its original state of homeostasis and adapts to mimic a state of homeostasis in the presence of the substance. In other words, the brain adjusts its operations to maximize functioning during states of intoxication, at the expense of becoming dysfunctional during states of withdrawal. Accordingly, withdrawal symptoms can increase drug seeking and drug taking via negative reinforcement (i.e., continued use of a substance to avoid distressing withdrawal symptoms). The sine qua non of substance dependence—impaired control over substance use—is thought to reflect changes in brain structure and function referred to as *neuroplasticity.*

From the perspective of neuroplasticity, the nature, strength, and balance of neural connections between different parts of the brain undergo marked change as a result of premorbid and genetic vulnerabilities, environmental and developmental factors, and direct pharmacological action of prolonged substance exposure. Impaired control can be understood as behavior resulting from central nervous system changes in which subcortical and limbic structures—involved in automatic and habitual actions (i.e., doing without having to think about it)—come to influence behavior more than does the prefrontal cortex (the center for conscious and executive decision making) (Kalivas and O'Brien 2008). Interestingly, compared with depressed patients without alcohol dependence, those with both major depression and alcohol dependence showed decreased metabolism in the prefrontal cortex (Sher et al. 2007).

Treatment

Treatment Models

We discuss two groups of models: 1) etiological models that have treatment implications and 2) health services models for delivering care to patients with co-occurring disorders. Among the etiological models, the *biological model* posits that addiction is a brain disease resulting from neuroadaptation and neuroplasticity in response to 1) direct physiological effects of chronic substance exposure, 2) genetic and premorbid vulnerabilities, and 3) environmental factors that shape learning and new behaviors. This model is similar to and compatible with a neurobiological model of depression. Moreover, comorbidity between SUDs and TRD is thought to result from shared genetic vulnerability as well as overlapping neurocircuitry and neurochemistry involved in the regulation of emotion and control of behavior (i.e., limbic system). The *self-medication model* of SUDs is a commonly held psychodynamic perspective that attributes substance use to a patient's attempts to ameliorate depressed mood and related symptoms.

Both the disease and the self-medication models can be useful clinically because they are intuitively sensible to patients. Patients readily understand, for example, that they do not feel well and hope that substances will improve their mood at least temporarily, even though they do not feel well overall or for extended periods. In the initial therapeutic visits, therefore, their attempts at self-medication can be framed as not working. Patients also readily understand that substances are chemicals that interact with chemicals in their own brains, which can sabotage their efforts to recover from depressive episodes. Thus, a therapeutic rationale for abstinence from addictive substances is firmly established.

Finally, the *dual-diagnosis model* is useful clinically because it deemphasizes the notion that whichever diagnosis had an earlier onset should be treated as the primary disorder. Instead, it implies that both disorders must be treated regardless of their chronological or etiological relations.

Among the health care service models for treating dual diagnoses are the sequential, parallel, and integrative care models. In the *sequential model,* patients first receive treatment in either a mental health or a substance abuse treatment program and then in the other type of program. Thus, each disorder is treated separately in series. In *parallel models,* patients receive simultaneous treatment for their disorders but by two different treatment teams or providers who may also be at different sites. In the *integrative care model,* both disorders are treated simultaneously by one treatment team that has training and experience to treat both disorders. The general consensus is that the integrative model is superior (Kleber et al. 2007) but not always available, depending on the resources of the community.

Treatment Goals

The goal of substance-related treatment in patients with TRD should be complete abstinence from all psychoactive substances not recommended by the treatment team. Although decreased use and controlled use are sometimes reasonable goals for patients without TRD, the need to optimally assess the contribution of substances to depressed mood requires their complete withdrawal to eliminate them from the "depressogenic equation." A treatment goal of abstinence is not always readily accepted by patients, who may either feel entitled to have a drink every now and then or believe that their substance use is not problematic. Thus, motivating patients and negotiating treatment goals are important elements of initial treatment (Kleber et al. 2007). Good outcomes of this initial treatment phase are for the patient and treatment professional to 1) share an understanding of substance use as an important factor that contributes to TRD and 2) accept the need for abstinence and treatment of both problems.

Treatment Sites and Levels of Care

Many treatment sites designed for treating mood disorders are not proficient in treating SUDs and vice versa. Treatment professionals also sort themselves into different types of practice at various sites, depending on their training and interests. Although sites with dual expertise that offer integrated treatment for both disorders are increasing, they are not readily available in all communities. As mentioned earlier, integrated care is preferred for patients with TRD and SUDs (Kleber et al. 2007). Two other models of care, sequential and parallel treatment, have the disadvantage of providing conflicting or contradictory messages to the patient because of differing treatment philosophies. Unfortunately, care that tries to treat one disorder selectively while ignoring the other is likely to increase rates of TRD at a systems level.

The major levels of care have been classified by the American Society of Addiction Medicine (2001). These include regular outpatient care, intensive outpatient care, partial hospitalization, short- and long-term residential treatment, and medically monitored intensive inpatient care. The criteria for determining an optimal level of care take the following into consideration: the likelihood of life-threatening intoxication or withdrawal, severity of comorbid medical and psychiatric disorders, environmental and social support for recovery, treatment acceptance or resistance, and potential for initiating abstinence and relapse. In clinical practice, level of care also depends on available and accessible resources for treatment.

Treatment Priorities and Timing of Interventions

The patient with TRD will by definition already have started treatment for depression. To the extent that an active SUD contributes to TRD, adding clinical focus to treat the SUD is logical. Timing of psychosocial interventions (initial focus on depression or substance use) may be less important than delivering both in an integrated fashion. In the interim, what medication treatment for depression should continue? There is no single answer. In general, maintaining the depression treatment while introducing substance-focused therapy allows the best assessment of the contribution of substances to TRD. Accordingly, the current regimen of antidepressants is continued. Other clinicians may prefer to discontinue antidepressant treatment at the start of treatment for SUDs for the following reasons: 1) substance-induced MDEs are likely to remit with 4 or more weeks of successful abstinence-based substance-focused therapy; 2) the current regimen of antidepressants is not working; 3) antidepressants may interact adversely with the substances being abused; and 4) their philosophy is to encourage patients to seek nonchemical solutions to their problems. All of these reasons should be considered. However, some depressions may worsen after discontinuation of medication, and current or past suicidality is always important to assess. In addition, some patients may believe that their depressive symptoms are being discounted if the psychiatrist discontinues antidepressant treatment. The best guidelines, therefore, are to individualize treatment and to do no harm. If evidence indicates that the current regimen has helped to some degree, and that the patient takes the medication responsibly without risk of adverse interactions, then maintaining that medication is prudent while augmenting it with substance-focused therapy.

Evidence-Based Addiction Pharmacotherapy

In patients with SUDs, medication may be used to treat states of intoxication and withdrawal or to prevent relapse (Kranzler and Ciraulo 2005). In this section, we focus on addiction pharmacotherapy for relapse prevention. At the start of 2010, approved and effective medications were available for treating alcohol, nicotine, and opioid dependence. No consistently effective medications are currently available for treating amphetamine, cannabis, cocaine, hallucinogen, inhalant, phencyclidine, or sedative-hypnotic dependence.

An important issue from the start is whether any of these medications are contraindicated in patients with comorbid major depression. The general answer is no, although there may be some exceptions. These are discussed by diagnosis in the following subsections.

Alcohol Dependence

Three medications are currently approved for alcohol dependence: disulfiram, naltrexone, and acamprosate (see Table 8–1). They can be distinguished on the basis of mechanism of action, mode of administration, half-life, metabolism, and side effects. Other medications such as topiramate and ondansetron are reviewed elsewhere (Johnson 2008).

Disulfiram.   Disulfiram works by inhibiting the enzyme aldehyde dehydrogenase, which mediates the second step of alcohol metabolism. After alcohol is metabolized to acetaldehyde, the second step metabolizes acetaldehyde to carbon dioxide and water. By inhibiting this step, disulfiram causes a toxic accumulation of acetaldehyde in the body, which causes several unpleasant physical symptoms, labeled the *disulfiram-ethanol reaction*. This reaction includes decreased blood pressure, flushing, dizziness, sweating, headache, and nausea and vomiting. To avoid these adverse symptoms, patients are cautioned not to drink. The usual dose is 250 mg orally once daily (range = 125–500 mg/day). Although the disulfiram-ethanol reaction is not generally life-threatening, it could be in patients with cardiac disease or those taking antihypertensive medication. Obviously, taking disulfiram with alcohol and other drugs impulsively as part of a suicide attempt also can be life-threatening and requires that patients be screened. In our experience, however, this is very uncommon unless the patient has comorbid Axis II disorders, probably because the physical symptoms are so unpleasant. Disulfiram has been associated with fulminant hepatitis, so monitoring of liver function tests is advised.

Disulfiram also inhibits the enzyme dopamine β-hydroxylase, leading to a relative increase in dopamine at the expense of norepinephrine. Two consequences have been attributed to this action. First are reports of disulfiram-induced psychosis, although these appear limited to doses exceeding 500 mg/day. Moreover, disulfiram has been reported to be relatively safe in patients with schizophrenia (Petrakis et al. 2005). Second are reports that disulfiram may decrease cocaine consumption among cocaine-dependent patients (Carroll et al. 2004). However, not all studies agree (Pettinati et al. 2008), and patients with comorbid alcohol and cocaine dependence may paradoxically fare worse than those with cocaine dependence alone (Carroll et al. 2004). Adherence is the greatest limitation to disulfiram use, and techniques to improve adherence improve effectiveness (Allen and Litten 1992).

Naltrexone.   Naltrexone works by blocking μ-opioid receptors, which are thought to mediate some of the reinforcing effects of alcohol. Another possible mechanism of action is its activation of an underreactive hypothalamic-pituitary-adrenal system. Naltrexone is available in both oral and extended-release intramuscular forms. The usual oral dose is 50 mg once daily (range = 25–100 mg/day). The dose for the extended-release intramuscular

TABLE 8–1. U.S. Food and Drug Administration (FDA)–approved medications for relapse prevention in 2010: alcohol dependence

Generic (brand) names	Typical dose (range)	Initiation issues	Monitoring issues	Proposed mechanism of action	Toxicity/adverse effects
Acamprosate (Campral)	666 mg orally three times a day (333–666 mg orally three times a day)	Best results if started when abstinent; excreted by kidneys; dose titration not needed	Contraindicated if creatinine clearance (CrCl) < 30 mL/min; reduced dose if CrCl = 30–50 mL/min	Glutamate modulator that reduces protracted withdrawal symptoms	Nausea, vomiting, bloating, diarrhea
Disulfiram (Antabuse)	250 mg/d orally (125–500 mg/d)	Must be abstinent (BAL = 0); metabolized by liver; obtain baseline LFTs; warn patient to avoid all alcohol; carry card for emergency department	Repeat LFTs in 1 wk if elevated, then every 1–6 mo; hold dose if LFTs are more than three times normal; supervised administration increases adherence	Inhibits breakdown of acetaldehyde, a toxic ethanol metabolite	Disulfiram-ethanol reaction of hypotension, dizziness, flushing, palpitations, headache, nausea
Naltrexone (oral) (ReVia)	50 mg/d (25–100 mg/d); start with 25-mg test dose	Drinking or abstinent; metabolized by liver; obtain baseline LFTs; must be opioid-free for 7–10 d; carry card for emergency department	Repeat LFTs in 1–2 wks if elevated, then every 6–12 mo once normalized; hold dose if LFTs are more than three times normal	Opioid antagonist that may block reinforcement by and craving for alcohol	Nausea, headache, nervousness, fatigue
Naltrexone (intramuscular) (Vivitrol)	380 mg monthly	Same as oral form	Same as oral form, except all injections are supervised in clinic	Same as oral form	Injection site pain or swelling, nausea, headache, nervousness, fatigue

Note. BAL = blood alcohol level; LFTs = liver function tests (alanine and aspartate aminotransferase and γ-glutamyltransferase).

form is 380 mg/month. Patients must be opioid-free as determined by self-report and a urine test, or naltrexone can precipitate a withdrawal response. Nausea is the major limiting side effect by either route of administration, and painful skin reactions can occur with injections. Because naltrexone is metabolized by the liver, it can be hepatotoxic in supratherapeutic doses (five to six times the usual range). When naltrexone works, patients will report decreased urges to drink alcohol and a muted reinforcing effect if they do drink. Good response to naltrexone is most likely among patients with a family history of alcoholism, early age at onset of drinking problems, high levels of naltrexone's active metabolite (β-naltrexol), and medication adherence. Response to extended-release naltrexone may be especially prominent in patients who abstained for at least 4 days prior to their first injection.

Acamprosate.   Acamprosate was approved for use in the United States in 2004 after about 20 years of availability in Europe. Acamprosate is a glutamate receptor modulator. The usual dose is 666 mg orally three times a day because of its short half-life. It can be started at full dose and does not require titration. The most common side effects are nausea and diarrhea. The dose may be decreased by 333–999 mg/day if side effects are poorly tolerated. Unlike disulfiram and naltrexone, acamprosate is not dependent on liver metabolism, so it may be preferred in patients with liver disease. It is contraindicated in patients with severe renal impairment (creatinine clearance≤30 mL/min), and dose reduction is usual practice when the creatinine clearance is 30–50 mL/min. Project COMBINE, a large multisite, randomized controlled trial in the United States, found that the combination of naltrexone and acamprosate was no more effective than naltrexone alone (Anton et al. 2006).

Nicotine Dependence

Three groups of medications are used for nicotine dependence, listed here in order of increasing efficacy: nicotine replacement therapy (NRT), bupropion, and varenicline (Eisenberg et al. 2008; Wu et al. 2006) (see Table 8–2).

Because of the well-known association between smoking and depressive symptoms, an important clinical finding is that smoking cessation among patients with depression does not necessarily worsen depression (Hall et al. 2006; Prochaska et al. 2008) and may even improve affect (Blalock et al. 2008). Alternatively, some patients may experience an increase in depressive symptoms with abstinence, which mediates in part their return to smoking (Catley et al. 2005). This variation in response is why a stepped-care approach may be most effective to treat nicotine dependence in patients with depression (Hall et al. 2006; Wilhelm et al. 2006).

NRT.   NRT includes several agents differentiated by their mode of administration: gum, patch, inhaler, nasal spray, and lozenges. Although depression has been associated with difficulty quitting, this was not the case in a recent trial with nicotine gum in which NRT was equally effective in both depressed and nondepressed smokers (Kinnunen et al. 2008).

Bupropion and other antidepressants.   Nicotine dependence is the only SUD for which antidepressants have a primary indication (Torrens et al. 2005). Bupropion appears equally effective in smoking cessation among patients with and without depressive symptoms (Brown et al. 2007; Catley et al. 2005; Torrens et al. 2005), and it has been associated with decreased depressive symptoms in highly dependent smokers. For smoking cessation, bupropion is administered orally for 1–2 weeks prior to a patient's targeted quit date in its sustained-released (SR) form starting at 150 mg/day for 3 days and then progressing to 150 mg orally twice a day for 7–12 weeks. Ongoing therapy may continue for as long as the patient benefits. Some evidence indicates that the tricyclic antidepressant nortriptyline is also effective for smoking cessation, and it may be considered a second-choice antidepressant for this indication. Dosing is generally in the 75–100 mg/day range, and nortriptyline may be therapeutic at plasma levels that are lower than those considered therapeutic for depression (Mooney et al. 2008). By contrast, selective serotonin reuptake inhibitors (SSRIs) may or may not decrease smoking among patients with major depression (Miyamoto et al. 2007; Spring et al. 2007). One potential strategy is to stabilize depressed patients with SSRIs and then add bupropion to aid smoking cessation. Although depression did not recur with this strategy, it was only modestly effective for smoking cessation in one study (Chengappa et al. 2001).

Varenicline.   Varenicline, a partial agonist at α_4-β_2 nicotinic acetylcholine receptors, was approved for use in 2006. Studies indicate that varenicline has greater efficacy than either NRT or bupropion for smoking cessation (Wu et al. 2006) and is equally effective in those with and without mental illness (Stapleton et al. 2008). Nevertheless, several published and unpublished case reports indicate the need for caution when varenicline is used in depressed patients (McIntyre 2008; Popkin 2008), and the U.S. Food and Drug Administration (FDA) label was changed in 2008 to include a warning about neuropsychiatric symptoms. Specifically, physicians and patients should monitor for any changes in symptoms of depressed mood, suicidal ideation or behavior, agitation, or changes in behavior that are unusual for the patient. If these symptoms occur, then stopping varenicline, at least temporarily, is advised. Of course, similar

TABLE 8–2. FDA-approved medications for relapse prevention in 2010: nicotine dependence

Generic (brand) names	Typical dose (range)	Initiation issues	Monitoring issues	Proposed mechanism of action	Toxicity/adverse effects
Bupropion SR (Zyban)	150 mg orally twice a day (start with 150 mg/d for first 3 days)	Start 1 week before quit date; contraindicated with seizure history or bulimia or anorexia nervosa; do not start during alcohol or sedative-hypnotic detoxification	Duration: 7–12 wks	Dopamine and norepinephrine reuptake inhibitor; nicotine receptor antagonist	Insomnia, dry mouth, nausea, dizziness, weight loss, increased risk of seizures
Nicotine replacement therapy		Choose preparation on the basis of patient preference, side effects, and prior effectiveness (if tried earlier)	Continue in select cases for as long as patient benefits and does not smoke; taper may help to discontinue	Nicotine receptor agonist	
Gum	2–4 mg every 1–2 h (with 2-mg dose for < 1 PPD smokers); maximum: 24 doses/24 h	Available over the counter	Duration: 2–3 mo		Hiccups, heartburn, nausea, stomach upset

TABLE 8–2. FDA-approved medications for relapse prevention in 2010: nicotine dependence *(continued)*

Generic (brand) names	Typical dose (range)	Initiation issues	Monitoring issues	Proposed mechanism of action	Toxicity/adverse effects
Lozenge	Same as gum but maximum is five lozenges per 6 h	Available over the counter	Duration: 12 wk		Hiccups, heartburn, nausea, stomach upset
Patch	14–21 mg/24 h with higher doses for > 10 cigarettes/d	Available over the counter	Duration: 8 wk		Skin reactions
Nasal spray	0.5 mg; start with 1–2 doses/nostril/h; maximum: 5 doses/h or 80 doses (40 mg)/d	By prescription only	Duration: 2–3 mo		Nasal irritation, runny nose, sneezing, cough
Inhaler	3–4 deep puffs/min for 20–30 min as needed = 1 cartridge; maximum: 16 cartridges/d	By prescription only	Duration: 2–3 mo		Cough; mouth and throat irritation
Varenicline (Chantix)	1 mg orally twice a day after eating, with full glass of water	Start 1 wk before quit date; days 1–3: 0.5 mg/d; days 4–7: 0.5 mg twice a day; days 8 and more: 1 mg twice a day	Duration: 12 wk with option to continue for another 12 wk	Partial agonist at α_4-β_2 nicotinic acetylcholine receptors that blocks craving for and effects of nicotine	Nausea, constipation, insomnia, abnormal dreams; some reports of increased depression and suicidal thoughts

Note. PPD = cigarette packs per day.

warnings regarding suicidal ideation and behavior have long been included for bupropion and all marketed antidepressant drugs in recipients younger than 25 years (U.S. Food and Drug Administration 2007). The most common side effects of varenicline are gastrointestinal symptoms (nausea in up to 30% of patients, vomiting, constipation, gas) and sleep disturbances, including insomnia and vivid dreams. Dosing for varenicline is designed to minimize side effects and starts at 0.5 mg/day orally for 3 days, then 0.5 mg orally twice a day for 4 days, and finally 1 mg orally twice a day for weeks 2 through 12. Varenicline may be continued for another 12 weeks according to its label, although in practice it is generally used for as long as the patient is benefiting.

Opioid Dependence

Opioid agonists, partial agonists, and antagonists are used to prevent relapse among opioid-dependent patients. They include naltrexone, methadone, and buprenorphine (see Table 8–3).

The use of medications with exactly opposite effects—that is, opioid receptor agonists and antagonists—to treat a single disorder is probably unique in medicine.

Naltrexone.   Naltrexone is the only currently approved opioid receptor antagonist for treating opioid dependence. Its use for the treatment of opioid dependence preceded its FDA approval to treat alcohol dependence by a decade. Unlike its proposed action for alcohol dependence, naltrexone does not act to reduce craving among opioid-dependent patients. By blocking opioid receptors, however, it blocks the psychoactive effects of any licit or illicit opioids that users might take. Theoretically, the paired association of opioids with no positive reinforcement over time should lead to extinction of opioid-taking behaviors. The desire for an opioid effect, however, makes adherence to naltrexone a treatment issue. This can be addressed in part by techniques similar to those recommended for disulfiram adherence (Allen and Litten 1992): by contingency management (Kleber et al. 2007) and by the extended-release intramuscular form, although the latter does not have formal FDA approval to treat opioid dependence as it does for alcohol dependence. Real-time monitoring of oral naltrexone ingestion also can be facilitated by thrice-weekly administration: 100 mg on Mondays, 100 mg on Wednesdays, and 150 mg on Fridays. This regimen is equivalent to 50 mg/day by mouth, a total of 350 mg/week, and is effective because of the long half-life and binding properties of naltrexone. Predictors of effectiveness include adherence monitoring, contingency management, and highly motivated opioid-dependent persons

TABLE 8–3. FDA-approved medications for relapse prevention in 2010: opioid dependence

Generic (brand) names	Typical dose (range)	Initiation issues	Monitoring issues	Proposed mechanism of action	Toxicity/adverse effects
Buprenorphine (Subutex)	8–16 mg/d sublingually (4–32 mg/d); M, W, F dosing also possible	Only during moderate opioid withdrawal or postwithdrawal; first dose: 2–4 mg; preferred form during pregnancy	Schedule III controlled substance; pill count at each visit; written monitoring agreement	Partial μ-opioid receptor agonist that decreases craving without inducing euphoria	Nausea, headache, anxiety, sedation, dizziness
Buprenorphine/ naloxone (Suboxone)	8/2–16/4 mg/d sublingually (4/1–32/8 mg); M, W, F dosing also possible	Only during moderate opioid withdrawal or postwithdrawal; first dose: 2/0.5–4/1 mg	Schedule III controlled substance; pill count at each visit; written monitoring agreement	Partial μ-opioid receptor agonist combined with full antagonist to block high if injected	Nausea, headache, anxiety, sedation, dizziness
Methadone (Dolophine)	80 mg/d orally (20–120 mg)	Prescription only by federally licensed methadone maintenance programs; check for CYP3A4-based drug interactions; perform baseline ECG	Schedule II controlled substance; daily witnessed administration until take-home privileges earned; perform ECG at 30 days and annually	Opioid agonist with slow onset and long duration that decreases craving without euphoria	Constipation, sexual dysfunction, sweating, ankle edema, drowsiness, respiratory depression
Naltrexone (ReVia, Trexan)	50 mg/d orally (or 100 mg orally on M, W; 150 mg orally on F) (25–50 mg/d)	Must be opioid-free for 7–10 days; metabolized by liver; obtain baseline LFTs; carry card for emergency department	Repeat LFTs in 1–2 wks if elevated, then every 6–12 mo once normalized; hold dose if LFTs are more than three times normal	Opioid antagonist that blocks the effects of abused opioids; does not block opioid craving	Nausea, headache, dizziness, nervousness, fatigue

Note. CYP = cytochrome P450; ECG = electrocardiogram; LFTs = liver function tests (alanine/aspartate aminotransferase; γ-glutamyltransferase). M, W, F = Monday, Wednesday, Friday.

such as health care practitioners. Side effects and precautions are the same as discussed earlier for treating alcohol dependence.

One important issue regarding the use of naltrexone is whether it may increase depressive symptoms by blocking the endogenous opioid system, which is involved in the experience of pleasure. The bulk of evidence suggests that naltrexone does not cause or worsen depression in either alcohol- or opioid-dependent patients (Dean et al. 2006; Petrakis et al. 2007). Nevertheless, some patients may be exceptions and warrant close monitoring (Schurks et al. 2005).

Methadone.   Methadone is a long-acting, orally active full agonist at opioid receptor sites. It is the only full agonist currently approved in the United States for treating opioid dependence. Another full agonist, L-α-acetylmethadol (LAAM), was removed from the market because of sudden deaths related to QT prolongation, despite superior outcomes for some patients. Since then, similar concerns about QT cardiotoxicity have surfaced with methadone. Informing patients of the cardiac risks is necessary, and guidelines recommend a screening electrocardiogram both before and 30 days after initiating treatment as well as annually thereafter (Krantz et al. 2008). Risk factors include preexisting heart disease and syncope, coadministration of drugs that either prolong the QT interval or inhibit the cytochrome P450 3A4 liver enzyme responsible for methadone metabolism, liver failure, hypokalemia, and high methadone doses. Critical to its efficacy is individualized dosing, although doses lower than 80 mg/day are considered subtherapeutic (Pollack and D'Aunno 2008). Methadone may be used for either detoxification or maintenance. Its efficacy for maintenance treatment is well established (Johansson et al. 2007). Although it is an effective detoxification agent as well, long-term outcomes are superior with maintenance treatment (Gruber et al. 2008). A more recently proposed benefit of methadone maintenance is improved regulation of mood compared with opioid-dependent patients who are opioid abstinent (Galynker et al. 2007; Schurks et al. 2005). Methadone is available to treat pain via parenteral administration, and the pill form is also used to treat pain, but the use of methadone for opioid dependence is limited to oral administration. Moreover, its use to treat opioid dependence is generally restricted to licensed outpatient methadone treatment programs, and it should not be used outside of specialized settings or specialty consultation for maintained patients in hospital settings. Common side effects include sedation, constipation, ankle edema, sweating, and change in libido.

Buprenorphine.   Buprenorphine was approved in 2002 for use in two sublingual forms for the treatment of opioid dependence. The two sublingual forms are buprenorphine alone and the combination of buprenorphine and naloxone in a 4:1 ratio. The sublingual buprenorphine/naloxone combination is available both as tablets and, since 2010, film. Buprenorphine is also available in intramuscular form for treating pain. Like methadone, buprenorphine may be used for either detoxification or maintenance. As a partial agonist, it is less likely than methadone to be abused and to cause respiratory depression, resulting in less overdose potential. Other advantages of buprenorphine compared with methadone include the option of daily or thrice-weekly administration and lessened withdrawal severity subsequent to its taper. Importantly, it may be prescribed in the office setting by qualified practitioners as opposed to only in licensed methadone treatment programs. Physicians in the United States qualify for a special waiver from the Drug Enforcement Administration to prescribe buprenorphine for opioid dependence in the office setting, contingent on completion of required buprenorphine training or addiction specialty certification. Training includes proper assessment of opioid withdrawal because buprenorphine should be administered only to newly abstinent physically dependent patients when they manifest a moderate degree of withdrawal symptoms, as determined by the Clinical Opiate Withdrawal Scale (Wesson and Ling 2003). Otherwise, buprenorphine can precipitate withdrawal because it binds to opioid receptors more strongly than the array of abused full agonists, thereby displacing full agonists from opioid receptors. Once patients have experienced buprenorphine-precipitated withdrawal in this manner, they will understandably be reluctant to receive further treatment with buprenorphine. Some controversy remains about the differential efficacy of methadone compared with buprenorphine maintenance treatment, which likely depends on dose and treatment retention (Mattick et al. 2008). Nevertheless, both are considered effective for some patients, although methadone is likely to be effective for most patients, especially those that require high-dose treatment. In this regard, it is noteworthy that the maximum daily dose of buprenorphine, 32 mg, is equivalent to only 60–70 mg of methadone, so patients requiring more than 60 mg/day of methadone may not do as well with buprenorphine. Given the advantages of buprenorphine, however, a stepped-care approach to treatment should be considered, in which patients are first given a trial of buprenorphine and subsequently transitioned to methadone if buprenorphine is not effective (Kakko et al. 2007).

Antidepressants for Substance Dependence, Co-Occurring Depression, or Both

The efficacy of antidepressants for treating substance dependence with and without co-occurring MDE has been reviewed (Nunes and Levin

2004; Torrens et al. 2005). In general, antidepressants have a modest benefit in decreasing depressive symptoms among patients with SUDs and co-occurring MDE, whereas the effects on SUDs are less impressive. Concomitant psychosocial therapy for SUDs improves outcomes and is thus routinely indicated (Nunes and Levin 2004). With the exception of nicotine dependence, as discussed earlier, antidepressant treatment of SUDs in the absence of MDE is not indicated (Torrens et al. 2005) until or unless subtype responders are established (Dundon et al. 2004). Indeed, some evidence suggests that high risk/severity (type B) alcoholic patients fare worse with SSRIs (Kranzler and Ciraulo 2005; Kranzler et al. 1996).

Evidence-Based Psychosocial Therapy for Addiction in Depressed Patients

For SUDs, the combination of psychosocial therapy and medication is increasingly common and preferred (Anton et al. 2006), whereas medication alone in the absence of addiction-focused psychotherapy is not recommended (Kleber et al. 2007). Some psychosocial therapies have been shown to be effective in treating SUDs (Kleber et al. 2007). They include motivational enhancement therapy, cognitive-behavioral therapy, 12-step facilitation, contingency management, and behavioral couples' therapy. Psychosocial therapy may be provided either individually or in a group setting. Group psychotherapy is commonly used to decrease feelings of shame, provide social support, and foster a sense of belonging with other patients similarly interested in recovery. Preliminary studies of cognitive-behavioral therapy and 12-step facilitation have reported beneficial effects on both depression and substance use outcomes, which were mediated by increases in self-efficacy (Brown et al. 2006; Glasner-Edwards et al. 2007). Overall, however, integrated psychosocial therapies for depression and SUDs are relatively new and not well studied (Carpenter et al. 2008; Carroll 2004).

Conclusion

Comorbidity rates for SUDs and depression are high in both general and clinical populations. TRD may result from unidentified and undiagnosed SUDs. Thus, SUDs are always part of the differential diagnosis for TRD.

All dependence-producing drugs, including alcohol, nicotine, prescription drugs, and illicit drugs, are capable of inducing both depression and co-occurring SUDs. The high comorbidity rates and potential of all these drugs to induce depression most likely result from both biological and psychosocial factors. Among the biological factors are 1) shared genetic vulnerability between the two disorders and 2) the pharmacological effects of drugs on brain systems that mediate hedonic and emotional regulation. Among the psychosocial factors are 1) guilt and shame, which lower self-esteem; 2) social isolation from significant losses, including marriages, friendships, and jobs, as a consequence of using substances; and 3) a substance-related chaotic lifestyle that interferes with adherence to depression treatments.

Depression that co-occurs with SUDs has been classified as either substance induced or substance independent. Substance-induced depression has its onset during the course of either intoxication with or withdrawal from a dependence-producing substance and usually remits within 4 weeks of abstinence. Substance-independent depression either precedes the onset of SUDs or persists during periods of prolonged abstinence. Both types of depression can result in serious consequences, including suicide. Moreover, a single patient can have episodes of both types of depression, occurring at different times during the course of the two disorders. It can be difficult to differentiate these two types of depression in the clinic. Therefore, both types of co-occurring depression require assessment, treatment, and monitoring. Finally, neither type should be considered less serious than the other.

Screening tools for SUDs should be routinely implemented in mental health settings, with awareness of their limitations and the defensive responses of patients. Sometimes an SUD is diagnosed in a depressed patient only after several visits during which a trusting therapeutic relationship is established. Biological models and self-medication models of SUDs can be used therapeutically to alleviate defensive guilt and shame by educating patients about etiologies that do not blame them for having SUDs. The dual-diagnosis model can help motivate the patient to accept treatment for both disorders when minimization of one disorder or the other is present.

Abstinence is the goal of treatment for SUDs in patients with TRD, both to assess the contribution of substances to depression and to eliminate a behavior that exacerbates, perpetuates, and is no longer effective at coping with depression. Targeting of both disorders is thought to be most effective within an integrated care model in which they are treated simultaneously by a single treatment team with dual expertise. Integrative treatment will include a combination of antidepressant medication, psychosocial therapy for both disorders, and substance-specific medication to prevent relapse. Safely initiating abstinence with medical detoxification may require inpatient or residential treatment, but detoxification is insufficient treatment of substance dependence. Acquiring the tools to maintain abstinence in an outpatient setting is both the challenge and the ultimate goal of treatment.

Key Clinical Concepts

- Comorbidity rates for substance use disorders (SUDs) and depression are high in both general and clinical populations. Thus, SUDs are always part of the differential diagnosis for Treatment Resistant Depression (TRD). Furthermore, comorbidity is high enough to justify screening all patients with major depression for SUDs, not just patients with TRD.

- Substance-induced major depressive episodes (MDEs) extend beyond those recognized officially in DSM-IV-TR (e.g., nicotine- and cannabis-induced MDEs can also occur). In clinical practice, therefore, all substances require an assessment for their effects on the development and course of TRD.

- The clinical utility of distinguishing between substance-induced and substance-independent co-occurring depressions remains to be established. In both types, each disorder adversely affects the course of the other, including an increased risk for suicide.

- The goal of substance-related treatment in patients with TRD should be complete abstinence from all psychoactive substances not recommended by the treatment team.

- Integrated care is preferred for patients with TRD and SUDs. Split care that tries to treat selectively one disorder or the other is likely to increase rates of TRD at a systems level.

- Although hospitalization or residential treatment may be necessary to initiate abstinence safely, maintaining abstinence in the outpatient setting is the ultimate treatment goal.

- Antidepressants should be continued even if a patient is abusing drugs, as long as adverse interactions do not occur.

- Addiction treatment consists of evidence-based psychosocial therapies. Combining psychosocial therapy and medication is preferred, whereas using medication alone in the absence of addiction-focused psychotherapy is not recommended.

- All of the U.S. Food and Drug Administration–approved medications for treating substance dependence may be safely used in patients with depression. Nevertheless, potential for overdose, especially with opioid agonists; deliberate or impulsive drinking while taking disulfiram; and worsening depression with naltrexone or varenicline should be considered and monitored.

References

Allen JP, Litten RZ: Techniques to enhance compliance with disulfiram. Alcohol Clin Exp Res 16:1035–1041, 1992

American Psychiatric Association: Diagnostic and Statistical Manual of Mental Disorders, 4th Edition, Text Revision. Washington, DC, American Psychiatric Association, 2000

American Society of Addiction Medicine: ASAM Patient Placement Criteria for the Treatment of Substance-Related Disorders. Chevy Chase, MD, American Society of Addiction Medicine, 2001

Anton RF, O'Malley SS, Ciraulo DA, et al: Combined pharmacotherapies and behavioral interventions for alcohol dependence: the COMBINE study: a randomized controlled trial. JAMA 295:2003–2017, 2006

Beullens J, Aertgeerts B: Screening for alcohol abuse and dependence in older people using DSM criteria: a review. Aging Ment Health 8:76–82, 2004

Blalock JA, Robinson JD, Wetter DW, et al: Nicotine withdrawal in smokers with current depressive disorders undergoing intensive smoking cessation treatment. Psychol Addict Behav 22:122–128, 2008

Breslau N, Schultz LR, Johnson EO, et al: Smoking and the risk of suicidal behavior: a prospective study of a community sample. Arch Gen Psychiatry 62:328–334, 2005

Brown RA, Niaura R, Lloyd-Richardson EE, et al: Bupropion and cognitive-behavioral treatment for depression in smoking cessation. Nicotine Tob Res 9:721–730, 2007

Brown SA, Glasner-Edwards SV, Tate SR, et al: Integrated cognitive behavioral therapy versus twelve-step facilitation therapy for substance-dependent adults with depressive disorders. J Psychoactive Drugs 38:449–460, 2006

Carpenter KM, Smith JL, Aharonovich E, et al: Developing therapies for depression in drug dependence: results of a stage 1 therapy study. Am J Drug Alcohol Abuse 34:642–652, 2008

Carroll KM: Behavioral therapies for co-occurring substance use and mood disorders. Biol Psychiatry 56:778–784, 2004

Carroll KM, Fenton LR, Ball SA, et al: Efficacy of disulfiram and cognitive behavior therapy in cocaine-dependent outpatients: a randomized placebo-controlled trial. Arch Gen Psychiatry 61:264–272, 2004

Catley D, Harris KJ, Okuyemi KS, et al: The influence of depressive symptoms on smoking cessation among African Americans in a randomized trial of bupropion. Nicotine Tob Res 7:859–870, 2005

Center for Substance Abuse Treatment: Substance Abuse Treatment for Persons With Co-Occurring Disorders. Treatment Improvement Protocol (TIP) Series 42 (DHHS Publ No SMA-05-3922). Rockville, MD, Substance Abuse and Mental Health Services Administration, 2005

Chengappa KN, Kambhampati RK, Perkins K, et al: Bupropion sustained release as a smoking cessation treatment in remitted depressed patients maintained on treatment with selective serotonin reuptake inhibitor antidepressants. J Clin Psychiatry 62:503–508, 2001

Connors G, Volk RJ: Self-report screening for alcohol problems among adults, in Assessing Alcohol Problems: A Guide for Clinicians and Researchers, 2nd Edition (NIH Publ No 03-3745). Edited by Allen JP, Wilson VB. Washington, DC, U.S. Department of Health and Human Services, Public Health Service, 2003, pp 21–35

Davis L, Uezato A, Newell JM, et al: Major depression and comorbid substance use disorders. Curr Opin Psychiatry 21:14–18, 2008

Dean AJ, Saunders JB, Jones RT, et al: Does naltrexone treatment lead to depression? Findings from a randomized controlled trial in subjects with opioid dependence. J Psychiatry Neurosci 31:38–45, 2006

Dundon W, Lynch KG, Pettinati HM, et al: Treatment outcomes in type A and B alcohol dependence 6 months after serotonergic pharmacotherapy. Alcohol Clin Exp Res 28:1065–1073, 2004

Eisenberg MJ, Filion KB, Yavin D, et al: Pharmacotherapies for smoking cessation: a meta-analysis of randomized controlled trials. CMAJ 179:135–144, 2008

Galynker II, Eisenberg D, Matochik JA, et al: Cerebral metabolism and mood in remitted opiate dependence. Drug Alcohol Depend 90:166–174, 2007

Glasner-Edwards S, Tate SR, McQuaid JR, et al: Mechanisms of action in integrated cognitive-behavioral treatment versus twelve-step facilitation for substance-dependent adults with comorbid major depression. J Stud Alcohol Drugs 68:663–672, 2007

Grant BF, Stinson FS, Dawson DA, et al: Prevalence and co-occurrence of substance use disorders and independent mood and anxiety disorders: results from the National Epidemiologic Survey on Alcohol and Related Conditions. Arch Gen Psychiatry 61:807–816, 2004

Gruber VA, Delucchi KL, Kielstein A, et al: A randomized trial of 6-month methadone maintenance with standard or minimal counseling versus 21-day methadone detoxification. Drug Alcohol Depend 94:199–206, 2008

Hall SM, Tsoh JY, Prochaska JJ, et al: Treatment for cigarette smoking among depressed mental health outpatients: a randomized clinical trial. Am J Public Health 96:1808–1814, 2006

Havard A, Teesson M, Darke S, et al: Depression among heroin users: 12-month outcomes from the Australian Treatment Outcome Study (ATOS). J Subst Abuse Treat 30:355–362, 2006

Johnson BA: Update on neuropharmacological treatments for alcoholism: scientific basis and clinical findings. Biochem Pharmacol 75:34–56, 2008

Johansson BA, Berglund M, Lindgren A: Efficacy of maintenance treatment with methadone for opioid dependence: a meta-analytical study. Nord J Psychiatry 61:288–295, 2007

Kakko J, Gronbladh L, Svanborg KD, et al: A stepped care strategy using buprenorphine and methadone versus conventional methadone maintenance in heroin dependence: a randomized controlled trial. Am J Psychiatry 164:797–803, 2007

Kalivas PW, O'Brien C: Drug addiction as a pathology of staged neuroplasticity. Neuropsychopharmacology 33:166–180, 2008

Kinnunen T, Korhonen T, Garvey AJ: Role of nicotine gum and pretreatment depressive symptoms in smoking cessation: twelve-month results of a randomized placebo controlled trial. Int J Psychiatry Med 38:373–389, 2008

Kleber HD, Weiss RD, Anton RF Jr, et al: Treatment of patients with substance use disorders, second edition: American Psychiatric Association. Am J Psychiatry 164 (suppl 4):5–123, 2007

Knight JR, Sherritt L, Harris SK, et al: Validity of brief alcohol screening tests among adolescents: a comparison of the AUDIT, POSIT, CAGE, and CRAFFT. Alcohol Clin Exp Res 27:67–73, 2003

Koob G, Kreek MJ: Stress, dysregulation of drug reward pathways, and the transition to drug dependence. Am J Psychiatry 164:1149–1159, 2007

Krantz MJ, Martin J, Stimmel B, et al: QTc interval screening in methadone treatment. Ann Intern Med 150:387–395, 2009

Kranzler HR, Ciraulo DA: Clinical Manual of Addiction Pharmacotherapy. Washington, DC, American Psychiatric Publishing, 2005

Kranzler HR, Burleson JA, Brown J, et al: Fluoxetine treatment seems to reduce the beneficial effects of cognitive-behavioral therapy in type B alcoholics. Alcohol Clin Exp Res 20:1534–1541, 1996

Mattick RP, Kimber J, Breen C, Davoli M. Buprenorphine maintenance versus placebo or methadone maintenance for opioid dependence. Cochrane Database of Systematic Reviews 2008, Issue 2. Art. No.: CD002207. DOI: 10.1002/14651858.CD002207.pub3

McIntyre RS: Varenicline and suicidality: a new era in medication safety surveillance. Expert Opin Drug Saf 7:511–514, 2008

Miyamoto K, Yoshimura R, Ueda N, et al: Effects of acute paroxetine treatment on the consumption of cigarette smoking and caffeine in depressed patients. Hum Psychopharmacol 22:483–490, 2007

Mooney ME, Reus VI, Gorecki J, et al: Therapeutic drug monitoring of nortriptyline in smoking cessation: a multistudy analysis. Clin Pharmacol Ther 83:436–442, 2008

Mueller TI, Lavori PW, Keller MB, et al: Prognostic effect of the variable course of alcoholism on the 10-year course of depression. Am J Psychiatry 151:701–706, 1994

Nunes EV, Levin FR: Treatment of depression in patients with alcohol or other drug dependence: a meta-analysis. JAMA 291:1887–1896, 2004

Pages KP, Russo JE, Roy-Byrne PP, et al: Determinants of suicidal ideation: the role of substance use disorders. J Clin Psychiatry 58:510–517, 1997

Petrakis I, Poling J, Levinson C, et al: Naltrexone and disulfiram in patients with alcohol dependence and comorbid psychiatric disorders. Biol Psychiatry 57:1128–1137, 2005

Petrakis I, Ralevski E, Nich C, et al: Naltrexone and disulfiram in patients with alcohol dependence and current depression. J Clin Psychopharmacol 27:160–165, 2007

Pettinati HM, Kampman KM, Lynch KG, et al: A double blind, placebo-controlled trial that combines disulfiram and naltrexone for treating co-occurring cocaine and alcohol dependence. Addict Behav 33:651–667, 2008

Pollack HA, D'Aunno T: Dosage patterns in methadone treatment: results from a national survey, 1988–2005. Health Serv Res 43:2143–2163, 2008

Popkin MK: Exacerbation of recurrent depression as a result of treatment with varenicline. Am J Psychiatry 165:774, 2008

Preuss UW, Schuckit MA, Smith TL, et al: A comparison of alcohol-induced and independent depression in alcoholics with histories of suicide attempts. J Stud Alcohol 63:498–502, 2002

Prochaska JJ, Hall SM, Tsoh JY, et al: Treating tobacco dependence in clinically depressed smokers: effect of smoking cessation on mental health functioning. Am J Public Health 98:446–448, 2008

Schuckit MA, Tipp JE, Bergman M, et al: Comparison of induced and independent major depressive disorders in 2,945 alcoholics. Am J Psychiatry 154:948–957, 1997

Schurks M, Overlack M, Bonnet U: Naltrexone treatment of combined alcohol and opioid dependence: deterioration of co-morbid major depression. Pharmacopsychiatry 38:100–102, 2005

Sher L, Milak MS, Parsey RV, et al: Positron emission tomography study of regional brain metabolic responses to a serotonergic challenge in major depressive disorder with and without comorbid lifetime alcohol dependence. Eur Neuropsychopharmacol 17:608–615, 2007

Sokero TP, Melartin TK, Rytsala HJ, et al: Suicidal ideation and attempts among psychiatric patients with major depressive disorder. J Clin Psychiatry 64:1094–1100, 2003

Spring B, Doran N, Pagoto S, et al: Fluoxetine, smoking, and history of major depression: a randomized controlled trial. J Consult Clin Psychol 75:85–94, 2007

Stapleton JA, Watson L, Spirling LI, et al: Varenicline in the routine treatment of tobacco dependence: a pre-post comparison with nicotine replacement therapy and an evaluation in those with mental illness. Addiction 103:146–154, 2008

Sullivan LE, Fiellin DA, O'Connor PG: The prevalence and impact of alcohol problems in major depression: a systematic review. Am J Med 118:330–341, 2005

Torrens M, Fonseca F, Mateu G, et al: Efficacy of antidepressants in substance use disorders with and without comorbid depression: a systematic review and meta-analysis. Drug Alcohol Depend 78:1–22, 2005

U.S. Food and Drug Administration: Questions and answers on antidepressant use in children, adolescents, and adults. May 2007. Available at: http://www.fda.gov/Drugs/DrugSafety/InformationbyDrugClass/ucm096321.htm. Accessed September 24, 2010.

Wesson DR, Ling W: The Clinical Opiate Withdrawal Scale (COWS). J Psychoactive Drugs 35:253–259, 2003

Wiesbeck GA, Kuhl HC, Yaldizli O, et al: Tobacco smoking and depression: results from the WHO/ISBRA study. Neuropsychobiology 57:26–31, 2008

Wilhelm K, Wedgwood L, Niven H, et al: Smoking cessation and depression: current knowledge and future directions. Drug Alcohol Rev 25:97–107, 2006

Wu P, Wilson K, Dimoulas P, et al: Effectiveness of smoking cessation therapies: a systematic review and meta-analysis. BMC Public Health 6:300, 2006

CHAPTER NINE

Sleep and Circadian Rhythms

An Understudied Area in Treatment Resistant Depression

Roseanne Armitage, Ph.D.
J. Todd Arnedt, Ph.D.

Sleep Disturbance as a Symptom of Depression and Bipolar Illness

Sleep disturbances are core features of depression; more than 80 % of patients with major depressive disorders (MDDs) report insomnia, hypersomnia, or insufficient sleep (Birmaher and Heydl 2001; Reynolds et al. 1987). Bipolar illness is accompanied by extreme insomnia in the manic phase and extreme hypersomnia in the depressed phase of the illness. It is also estimated that some 10 % of depressed adolescent patients experience simultaneous insomnia and hypersomnia (Liu et al. 2005).

Laboratory sleep studies confirm sleep abnormalities in unipolar and bipolar mood disorders (Armitage 2007; Benca et al. 1992; Perlis et al. 1997; Peterson and Benca 2006; Tsuno et al. 2005). Increased sleep latency (sleep-onset insomnia), nighttime or early awakening, increased light sleep, shifts in the occurrence of rapid eye movement (REM) sleep, and decreased deep sleep or impaired homeostatic drive for sleep all have been reported. These findings have been bolstered by a study of sleep microarchitecture that used quantitative electroencephalogram (EEG) analyses (e.g., power spectral analysis, period amplitude analysis), reporting increased fast-frequency beta and alpha activity, decreased delta activity (especially in males), and poor synchronization of sleep EEG rhythms between and within the right and left hemispheres (Armitage et al. 1999).

However, no single subjective or objective sleep EEG variable is likely to reliably distinguish patients from control subjects or individuals with depression or bipolar illness from those with other psychiatric disorders. Nevertheless, in mood disorders it is clear that the timing of the REM/ non-REM sleep cycle and the basic drive for sleep are no longer in alignment with 24-hour circadian organization of sleep and wakefulness (Armitage 2007).

Circadian Abnormalities in Depression and Bipolar Illness

The suggestion that mood disorders may be associated with circadian dysregulation was introduced more than 30 years ago and continues to be a popular theme in circadian and sleep deprivation research (Wirz-Justice 2007). Both an advance and a delay in circadian phase have been postulated to accompany depression and bipolar illness. Phase advances are associated with greater sleepiness early in the evening and early-morning awakenings, whereas phase delay is associated with sleepiness occurring well past midnight and an inability to awaken in the morning. However, more recent work has suggested that it is either a misalignment of sleep and circadian phase (Lewy et al. 2007) or an instability in circadian phase or amplitude (Armitage et al. 2004; Teicher et al. 1997) that is characteristic of mood disorders. Zeitgebers or circadian entrainers such as light, melatonin, and social cues interacting with genetic phase preferences or vulnerabilities; hypothalamic-pituitary-adrenal axis dysregulation; and the consequences of sleep loss all could contribute to the expression of circadian abnormalities in mood disorders (Harvey 2008).

Sleep and Circadian Rhythm Abnormalities as Risk Factors for Depression

Good evidence indicates that changes in sleep-wake cycles are prodromal symptoms of mood disorders, heralding the onset of a new episode of depression or mania in those with recurrent illness (Harvey et al. 2007; Liu et al. 2007). Furthermore, there is general agreement that persistent sleep disturbances increase the risk of relapse and recurrence of depression and are associated with greater suicidality (Barbe et al. 2005; Fawcett et al. 1990; Ford and Kamerow 1989; Wingard and Berkman 1983). Persistent sleep disturbances are extremely common in mood disorders and are often the number one residual symptom even after an adequate course of antidepressant treatment (Kennard et al. 2006; Liu et al. 2007). In addition, sleep EEG variables collected at baseline may identify those individuals at greatest risk for recurrence in 1–3 years of follow-up (Armitage et al. 2002; Emslie et al. 2001).

Most important, sleep and circadian rhythm abnormalities are also evident in the as-yet-unaffected relatives of depressed patients (Fulton et al. 2000; Morehouse et al. 2002). Furthermore, in Morehouse and colleagues' study (2002), those with a history of maternal depression and the most disrupted sleep were at greatest risk for developing depression within 3–5 years. This study provides strong evidence that sleep EEG abnormalities may reflect antecedent risk for mood disorders. More recently, we have shown that sleep and circadian rest-activity cycles are slower to entrain in infants who have depressed mothers (Armitage et al. 2009).

Taken together, these data clearly identify sleep and circadian dysregulation as a characteristic of mood disorders, a marker of increased risk of relapse and recurrence in those who are already ill, and a prospective predictor of those at greatest risk for developing a first episode. Given that depression and bipolar illness become more chronic with inadequate treatment or persistent symptoms (Mathew et al. 2008), we suggest that sleep and circadian dysregulation may contribute to increased risk of developing Treatment Resistant Depression (TRD), either via a mechanism similar to the contribution of serotonin type 1A ($5-HT_{1A}$) receptor and brain-derived neurotrophic factor genotypes (Anttila et al. 2007) or through more direct effects on adaptation and homeostasis (Shaffery et al. 2002).

Sleep in Patients With Treatment Resistant Depression

Evidence indicates that sleep and circadian dysregulation is more severe in TRD (Sharpley et al. 2005; Terman 2007), although substantially fewer sleep studies have been done in TRD patients than in other populations. When compared with patients without TRD, those with TRD show dampening of delta rhythm amplitude during sleep (Armitage et al.

2003). Because the organization of delta rhythms is believed to be the key to the restorative function of sleep, one would expect that interventions that target delta sleep abnormalities would be particularly beneficial in TRD. Vagus nerve stimulation, and perhaps other methods of brain stimulation, may enhance the amplitude of delta rhythms and improve the restorative function of sleep (Armitage et al. 2003). Early work also suggests that repetitive transcranial magnetic stimulation may normalize the timing of the REM/non-REM sleep cycle and, by inference, improve sleep regulation (Hajak et al. 1999). One ongoing study in our laboratory supports this view, indicating that bilateral electroconvulsive therapy may enhance delta rhythms.

Studies also have found an increased prevalence of sleep-disordered breathing in depressed individuals (Sharafkhaneh et al. 2005), and abnormal respiration distinguished individuals with MDD from control subjects with 80% accuracy in one study (Deldin et al. 2006). Thus, the failure to treat sleep-disordered breathing could either result in a more protracted episode of depression or increase the risk for relapse or recurrence. It is quite likely that untreated sleep-disordered breathing may further increase the risk for developing TRD.

Chronotherapeutics, interventions that target biological rhythm disturbances, are increasing in prevalence in the treatment of psychiatric disorders (Benedetti et al. 2007; Lewy et al. 2007). In particular, light and dark therapy, sleep deprivation, and melatonin are becoming a focus of intervention development and treatment augmentation in depression. Unfortunately, the role of sleep and circadian rhythm disturbances in developing treatment resistance per se has not been fully explored. Whether the improvement in sleep is part of the mechanism of action of antidepressant treatments has not yet been established. As clinical evidence suggests is the case in vagus nerve stimulation treatment, improving sleep and circadian rhythms may contribute to increased quality of life and sustained functioning over time rather than directly affecting depressed mood (Daban et al. 2008). Regardless of the precise mechanism of action, the evidence is clear that clinical course is improved when sleep problems are managed.

Options for Treating Sleep Disturbances in Depression

Available treatments for sleep disturbances in depression include hypnotics and nonpharmacological treatments. Benzodiazepine receptor agonists (e.g., zolpidem, eszopiclone) and one melatonin receptor agonist (ramelteon) are U.S. Food and Drug Administration–approved medications for insomnia. Antidepressant and atypical antipsychotic agents, despite not having an official indication for sleep disturbances, are frequently used in psychiatric settings for their hypnotic properties and relatively limited abuse potential. Patients also may use over-the-counter agents (e.g., melatonin, diphenhydramine) to self-treat sleep problems. Nonpharmacological sleep treatments, such as cognitive-behavioral therapy for insomnia, sleep deprivation, and light therapy, may be preferred by some patients, although these modalities are used less commonly and are less widely available. With few exceptions, the efficacy and safety of pharmacological and nonpharmacological sleep treatments remain to be established in patients with TRD.

Pharmacological Treatment Options

Benzodiazepine receptor agonists, including newer agents such as zolpidem, zolpidem modified-release formula, and eszopiclone, are widely considered first-line treatments for improving sleep quality in individuals without depression on the basis of the available scientific evidence and their relatively favorable side-effect profiles (Nowell et al. 1997; Smith et al. 2002). The newer agents are also unlikely to disrupt sleep architecture during the night and are generally easier to discontinue than more traditional benzodiazepines used for sleep (e.g., temazepam). Studies have evaluated mood improvement in depressed patients receiving both mood- and sleep-focused treatment (Asnis et al. 1999; Fava et al. 2006). In a randomized controlled trial, individuals with depression and insomnia who received a combination of fluoxetine with 3 mg/day eszopiclone showed greater sleep improvements and were more likely to achieve remission from depression than were those receiving fluoxetine and placebo (Fava et al. 2006).

Despite evidence favoring benzodiazepine receptor agonists as first-line treatments, trazodone is the most commonly prescribed hypnotic for depressed patients with sleep problems. Early controlled studies showed improved subjective sleep quality in patients receiving trazodone for antidepressant-associated insomnia (Nierenberg et al. 1994), but impairments in next-day functioning, such as sedation, are common, and efficacy over the longer term is unclear (Mendelson 2005). Open-label small-scale trials have shown improvements in Hamilton Rating Scale for Depression (Ham-D) scores in patients with TRD following augmentation therapy with nightly risperidone (0.5–1 mg/day; Sharpley et al. 2003), olanzapine (2.5–10 mg; Sharpley et al. 2005), or quetiapine (50–800 mg/day; mean = 340 mg/day; Baune et al. 2007) administered for 2–4 weeks.

Improvements in Ham-D scores and sleep continuity were correlated in one study (Sharpley et al. 2003) but not in another (Sharpley et al. 2005). These findings require replication in larger randomized trials in which safety end points are also evaluated, because atypical antipsychotics are well known to produce a variety of adverse effects, including extrapyramidal and cardiovascular abnormalities.

Four weeks of augmentation therapy with slow-release melatonin 5–10 mg/day failed to substantially improve Ham-D-rated mood in patients with TRD, although subjective improvements in sleep were reported (Dalton et al. 2000). In a 6-week randomized placebo-controlled trial, patients with MDD taking agomelatine 25–50 mg/day, a potent melatonin receptor agonist (MT_1 and MT_2) and $5\text{-}HT_{2C}$ antagonist, showed a higher response rate and faster time to first response compared with those given placebo, with no differences in side effects and greater improvement in Ham-D-rated sleep quality (Olie and Kasper 2007). Agomelatine may have antidepressant properties similar to those of more commonly used antidepressant agents (e.g., venlafaxine) but with earlier and greater benefits to subjective sleep quality (Lemoine et al. 2007). Its phase-shifting properties (Leproult et al. 2005), in addition to its beneficial effects on sleep disruption (Lopes et al. 2007), make it particularly well suited for further study in TRD patients.

Nonpharmacological Treatment Options

Cognitive-behavioral therapy for insomnia (CBT-I), delivered in individual or group format, can improve sleep and mood in individuals with MDD, but no studies have included TRD patients. CBT-I targets cognitive (e.g., worry, beliefs, apprehension about sleep) and behavioral (e.g., maladaptive sleep habits, irregular sleep scheduling) factors that are believed to perpetuate insomnia. For patients with chronic insomnia without psychiatric comorbidity, CBT-I produces moderate to large treatment effects across most sleep parameters, with treatment gains maintained over follow-up periods ranging from 3 weeks to 3 years (Morin et al. 1994; Murtagh and Greenwood 1995; Smith et al. 2002). A recent controlled trial found that two-thirds of patients with MDD and insomnia who received CBT-I plus escitalopram 10–20 mg/day achieved remission (Ham-D score ≤7), compared with one-third of patients who received escitalopram plus placebo (Manber et al. 2008). Alterations in format and content of CBT-I may be important to optimize outcomes in TRD patients.

Other sleep-focused treatments for mood disorders include sleep deprivation and light therapy. Sleep deprivation has long been known to benefit approximately 60% of mood disorder patients, but its clinical utility has been limited by a reversal of treatment effects with subsequent sleep (for review, see Wu and Bunney 1990). Mood benefits from light therapy, which can be marked especially when combined with selective serotonin reuptake inhibitor treatment, may be mediated through modification of circadian rhythms (Wirz-Justice 2006). One study found that 1 week of adjunctive total sleep deprivation and light therapy (30 minutes daily of 400-lux green light in the morning) produced acute, but not sustained, mood improvement in patients with drug-resistant bipolar depression (Benedetti et al. 2005). Nonpharmacological approaches to sleep disturbances have several potential advantages over pharmacological treatments, including greater patient acceptance and fewer adverse side effects, but they require further study in TRD patients.

Key Clinical Concepts

- ▪ Sleep and circadian rhythm disturbances are key features of depression and bipolar illness.

- ▪ Persistent sleep problems increase the risk of relapse and recurrence of depression and may increase the likelihood of developing treatment resistance.

- ▪ Patients with Treatment Resistant Depression (TRD) show more severe circadian dysregulation and delta sleep abnormalities. Interventions that enhance the amplitude of delta rhythms may be of particular benefit in TRD.

- ▪ Sleep agents such as benzodiazepine receptor agonists, melatonin agonists, and serotonin type 2C receptor antagonists have been shown to be effective in treating sleep problems in depression.

- ▪ Cognitive-behavioral therapy for insomnia is effective in treating sleep problems in depression, particularly when used in combination with antidepressant medications.

References

Anttila S, Huuhka K, Huuhka M, et al: Interaction between 5-HT1A and BDNF genotypes increases the risk of treatment-resistant depression. J Neural Transm 114:1065–1068, 2007

Armitage R: Sleep and circadian rhythms in mood disorders. Acta Psychiatr Scand Suppl (433):104–115, 2007

Armitage R, Hoffmann RF, Rush AJ: Biological rhythm disturbance in depression: temporal coherence of ultradian sleep EEG rhythms. Psychol Med 29:1435–1448, 1999

Armitage R, Hoffmann RF, Emslie GJ, et al: Sleep microarchitecture as a predictor of recurrence in children and adolescents with depression. Int J Neuropsychopharmacol 5:217–228, 2002

Armitage R, Husain M, Hoffmann R, et al: The effects of vagus nerve stimulation on sleep EEG in depression: a preliminary study. J Psychosom Res 54:475–482, 2003

Armitage R, Cole D, Suppes T, et al: Effects of clozapine on sleep in bipolar and schizoaffective disorders. Prog Neuropsychopharmacol Biol Psychiatry 28:1065–1070, 2004

Armitage R, Landis C, Hoffmann R, et al: Power spectral analysis of sleep EEG in twins discordant for chronic fatigue syndrome. J Psychosom Res 66:51–57, 2009

Asnis GM, Chakraburtty A, DuBoff EA, et al: Zolpidem for persistent insomnia in SSRI-treated depressed patients. J Clin Psychiatry 60:668–676, 1999

Barbe RP, Williamson DE, Bridge JA, et al: Clinical differences between suicidal and non suicidal depressed children and adolescents. J Clin Psychiatry 66:492–498, 2005

Baune BT, Caliskan S, Todder D: Effects of adjunctive antidepressant therapy with quetiapine on clinical outcome, quality of sleep and daytime motor activity in patients with treatment-resistant depression. Hum Psychopharmacol 22:1–9, 2007

Benca RM, Obermeyer WH, Thisted RA, et al: Sleep and psychiatric disorders: a meta-analysis. Arch Gen Psychiatry 49:651–668; discussion 669–670, 1992

Benedetti F, Barbini B, Fulgosi MC, et al: Combined total sleep deprivation and light therapy in the treatment of drug-resistant bipolar depression: acute response and long-term remission rates. J Clin Psychiatry 66:1535–1540, 2005

Benedetti F, Bernasconi A, Blasi V, et al: Neural and genetic correlates of antidepressant response to sleep deprivation: a functional magnetic resonance imaging study of moral valence decision in bipolar depression. Arch Gen Psychiatry 64:179–187, 2007

Birmaher B, Heydl P: Biological studies in depressed children and adolescents. Int J Neuropsychopharmacol 4:149–157, 2001

Daban C, Martinez-Aran A, Cruz N, et al: Safety and efficacy of vagus nerve stimulation in treatment-resistant depression: a systematic review. J Affect Disord 110:1–15, 2008

Dalton EJ, Rotondi D, Levitan RD, et al: Use of slow-release melatonin in treatment-resistant depression. J Psychiatry Neurosci 25:48–52, 2000

Deldin PJ, Phillips LK, Thomas RJ: A preliminary study of sleep-disordered breathing in major depressive disorder. Sleep Med 7:131–139, 2006

Emslie GJ, Armitage R, Weinberg WA, et al: Sleep polysomnography as a predictor of recurrence in children and adolescents with major depressive disorder. Int J Neuropsychopharmacol 4:159–168, 2001

Fava M, McCall WV, Krystal A, et al: Eszopiclone co-administered with fluoxetine in patients with insomnia coexisting with major depressive disorder. Biol Psychiatry 59:1052–1060, 2006

Fawcett J, Scheftner WA, Fogg L, et al: Time-related predictors of suicide in major affective disorder. Am J Psychiatry 147:1189–1194, 1990

Ford DE, Kamerow DB: Epidemiologic study of sleep disturbances and psychiatric disorders: an opportunity for prevention? JAMA 262:1479–1484, 1989

Fulton MK, Armitage R, Rush AJ: Sleep electroencephalographic coherence abnormalities in individuals at high risk for depression: a pilot study. Biol Psychiatry 47:618–625, 2000

Hajak G, Cohrs S, Tergau F, et al: Sleep and rTMS: investigating the link between transcranial magnetic stimulation, sleep, and depression. Electroencephalogr Clin Neurophysiol Suppl 51:315–321, 1999

Harvey AG: Sleep and circadian rhythms in bipolar disorder: seeking synchrony, harmony, and regulation. Am J Psychiatry 165:820–829, 2008

Harvey PD, Hassman H, Mao L, et al: Cognitive functioning and acute sedative effects of risperidone and quetiapine in patients with stable bipolar I disorder: a randomized, double-blind, crossover study. J Clin Psychiatry 68:1186–1194, 2007

Kennard B, Silva S, Vitiello B, et al: Remission and residual symptoms after short-term treatment in the treatment of adolescents with depression study (TADS). J Am Acad Child Adolesc Psychiatry 45:1404–1411, 2006

Lemoine P, Guilleminault C, Alvarez E: Improvement in subjective sleep in major depressive disorder with a novel antidepressant, agomelatine: randomized, double-blind comparison with venlafaxine. J Clin Psychiatry 68:1723–1732, 2007

Leproult R, Van Onderbergen A, L'Hermite-Baleriaux M, et al: Phase-shifts of 24-h rhythms of hormonal release and body temperature following early evening administration of the melatonin agonist agomelatine in healthy older men. Clin Endocrinol (Oxf) 63:298–304, 2005

Lewy AJ, Rough JN, Songer JB, et al: The phase shift hypothesis for the circadian component of winter depression. Dialogues Clin Neurosci 9:291–300, 2007

Liu X, Liu L, Owens JA, et al: Sleep patterns and sleep problems among school-children in the United States and China. Pediatrics 115:241–249, 2005

Liu X, Buysse DJ, Gentzler AL, et al: Insomnia and hypersomnia associated with depressive phenomenology and comorbidity in childhood depression. Sleep 30:83–90, 2007

Lopes MC, Quera-Salva MA, Guilleminault C: Non-REM sleep instability in patients with major depressive disorder: subjective improvement and improvement of non-REM sleep instability with treatment (Agomelatine). Sleep Med 9:33–41, 2007

Manber R, Edinger JD, Gress JL, et al: Cognitive behavioral therapy for insomnia enhances depression outcome in patients with comorbid major depressive disorder and insomnia. Sleep 31:489–495, 2008

Mathew SJ, Manji HK, Charney DS: Novel drugs and therapeutic targets for severe mood disorders. Neuropsychopharmacology 33:2080–2092, 2008

Mendelson WB: A review of the evidence for the efficacy and safety of trazodone in insomnia. J Clin Psychiatry 66:469–476, 2005

Morehouse RL, Kusumakar V, Kutcher SP, et al: Temporal coherence in ultradian sleep EEG rhythms in a never-depressed, high-risk cohort of female adolescents. Biol Psychiatry 51:446–456, 2002

Morin CM, Culbert JP, Schwartz SM: Nonpharmacological interventions for insomnia: a meta-analysis of treatment efficacy. Am J Psychiatry 151:1172–1180, 1994

Murtagh DR, Greenwood KM: Identifying effective psychological treatments for insomnia: a meta-analysis. J Consult Clin Psychol 63:79–89, 1995

Nierenberg AA, Adler LA, Peselow E, et al: Trazodone for antidepressant-associated insomnia. Am J Psychiatry 151:1069–1072, 1994

Nowell PD, Mazumdar S, Buysse DJ, et al: Benzodiazepines and zolpidem for chronic insomnia: a meta-analysis of treatment efficacy. JAMA 278:2170–2177, 1997

Olie JP, Kasper S: Efficacy of agomelatine, a MT1/MT2 receptor agonist with 5-HT2C antagonistic properties, in major depressive disorder. Int J Neuropsychopharmacol 10:661–673, 2007

Perlis ML, Giles DE, Buysse DJ, et al: Self-reported sleep disturbance as a prodromal symptom in recurrent depression. J Affect Disord 42:209–212, 1997

Peterson MJ, Benca RM: Sleep in mood disorders. Psychiatr Clin North Am 29:1009–1032; abstract ix, 2006

Reynolds CF III, Kupfer DJ, Hoch CC, et al: Sleep deprivation as a probe in the elderly. Arch Gen Psychiatry 44:982–990, 1987

Shaffery JP, Sinton CM, Bissette G, et al: Rapid eye movement sleep deprivation modifies expression of long-term potentiation in visual cortex of immature rats. Neuroscience 110:431–443, 2002

Sharafkhaneh A, Giray N, Richardson P, et al: Association of psychiatric disorders and sleep apnea in a large cohort. Sleep 28:1405–1411, 2005

Sharpley AL, Bhagwagar Z, Hafizi S, et al: Risperidone augmentation decreases rapid eye movement sleep and decreases wake in treatment-resistant depressed patients. J Clin Psychiatry 64:192–196, 2003

Sharpley AL, Attenburrow ME, Hafizi S, et al: Olanzapine increases slow wave sleep and sleep continuity in SSRI-resistant depressed patients. J Clin Psychiatry 66:450–454, 2005

Smith MT, Perlis ML, Park A, et al: Comparative meta-analysis of pharmacotherapy and behavior therapy for persistent insomnia. Am J Psychiatry 159:5–11, 2002

Teicher MH, Glod CA, Magnus E, et al: Circadian rest-activity disturbances in seasonal affective disorder. Arch Gen Psychiatry 54:124–130, 1997

Terman M: Evolving applications of light therapy. Sleep Med Rev 11:497–507, 2007

Tsuno N, Besset A, Ritchie K: Sleep and depression. J Clin Psychiatry 66:1254–1269, 2005

Wingard DL, Berkman LF: Mortality risk associated with sleeping patterns among adults. Sleep 6:102–107, 1983

Wirz-Justice A: Biological rhythm disturbances in mood disorders. Int Clin Psychopharmacol 21 (suppl 1):S11–S15, 2006

Wirz-Justice A: Chronobiology and psychiatry. Sleep Med Rev 11:423–427, 2007

Wu JC, Bunney WE: The biological basis of an antidepressant response to sleep deprivation and relapse: review and hypothesis. Am J Psychiatry 147:14–21, 1990

CHAPTER TEN

Psychotherapy Strategies for Treatment Resistant Depression

Heather A. Flynn, Ph.D.
Joseph Himle, Ph.D.

CURRENT CONCEPTUALIZATIONS and operational definitions of treatment-refractory depression or Treatment Resistant Depression (TRD) are based exclusively on lack of expected response to pharmacotherapy (European Medicines Agency Committee for Medicinal Products for Human Use [CHMP] 2010; Fava 2003; Souery et al. 1999; Thase et al. 1997). Four of the most accepted definitions of TRD, including the Thase and Rush staging method, the Committee for Medicinal Products for Human Use definition, the Massachusetts General Hospital Staging Method, and the Souery and colleagues criteria, describe *depression treatment resistance* as some degree of inadequate response to antidepressant medications. This conceptualization omits a vast and growing research literature that supports the efficacy of psychotherapeutic treatments for chronic, recurrent depression. The exclusive focus on medication treatment is problematic to the extent that it perpetuates the omission of psychotherapeutic treatments either as a viable option for depressed patients or in the training of clinicians, or both. Definitions that stage treatment "failure" based entirely on medication trials run the risk of implying a treatment strategy or algorithm that excludes psychotherapy and other nonpharmacological treatment options. More recent depression treatment algorithms tested in randomized clinical trials such as the Sequenced Treatment Alternatives to Relieve Depression (STAR*D) and the Texas Medication Algorithm Project (Adli et al. 2003; Thase et al. 2007) have shown some support for inclusion of psychotherapy as an effective switching or augmentation strategy.

In this chapter, we briefly review evidence supporting the role of psychotherapy in the conceptualization and treatment of TRD. Depression-specific psychotherapies, including cognitive-behavioral therapy (CBT), interpersonal psychotherapy (IPT), and Cognitive Behavioral Analysis System of Psychotherapy (CBASP—specifically developed and tested for the treatment of chronic depression), all have been studied in samples of patients with recurrent depression of at least moderate severity. These treatments have been studied both as monotherapies and in combination with pharmacotherapy. We also present evidence that psychotherapy may effectively target and treat specific residual symptoms that leave patients prone to relapse. Evidence for the overall prophylactic effect of psychotherapy for chronic depression also is reviewed. The chapter culminates in a "call to action" to revise the current conceptualizations of TRD to include psychotherapeutic treatment response and outlines an accompanying clinical research agenda.

We begin with a clinical vignette of a patient typical of those presenting for psychiatry specialty care who would be considered treatment resistant on the basis of existing definitions.

Clinical Vignette

Mr. H, a 48-year-old married man, was referred to a depression specialty outpatient clinic by his community psychiatrist for nonresponse to several trials of antidepressant medication. Mr. H had a history of panic attacks and anxiety symptoms dating back to school age. His first discernible major depressive episode (MDE) occurred in high school around the time of his parents' separation and eventual divorce. His depression was not treated at that time and did not fully remit. He reported residual symptoms of anhedonia, sleep disturbance, and anxiety, including recurrence of intermittent panic attacks. In college, he experienced his second full episode of major depressive disorder (MDD). At that time, a physician at the student health center prescribed fluoxetine, which was titrated up to 60 mg/day. He reported taking fluoxetine at the prescribed dose for 6–8 months and discontinuing it after some symptom relief. Into adulthood, he reported never feeling "quite right," with clear periods of worsening around life transitions such as being fired from a job and difficulties in his marriage.

Mr. H was seen in and out of specialty care and received several antidepressants and combinations on and off over the years. He had trials of fluoxetine (40 mg/day, 6 months), paroxetine (20 mg/day, 4 months), bupropion (150 mg/day, 4 months), and sertraline (up to 300 mg/day, 1 year). His history showed evidence that his adherence was at times sporadic.

Mr. H's current presenting symptoms include irritable and depressed mood most days per week; little interest or pleasure from his work or interacting with his children; delayed sleep latency most nights, requiring an average of 1–2 hours to fall asleep; and not feeling rested. Mr. H reported feelings of just "going through the motions" each day, feeling passively suicidal without intent or plan. Specifically, he indicated that he "would rather not be here" but would never harm himself because of his children. He expressed frustration with treatment, indicating that he had tried everything but never felt much better. He felt like he was "defective" and a failure as a husband, father, and employee. He had been told by his clinician that he was not adequately responding to treatment. He reported feeling demoralized and did not expect to get better but was willing to remain in treatment and "give it another try." Mr. H had not previously been offered depression-specific psychotherapy.

Role of Psychotherapy in Treatment Resistant Depression

Brief Review of Psychotherapy for Depression Treatment

Depression-specific psychotherapies alone are significantly more effective than placebo or waiting-list or minimal-contact control treatment and typically produce response rates in randomized controlled trials (RCTs) similar to those for pharmacotherapy for the acute-phase treatment of moderate to severe unipolar depression (Thase et al. 2001; U.S. Department of Health and Human Services 1993). For example, DeRubeis et al. (1999) conducted a mega-analysis of four RCTs comparing acute-phase outcomes of medication and CBT in severely depressed outpatients. Severe depression was defined as scores greater than 20 on the Hamilton Rating Scale for Depression (Ham-D; Hamilton 1960) or scores greater than 30 on the Beck Depression Inventory (BDI; Beck et al. 1961). Results of the analyses indicated equal reduction in depression for CBT and medications, with a slight edge found for CBT based on pooled data. A more recent trial (DeRubeis et al. 2005) randomly assigned 240 moderately to severely depressed outpatients to 16 weeks of cognitive therapy, 16 weeks of medications, or 8 weeks of pill placebo. Similar remission rates were found at 16 weeks for the two active treatments (46% for medications and 40% for cognitive therapy; both superior to placebo). In that study, effectiveness of cognitive therapy depended on level of therapist experience.

IPT similarly has been shown to produce depression outcomes (remission and response rates) comparable to those for antidepressant medications in several RCTs (de Mello et al. 2005) of samples composed of patients with recurrent depression of at least moderate severity (Frank et al. 1990). RCTs comparing CBASP with antidepressant medication treatment in the acute phase of chronic depression also found statistically indistinguishable depression outcomes for the two treatments, with combination medication-psychotherapy producing significantly greater response rates (Keller et al. 2000). In summary, the current evidence demonstrates comparable efficacy for depression-specific psychotherapy and antidepressant pharmacotherapy in the treatment of recurrent depression.

Symptoms and Features of TRD Targeted by Psychotherapy

Stress has been closely linked with depression throughout the clinical, psychological, and biological research literature. Both physical and psychological stressors are temporally (and perhaps causally) related to the onset of depressive episodes (Post 1992). Some studies have suggested that, at least for recurrent depression, stressful life events are more common in "nonendogenous depression" (Frank et al. 1994). Regardless of causality, stress very likely interacts with genetic predisposition, such that in some vulnerable individuals, a stressor can precipitate a mood disorder. For example, studies by Kendler et al. (1993) and by Caspi et al. (2003) have identified a clear interaction between genetic substrate and stressful life events in the precipitation of a depressive episode. The presence of specific psychosocial factors that can be construed as chronic "stressors," including poor social support, long-standing marital discord, and social isolation, also have been associated with antidepressant nonresponse (Thase and Howland 1994; Thase et al. 2001). Neuroticism (a pattern of heightened emotional and physiological reactivity) and excessive pessimistic and negative thinking also have been implicated in treatment nonresponse (Thase et al. 2001). In fact, it has been argued that the additive or interactive effect of external and perceived stressors will reinforce negative thinking and will enhance hopelessness, helplessness, and anhedonia in treatment-refractory depression (Thase et al. 2001). Given the central role of stress in depression, it is important to understand the mechanisms whereby stress can trigger and maintain a depressive episode and to establish whether direct intervention on stress will improve outcomes. Basic and clinical data point to the hypothalamic-pituitary-adrenal (HPA) axis as one of the possible neurobiological mediators of stress effects on mood.

On the basis of existing research literature and current understanding of the mechanisms underlying TRD, a strong case can be made for the utility of trials of evidence-based psychotherapies for this population (Stimpson et al. 2002; Thase et al. 2001). That is, it can be argued that complete treatment of refractory depression must intervene at both the biomedical and the psychosocial level (Pizzagalli et al. 2004).

Time-limited, depression-specific psychotherapies such as CBT and IPT have been found to produce remission rates similar to those of pharmacotherapy for the treatment of MDD in dozens of clinical trials (Hollon et al. 2002). Reviews have suggested an urgent need for trials of TRD to investigate the effectiveness of psychotherapy in conjunction with medication (Kupfer and Frank 2001; Thase 2003). The rationale for this recommendation is based primarily on the prominence of ongoing psychosocial difficulties in the lives of patients with TRD. In addition, compelling evidence indicates that patients with chronic depression with a history of childhood trauma respond significantly better to psychotherapy than to medication treatment (Heim et al. 2008).

IPT, for example, directly targets psychosocial factors that have been specifically implicated in nonresponse or partial response to antidepressant treatment, such as poor social support, ongoing psychosocial stress, marital or interpersonal conflict, and poor treatment alliance (Thase et al. 2001). IPT is a relatively short-term psychotherapy (12–16 sessions) that aims to improve interpersonal functioning in psychosocial domains relevant to the onset and perpetuation of depression. IPT has been found to lead to significant symptom reduction in several clinical trials for MDD, comparable to results with antidepressant medications (Elkin et al. 1989; Frank et al. 1990). IPT was developed as a pragmatic treatment designed to address depression directly as part of the medical model while recognizing the complex biological and psychosocial etiology of the illness. There is evidence that the primary mechanism of action of IPT is the alteration of social circumstances and relationships, but this mechanism is not fully understood (Thase et al. 2001; Weissman et al. 2000). IPT directly and primarily intervenes with social behavior to improve communication and social support. By means of these changes, the individual directly attenuates environmental stress. In fact, successful response to IPT in patients with MDD has been found to decrease the potency of stressful life events in provoking depression recurrence (Harkness et al. 2002). Specific to TRD, the process of failure to respond to treatment may worsen social stress by taxing social supports and fostering pessimism. Therefore, the explicit focus in IPT on instilling optimism (even in the face of previous treatment failure) (Markowitz 2003) and on successful negotiation of social support may be particularly effective for TRD.

Psychotherapy also can specifically and effectively target other symptoms of depression and may affect treatment response and relapse. Residual sleep abnormalities, for example, have been associated with risk for relapse following antidepressant medication treatment (Armitage et al. 2002; Emslie et al. 2001). CBT for insomnia has been found to improve sleep and depression outcomes when combined with medication in acute-phase treatment (Manber et al. 2008a). Some research supports clinical trials indicating that behavioral activation, a specific component of CBT that emphasizes engagement in reinforcing "antidepressant" behaviors, may be particularly useful in treating difficult-to-treat depression associated with greater functional impairment, especially in the social domain (Coffman et al. 2007).

Evidence supports the effectiveness of combination treatment for severe, chronic depression in improving treatment response and preventing relapse. What further treatments are needed when treatment with established efficacy is delivered but response is inadequate? Little empirical evidence and practice consensus exist on strategies to combine, sequence, and select psychotherapy in conjunction with medication treatment. Understanding the current state of the evidence on combining and sequencing treatments will aid in establishing a research agenda and in guiding treatment selection strategies. Combination medication-psychotherapy may be effective because of synergistic effects in that each treatment enhances the other to achieve better effectiveness than with monotherapy. Alternatively, the advantage of combination treatment may be that it increases the likelihood that any given patient will receive some type of treatment to which his or her depression will respond. Although no studies to date have directly tested these models, the research on combination psychotherapy to date has shown strong support for treatment of recurrent depression.

Although earlier meta-analyses (Conte et al. 1986; Gaffan et al. 1995; Robinson et al. 1990) found no difference between combination therapy and either treatment alone, more recent studies have provided support. For example, Pampallona et al. (2004) conducted a systematic review of studies from 1980 to 2002 to determine the relation between adherence to use and efficacy of antidepressant medications plus psychological treatments, as compared with medication treatment alone, in depressive disorders. That analysis found that psychotherapy combined with medication treatment was associated with a higher response rate than was medication alone. The addition of psychotherapy was found to improve overall treatment adherence. For shorter treatment (12 weeks), combined treatment may be more effective for depression that would not have responded to medications alone; for longer treatments, combination therapy may induce stronger compliance with both treatments.

Hegerl et al. (2004) performed a qualitative review of RCTs conducted in the 1990s to evaluate the efficacy of the combination of psychotherapy and pharmacotherapy compared with either alone. For severe or persisting MDD, MDD plus dysthymia, or partially remitted MDD with poor interepisode recovery, patients were found to benefit more from combination treatment than from psychotherapy alone. For milder and more uncomplicated MDD, combination treatment was not found to be superior to medications or psychotherapy alone. Jindal and Thase (2003) conducted a review of methodological issues involved in studies of combining psychotherapy and medications and reexamined the evidence in light of those issues. Their review concluded that greater symptom severity should be used to select patients for whom combined treatment may be most cost-effective. They also concluded that combination treatment may be especially useful for patients during and after an acute hospitalization and to prevent recurrences. A reanalysis of data from a combination treatment trial of patients with chronic depression found that the combination of medications and CBASP achieved significantly faster remission than did either treatment alone (Manber et al. 2008b). Although that analysis found the best remission rates among patients with lower Ham-D scores (<26) and among those with higher Ham-D scores (≥26) but lower anxiety, more research is needed on patient predictors of response to combination treatment.

Evidence for Switching to or Augmenting Pharmacotherapy With Psychotherapy

Schatzberg and colleagues (2005) found a strong benefit of switching patients whose chronic depression did not respond to 12 weeks of treatment with either medication (nefazodone) or psychotherapy to crossover treatment. Original treatment was discontinued at the point of crossover. Response rates were higher for patients who were switched to psychotherapy from medications (57%) than for patients who were switched to medications from psychotherapy (42%). In that study, attrition also was found to be lower when psychotherapy was added after a failed trial of medications. Thus, medication failure may result in better participation in psychotherapy, but not vice versa. Frank and colleagues (2000) evaluated a sequential treatment strategy in women with recurrent MDD and found a significantly higher (79%) remission rate in patients who received IPT alone as an initial treatment strategy, then *subsequently* received medication because of inadequate response, compared with those who received IPT in combination with pharmacotherapy *simultaneously* at the outset of treatment (66% remission rate). A more recent trial showed faster time to remission among patients with chronic depression who received combination psychotherapy with medication as compared with either treatment alone (Manber et al. 2008b).

Psychotherapy to Prevent Recurrence

The addition of psychotherapy to pharmacotherapy has been found to reduce recurrence rates for patients with chronic, recurrent depression and nonresponse or partial response to medication treatment (Fava et al. 1997; Thase et al. 1997). Whereas medication treatment has no known enduring effect on relapse after discontinuation, cognitive therapy given either alone or in combination with medication during acute-phase treatment of moderate to severe MDD in outpatients may prevent relapse or recurrence. Some studies show superiority of cognitive therapy for relapse prevention compared with clinical management or active maintenance pharmacotherapy (Dobson et al. 2008; Hollon et al. 2005). Several studies have shown prophylactic effects of psychotherapy for patients with recurrent depression of at least moderate severity. In an earlier study by Kovacs and colleagues (1981), depressed patients receiving prior (acute phase over 12 weeks) cognitive therapy showed lower BDI scores than did patients receiving imipramine after 1 year. The medication group's relapse rate was close to twice the rate of the cognitive therapy group. Other early studies similarly have shown that treatment groups with a cognitive therapy arm (with or without medication) sustained remission at 1, 6, and 12 months after treatment (Blackburn et al. 1986).

Studies that have included longer follow-up periods also have shown support for acute-phase depression-specific psychotherapy as preventive for relapse over several years. In one study, 40 patients with MDD successfully treated with medications were randomly assigned either to CBT for residual symptoms or to clinical management. Medications were gradually tapered or discontinued (Fava and Davidson 1996). A 4-year follow-up assessment showed lower relapse rates in the CBT group (35%) compared with the clinical management group (70%). A 6-year continuation (Fava et al. 1998) found that the CBT group had significantly fewer relapses than did the clinical management group. Studies with larger sample sizes have replicated the prophylactic effect of continuation therapy with CBT, as compared with medications alone, on depression outcomes (Paykel et al. 1999). More recently, Hollon and colleagues (2005) compared moderate to severe MDD that responded to cognitive therapy or medications after 12 months of continuation-phase treatment with either the same medication and dosage that produced initial response or three booster cognitive therapy sessions over 12 months. Patients withdrawn from cognitive therapy were less likely to relapse than were patients withdrawn from medications (31% vs. 76%) and were no more likely to relapse than were patients who continued taking medications (31% vs. 47%). Prior cognitive therapy with limited booster sessions, therefore, was found to be as protective against relapse as were maintenance medications. This finding has been replicated in several trials (DeRubeis et al. 2008).

Hollon and colleagues (2005) have reviewed evidence of the neural mechanisms involved in depression recovery through psychotherapy and medication treatment. That review concluded that decreased prefrontal function associated with depressed patients' difficulties in emotion regulation may benefit more from cognitive therapy than from medication treatments.

Taken together, this research supports the role of psychotherapy in combination with medication treatment as an effective treatment strategy for moderate to severe recurrent depression. Importantly, the evidence-based psychotherapies lengthen interepisode recovery, prevent recurrences, and dampen severity of subsequent episodes. Less time experiencing depression across the life span may prevent treatment resistance through modification of stressors or through alleviation of neurological risk.

Practical Issues in Psychotherapy Delivery

Because earlier detection of depression must occur in nonspecialty settings (such as primary care, school-based settings, emergency department, obstetrics/gynecology), we must improve access to and availability of quality psychotherapy in these contexts. Although evidence-based psychotherapies such as cognitive therapy, behavioral activation, CBT, CBASP, and IPT are all potentially useful in addressing TRD (Cuijpers et al. 2009; Dunner et al. 2006), most persons with depression do not receive these services (Wang et al. 2000). Data from the National Comorbidity Survey indicate that only 20.1% of persons with severe depression sought help for their condition in a specialty mental health setting, the only place where evidence-based psychosocial interventions for depression are likely to be available (Roy-Byrne et al. 2000). Even in the rare circumstances in which evidence-based psychotherapies are offered to depressed patients, many therapists offering these services probably are not sufficiently trained to deliver these interventions with adequate fidelity to the model (Stuart et al. 2004).

Many practicing clinicians simply have not had adequate training in evidence-based psychotherapies. In a review of psychology training programs, Barlow and colleagues (1999) concluded that clinical psychology training programs are not attentive enough to teaching data-based treatments (Barlow et al. 1999). Crits-Christoph et al. (1995) conducted a survey of directors of American Psychological Association–approved clinical psychology training programs and internships and found that more than 20% of doctoral programs failed to provide minimal coverage of empirically supported treatments in didactic courses, and the vast majority of internship programs did not require that students be competent in any empirically supported treatments before completing their programs. In a survey of 428 American Psychological Association–approved internship program directors, only half of adult-only programs provided any meaningful training in empirically validated CBT or IPT for depression (Crits-Christoph et al. 1995). Clearly, a significant need exists to improve training in evidence-based psychotherapies for emerging mental health practitioners (Barlow et al. 1999), and recent evidence suggests many programs are making positive steps toward this goal (Steinfeld et al. 2009).

Another potential remedy for the limited availability of evidence-based psychotherapy resources is to encourage existing practitioners to seek training in empirically supported psychotherapy for depression. Barlow et al. (1999) recommended that practitioners aiming to acquire competency in a particular empirically supported psychosocial treatment begin by studying an available treatment manual, attending a lengthy didactic presentation, and treating one (or more) pilot cases with direct supervision. They indicated that this training standard clearly exceeds the type of training included in typical continuing education programs. A typical half-day workshop is not known to significantly change the behavior of practitioners in attendance (Davis et al. 1992). Obtaining the training recommended by Barlow et al. would likely involve significant time and expense. Another significant barrier to improving access to state-of-the-art psychotherapies concerns practitioner opinions about manualized treatments. Addis and Krasnow (2000) reported that many practitioners hold negative opinions about the value of manualized treatments. Some practitioners believe that manuals have a dehumanizing effect on the therapeutic process. Despite these significant barriers, several innovative training and certification programs have emerged that provide both didactic instruction and critically needed ongoing supervision for practitioners seeking skills in evidence-based psychotherapy (Beck Institute for Cognitive Therapy and Research 2009; Behavioral Tech 2010; International Society for Interpersonal Therapy 2011).

Because training existing practitioners and producing trainees with solid skills in evidence-based interventions for depression will take considerable time to have a meaningful effect on the availability of these treatments, creative strategies are needed to bridge the treatment access gap. Strategies generally placed under the heading of "telemedicine" hold considerable promise as methods to address unmet needs for evidence-based psychotherapy. Anecdotal and group trials reports over the past decade specifically support the use of videoconferencing (Frueh et al. 2000), telephone (Baquet 1997), and computer-driven (Christensen et al. 2002) therapy as methods to efficiently deliver evidence-based psychotherapy for depression. Unfortunately, most of this research has been limited to persons experiencing mild to moderate depression (Mohr et al. 2008). The efficacy of telemedicine strategies for treatment-resistant and severe depression is largely unknown (Mohr et al. 2008). Another important issue related to the expansion of telemedicine-delivered psychotherapy is limited insurance reimbursement, but some progress has been made in addressing this problem. Studies have, however, reported cost savings attributable to telemedicine (Ruskin et al. 2004).

Another strategy for improving access to evidence-based psychotherapies for depression involves providing these services in nontraditional settings. Primary care settings have received considerable attention from depression researchers as sites to improve access to evidence-based treatment for depression (Uebelacker et al. 2009). Cognitive (Scott et al. 1997), behavioral (Uebelacker et al. 2009), and interpersonal (Raue et al. 2009) therapies all have been shown to be delivered effectively in primary care offices. Primary care sites offer several advantages in terms of therapy delivery, including reduced stigma, convenience, coordination of care (Uebelacker et al. 2009), and consideration of co-occurring medical conditions. These settings are particularly promising for persons residing in rural or underserved urban areas because access to specialty mental health settings is very limited (Gamm et al. 2003). However, research involving the provision of evidence-based psychotherapies for depression in primary care settings indicates several important shortcomings. First, most of these studies include only participants with mild to moderate depression (Bortolotti et al. 2008), and data regarding the effect of primary care–delivered psychotherapy on recurrent TRD are highly limited (Bortolotti et al. 2008). One of the most challenging aspects of primary care–delivered psychotherapy involves the considerable challenge of maintaining treatment programs after research protocols are completed (Blasinsky et al. 2006). Funding and reimbursement issues have proved to be a challenge in the ongoing delivery of evidence-based psychotherapies in primary care settings (Blasinsky et al. 2006). These considerations notwithstanding, providing evidence-based psychotherapies in primary care settings holds great promise as a method to attract patients to treatment before severity and recurrence result in treatment resistance.

Other nontraditional settings hold promise as potential venues to deliver evidence-based psychotherapies. Obstetrics/gynecology clinics have emerged as highly promising sites to deliver CBT (Faramarzi et al. 2008) and IPT (Grote et al. 2009). Obstetrics/gynecology settings are particularly promising delivery sites given the considerable time and access barriers that many expectant and new mothers experience (Scholle et al. 2003). Despite these advantages, placing well-trained psychotherapists in these settings has proven to be challenging (Scholle et al. 2003), and researchers have suggested that the obstetrics/gynecology site may not be suitable for the provision of psychotherapy for severe TRD. Conversely, the obstetrics/gynecology clinic has clear advantages in terms of capturing depressed women early in the course of their illness, before high severity and recurrence have occurred.

In keeping with the early intervention and prevention opportunities present in primary care and obstetrics/gynecology settings, schools have high potential as a delivery site for evidence-based psychotherapy for depression. Small-scale studies involving both individual and group-based interventions based on CBT (Ruffolo and Fischer 2009; Shirk et al. 2009) and IPT (Mufson et al. 2004) principles have yielded promising outcomes for youths at risk for or experiencing depressed mood. Although schools are not likely appropriate delivery sites for youths experiencing severe, treatment-resistant symptoms, these settings hold great promise as sites to teach youths about strategies for treating low mood and responding to life stressors.

Although increasing the number of practitioners trained in evidence-based psychotherapies and moving delivery to nontraditional settings can increase the availability of treatment for depression, the gap between the need for and the availability of evidence-based psychotherapy will likely remain large for many years to come. One interesting method to address this problem involves simplifying CBT-related and IPT treatment strategies. The duration of treatment varies considerably among studies of depressed patients receiving CBT-related interventions. In a meta-analysis, length of treatment did not predict outcome, suggesting that CBT-related interventions may be effective with a modest number of sessions (Ekers et al. 2008).

Recent research also suggests that the simpler-to-administer behavioral activation component of CBT may be especially efficacious in the treatment of major depression (Dimidjian et al. 2006). The training burden associated with learning how to administer behavioral activation is lighter than for other CBT strategies (e.g., cognitive restructuring), suggesting that behavioral activation may be a particularly promising technique for broadening the availability of evidence-based interventions for major depression. Of particular relevance to this chapter, research indicates that behavioral activation may be more effective than other CBT-related strategies in treating severely depressed adults (Dimidjian et al. 2006).

Future Directions

Despite strong empirical support for the efficacy of depression-specific psychotherapy for recurrent depression that might otherwise be labeled as TRD, challenges in psychotherapy implementation and prediction of treatment response remain. One of the key questions to be addressed with clinical research involves mechanisms of action. Why is combination treatment superior to monotherapy for chronic depression? What are the mechanisms? Several possibilities exist. For example, particular residual symptoms, especially certain clusters of symptoms conferring relapse risk (e.g., low self-esteem, sleep disturbance, anhedonia), may be targeted to ensure complete remission and perhaps prevent or prolong relapse. To address this, studies must track and report residual symptoms and compare residual symptoms resulting from combination therapy and monotherapy with state-of-the-art assessments, particularly in the area of sleep. Another question involves the extent to which psychotherapy in combination with medications exerts a direct effect on depression recovery and relapse or whether the effect is mediated by overall treatment adherence. For example, combination treatment trials have found evidence that the addition of psychotherapy was associated with lower study attrition and greater medication compliance (Hollon et al. 2005). To provide information on the mediating effect of adherence, future studies should separate medication effects by adherence (Hollon et al. 2005). Also, psychotherapy may affect broader outcomes such as social and occupational functioning (Harkness et al. 2002). Future studies must assess and report functioning measures when evaluating the relative efficacy of combined therapy and monotherapy. Finally, different neural mechanisms may be affected by psychotherapy as compared with medication treatment (DeRubeis et al. 2008) and may confer risk for treatment nonresponse or relapse. Fortunately, neurobiological and neuroimaging research into such mechanisms of action and predictors of response is ongoing.

Questions also remain about the effects of therapist competence and adherence to the evidence-based, depression-specific psychotherapies such as CBT and IPT. Studies that have used well-trained cognitive-behavioral and interpersonal therapists with fidelity monitoring have shown evidence of a therapist training effect (DeRubeis et al. 2005). Studies with sufficient sample sizes to compare acute and longer-term depression and functioning outcomes after treatment by therapists with varying levels of training would be useful. Finally, RCTs that have proscribed dosages of psychotherapy (such as weekly for 16 weeks) have provided information on the efficacy of treatment. However, the precise dosing of psychotherapy (e.g., amount of contact) needed to maximize prevention of relapse is not known. Studies must compare varying doses of psychotherapy contact in continuation and maintenance phases to maximize the cost-effectiveness and potency of psychotherapy in TRD. Modifications of psychotherapy and innovations in the delivery and training of psychotherapy will improve effectiveness and widespread access to this viable treatment for depression.

The evidence shows that psychotherapeutic treatments are equally as effective for recurrent MDD of at least moderate severity as is medication treatment and that, unlike medications, psychotherapies have enduring preventive effects. Psychotherapies directly target symptoms and features of depression, such as stress, social isolation, deficient cognitive or emotional processing, and sleep disturbance, that may, over time, confer risk for treatment nonresponse. Depressed patients with dysregulated neuroendocrine stress response associated with childhood trauma, in particular, may show superior treatment response to psychotherapy as compared with medication treatment. As a result, psychotherapy alone or in combination with medications is the recommended, evidence-based treatment for unipolar depression.

Therefore, conceptualization of patients as treatment nonresponders (TRD) based exclusively on prior response to medication treatment is not useful in that it ignores information on trials of and response to an equally effective treatment option. The definition of treatment resistance should be revised to include prior response to depression-specific psychotherapies such as CBT, IPT, and CBASP. Clinicians then may be able to more thoroughly evaluate effective treatment alternatives. For example, symptoms that have not responded adequately to sufficient trials of antidepressant medications alone should not be considered treatment resistant until an adequate trial of a depression-specific psychotherapy has been tried. In particular, patients with a history of childhood trauma or the presence of psychosocial stress that significantly affects their symptoms should be referred for a course of psychotherapy either alone or in combination. Revision of TRD definitions that incorporate psychotherapy trials will provide needed guidance for clinicians and testable strategies for clinical researchers.

Key Clinical Concepts

∎ Depression-specific psychotherapies (e.g., cognitive-behavioral and interpersonal psychotherapies) have been found to have outcomes comparable to those of antidepressant medications for recurrent major depressive disorder. These therapies should be routinely offered and should be considered in the conceptualization of Treatment Resistant Depression (TRD).

∎ Evidence supports the effectiveness of combination treatment (depression-specific psychotherapy plus antidepressant medications) for severe, chronic depression in improving treatment response and preventing relapse.

∎ Combination treatment with psychotherapy may improve adherence and overall response to other TRD treatments.

∎ Mechanisms of action of psychotherapy may be complementary to medication mechanisms and thus may have a synergistic effect on symptom improvement.

∎ The availability and accessibility of clinicians who are well trained in depression-specific psychotherapies must be expanded to primary care and community settings to avoid having patients receive multiple trials of antidepressant medication without combination psychotherapy.

References

Addis ME, Krasnow AD: A national survey of practicing psychologists' attitudes toward psychotherapy treatment manuals. J Consult Clin Psychol 68:331–339, 2000

Adli M, Rush AJ, Moller HJ, et al: Algorithms for optimizing the treatment of depression: making the right decision at the right time. Pharmacopsychiatry 36 (suppl 3):222–229, 2003

Armitage R, Hoffmann RF, Emslie G, et al: Sleep microarchitecture as a predictor of recurrence in children and adolescents with depression. Int J Neuropsychopharmacol 5:217–228, 2002

Baquet CR: An overview of telemedicine. J Assoc Acad Minor Phys 8:2–10, 1997

Barlow D, Levitt JT, Bufka LF: The dissemination of empirically supported treatments: a view to the future. Behav Res Ther 37:S147–S162, 1999

Beck Institute for Cognitive Therapy and Research: Training. 2009. Available at: http://www.beckinstitute.org/FolderID/235/SessionID/%7B833E476B-52FC-4EDD-87A9-E5CFC6A66832%7D/PageVars/Library/InfoManage/Guide.htm. Accessed September 28, 2010.

Beck AT, Ward CH, Mendelson M, et al: An inventory for measuring depression. Arch Gen Psychiatry 4:561–571, 1961

Behavioral Tech: Training. 2010. Available at: http://behavioraltech.org/training/ . Accessed September 28, 2010.

Blackburn IM, Eunson KM, Bishop S: A two-year naturalistic follow-up of depressed patients treated with cognitive therapy, pharmacotherapy, and a combination of both. J Affect Disord 10:67–75, 1986

Blasinsky M, Goldman HH, Unützer J: Project IMPACT: a report on barriers and facilitators to sustainability. Adm Policy Ment Health 33:718–729, 2006

Bortolotti B, Menchetti M, Bellini F, et al: Psychological interventions for major depression in primary care: a meta-analytic review of randomized controlled trials. Gen Hosp Psychiatry 30:293–302, 2008

Caspi A, Sugden K, Moffitt TE, et al: Influence of life stress on depression: moderation by a polymorphism in the 5-HTT gene. Science 301:386–389, 2003

Christensen H, Griffiths KM, Korten A: Web-based cognitive behavior therapy: analysis of site usage and changes in depression and anxiety scores. J Med Internet Res 4:E3, 2002

Coffman SJ, Martell CR, Dimidjian S, et al: Extreme nonresponse in cognitive therapy: can behavioral activation succeed where cognitive therapy fails? J Consult Clin Psychol 75:531–541, 2007

Conte HR, Plutchik R, Wild KV, et al: Combined psychotherapy and pharmacotherapy for depression: a systematic analysis of the evidence. Arch Gen Psychiatry 43:471–479, 1986

Crits-Christoph P, Frank E, Chambless DL, et al: Training in empirically validated treatments: what are clinical psychology students learning? Prof Psychol Res Pr 26:514–522, 1995

Cuijpers P, van Straten A, Warmerdam L, et al: Psychotherapy versus the combination of psychotherapy and pharmacotherapy in the treatment of depression: a meta-analysis. Depress Anxiety 26:279–288, 2009

Davis DA, Thomson MA, Oxman AD, et al: Evidence for the effectiveness of CME. JAMA 268:1111–1117, 1992

de Mello MF, de Jesus Mari J, Bacaltchuk J, et al: A systematic review of research findings on the efficacy of interpersonal therapy for depressive disorders. Eur Arch Psychiatry Clin Neurosci 255:75–82, 2005

DeRubeis RJ, Gelfand LA, Tang TZ, et al: Medications versus cognitive behavior therapy for severely depressed outpatients: mega-analysis of four randomized comparisons. Am J Psychiatry 156:1007–1013, 1999

DeRubeis RJ, Hollon S, Amsterdam JD, et al: Cognitive therapy vs medication in the treatment of moderate to severe depression. Arch Gen Psychiatry 62:409–416, 2005

DeRubeis RJ, Siegle GJ, Hollon SD: Cognitive therapy versus medication for depression: treatment outcomes and neural mechanisms. Nat Rev Neurosci 9:788–796, 2008

Dimidjian S, Hollon SD, Dobson KS, et al: Randomized trial of behavioral activation, cognitive therapy, and antidepressant medication in the acute treatment of adults with major depression. J Consult Clin Psychol 74:658–670, 2006

Dobson KS, Hollon SD, Dimidjian S, et al: Randomized trial of behavioral activation, cognitive therapy, and antidepressant medication in the prevention of relapse and recurrence in major depression. J Consult Clin Psychol 76:468–477, 2008

Dunner DL, Rush AJ, Russell JM, et al: Prospective, long-term, multicenter study of the naturalistic outcomes of patients with treatment-resistant depression. J Clin Psychiatry 67:688–695, 2006

Ekers D, Richards D, Gilbody S: A meta-analysis of randomized trials of behavioural treatment of depression. Psychol Med 38:611–623, 2008

Elkin I, Shea MT, Watkins JT, et al: National institute of mental health treatment of depression collaborative research program: general effectiveness of treatments. Arch Gen Psychiatry 46:971–982, 1989

Emslie G, Armitage R, Weinberg WA, et al: Sleep polysomnography as a predictor of recurrence in children and adolescents with major depressive disorder. Int J Neuropsychopharmacol 4:159–168, 2001

European Medicines Agency Committee for Medicinal Products for Human Use (CHMP): Concept paper on revision of note for guidance on the clinical investigation of human normal immunoglobulin for subcutaneous and intramuscular use] (CPMP/BPWG/283/00) (2005). London, November 26, 2010. Available at: http://www.ema.europa.eu/docs/en_GB/document_library/Scientific_guideline/2010/12/WC500099995.pdf. Accessed February 8, 2011.

Faramarzi M, Alipor A, Esmaelzadeh S, et al: Treatment of depression and anxiety in infertile women: cognitive behavioral therapy versus fluoxetine. J Affect Disord 108:159–164, 2008

Fava M: Diagnosis and definition of treatment-resistant depression. Biol Psychiatry 53:649–659, 2003

Fava GA, Rafanelli C, Grandi S, et al: Six-year outcome for cognitive behavioral treatment of residual symptoms in major depression. Am J Psychiatry 155:1443–1445, 1998

Fava M, Davidson KG: Definition and epidemiology of treatment-resistant depression. Psychiatr Clin North Am 19:179–200, 1996

Fava M, Uebelacker LA, Alpert JE, et al: Major depressive subtypes and treatment response. Biol Psychiatry 42:568–576, 1997

Frank E, Kupfer DJ, Perel JM, et al: Three-year outcomes for maintenance therapies in recurrent depression. Arch Gen Psychiatry 47:1093–1099, 1990

Frank E, Anderson B, Reynolds CF, et al: Life events and the research diagnostic criteria endogenous subtype: a confirmation of the distinction using the Bedford College methods. Arch Gen Psychiatry 51:519–524, 1994

Frank E, Grochocinski VJ, Spanier CA, et al: Interpersonal psychotherapy and antidepressant medication: evaluation of a sequential treatment strategy in women with recurrent major depression. J Clin Psychiatry 61:51–57, 2000

Frueh FC, Santos AB, Johnson MR, et al: Procedural and methodological issues in telepsychiatry research and program development. Psychiatr Serv 51:1522–1527, 2000

Gaffan EA, Tsaousis I, Kemp-Wheeler SM: Researcher allegiance and meta-analysis: the case of cognitive therapy for depression. J Consult Clin Psychol 63:996, 1995

Gamm L, Stone S, Pittman S: Mental health and mental disorders—a rural challenge: a literature review, in Rural Healthy People 2010: A Companion Document to Rural Healthy People 2010, Vol 2. Edited by Gamm LD, Hutchison LL, Dabney BJ, et al. College Station, TX, The Texas A&M University System Health Science Center, School of Rural Public Health, Southwest Rural Health Research Center, 2003, pp 165–170

Grote NK, Swartz HA, Geibel SL, et al: A randomized controlled trial of culturally relevant, brief interpersonal psychotherapy for perinatal depression. Psychiatr Serv 60:313–321, 2009

Hamilton M: A rating scale for depression. J Neurol Neurosurg Psychiatry 23:56–62, 1960

Harkness KL, Frank E, Anderson B, et al: Does interpersonal psychotherapy protect women from depression in the face of stressful life events? J Consult Clin Psychol 70:908–915, 2002

Hegerl U, Plattner A, Moller HJ: Should combined pharmaco- and psychotherapy be offered to depressed patients? A qualitative review of randomized clinical trials from the 1990s. Eur Arch Psychiatry Clin Neurosci 254:99–107, 2004

Heim C, Newport DJ, Mletzko T, et al: The link between childhood trauma and depression: insights from HPA axis studies in humans. Psychoneuroendocrinology 33:693–710, 2008

Hollon S, Thase ME, Markowitz JC: Treatment and prevention of depression. Psychological Science in the Public Interest 3:39–77, 2002

Hollon SD, Jarrett RB, Nierenberg AA, et al: Psychotherapy and medication in the treatment of adult and geriatric depression: which monotherapy or combined treatment? J Clin Psychiatry 66:455–468, 2005

International Society for Interpersonal Therapy: IPT Training and Events: 2011. Available at: http://www.interpersonalpsychotherapy.org. Accessed February 8, 2011.

Jindal RD, Thase ME: Integrating psychotherapy and pharmacotherapy to improve outcomes among patients with mood disorders. Psychiatr Serv 54:1484–1490, 2003

Keller MB, McCullough JP, Klein DN, et al: A comparison of nefazodone, the cognitive behavioral-analysis system of psychotherapy, and their combination for the treatment of chronic depression. N Engl J Med 342:1462–1470, 2000

Kendler KS, Kessler RC, Neale MC, et al: The prediction of major depression in women: toward an integrated etiological model. Am J Psychiatry 150:1139–1148, 1993

Kovacs M, Rush AJ, Beck AT, et al: Depressed outpatients treated with cognitive therapy or pharmacotherapy: a one-year follow-up. Arch Gen Psychiatry 38:33–39, 1981

Kupfer DJ, Frank E: The interaction of drug- and psychotherapy in the long-term treatment of depression. J Affect Disord 62:131–137, 2001

Manber R, Edinger JD, Gress JL, et al: Cognitive behavioral therapy for insomnia enhances depression outcome in patients with comorbid major depressive disorder and insomnia. Sleep 31:489–495, 2008a

Manber R, Kraemer HC, Arnow BA, et al: Faster remission of chronic depression with combined psychotherapy and medication than with each therapy alone. J Consult Clin Psychol 76:459–467, 2008b

Markowitz JC: Interpersonal psychotherapy for chronic depression. J Clin Psychol 59:847–858, 2003

Mohr DC, Vella L, Hart SL, et al: The effect of telephone-administered psychotherapy on symptoms of depression and attrition: a meta-analysis. Clinical Psychology: Science and Practice 15:243–253, 2008

Mufson LH, Dorta KP, Olfson M, et al: Effectiveness research: transporting interpersonal psychotherapy for depressed adolescents (IPT-A) from the lab to school-based health clinics. Clin Child Fam Psychol Rev 7:251–261, 2004

Pampallona S, Bollini P, Tibaldi G, et al: Combined pharmacotherapy and psychological treatment for depression: a systematic review. Arch Gen Psychiatry 61:714–719, 2004

Paykel ES, Scott J, Teasdale JD, et al: Prevention of relapse in residual depression by cognitive therapy: a controlled trial. Arch Gen Psychiatry 56:829–835, 1999

Pizzagalli DA, Oakes TR, Fox AS, et al: Functional but not structural subgenual prefrontal cortex abnormalities in melancholia. Mol Psychiatry 9:393–405, 2004

Post RM: Transduction of psychosocial stress into the neurobiology of recurrent affective disorder. Am J Psychiatry 149:999–1010, 1992

Raue PJ, Schulberg HC, Heo M, et al: Patients' depression treatment preferences and initiation, adherence, and outcome: a randomized primary care study. Psychiatr Serv 60:337–343, 2009

Robinson LA, Berman JS, Neimeyer RA: Psychotherapy for the treatment of depression: a comprehensive review of the controlled outcome research. Psychol Bull 108:30–49, 1990

Roy-Byrne PP, Stang P, Wittchen H, et al: Lifetime panic-depression comorbidity in the national comorbidity survey: association with symptoms, impairment, course and help-seeking. Br J Psychiatry 176:229–235, 2000

Ruffolo MC, Fischer D: Using an evidence-based CBT group intervention model for adolescents with depressive symptoms: lessons learned from a school-based adaptation. Child and Family Social Work 14:189–197, 2009

Ruskin PE, Silver-Aylaian M, Kling MA, et al: Treatment outcomes in depression: comparison of remote treatment through telepsychiatry to in-person treatment. Am J Psychiatry 161:1471–1476, 2004

Schatzberg AF, Rush AJ, Arnow BA, et al: Chronic depression: medication (nefazodone) or psychotherapy (CBASP) is effective when the other is not. Arch Gen Psychiatry 62:513–520, 2005

Scholle S, Haskett R, Hanusa B, et al: Addressing depression in obstetrics/gynecology practice. Gen Hosp Psychiatry 25:83–90, 2003

Scott C, Tacchi MJ, Jones R, et al: Acute and one year outcome of a randomized trial of brief cognitive therapy for major depressive disorder in primary care. Br J Psychiatry 171:131–134, 1997

Shirk SR, Kaplinski H, Gudmundsen G: School-based cognitive-behavioral therapy for adolescent depression: a benchmarking study. J Emot Behav Disord 17:106–117, 2009

Souery D, Amsterdam J, de Montigny C: Treatment resistant depression: method-
    ological overview and operational criteria. Eur Neuropsychopharmcol 9:83–
    91, 1999
Steinfeld BI, Coffman SJ, Keyes JA: Implementation of an evidence-based practice
    in a clinical setting: what happens when you get there? Prof Psychol Res Pr
    40:410–416, 2009
Stimpson N, Agrawal N, Lewis G: Randomised controlled trials investigating
    pharmacological and psychological interventions for treatment-refractory de-
    pression: systematic review. Br J Psychiatry 181:284–294, 2002
Stuart GW, Tondora J, Hoge MA: Evidence-based teaching practice: implications
    for behavioral health. Adm Policy Ment Health 32:107–130, 2004
Thase ME: Therapeutic alternatives for difficult to treat depression: what is the
    state of the evidence? Psychiatr Ann 33:813–821, 2003
Thase ME, Howland R: Refractory depression: relevance of psychosocial factors
    and therapies. Psychiatr Ann 24:232–240, 1994
Thase ME, Greenhouse JB, Frank E: Treatment of major depression with psycho-
    therapy or psychotherapy-pharmacotherapy combinations. Arch Gen Psychi-
    atry 54:1009–1015, 1997
Thase ME, Friedman ES, Howland R: Management of treatment resistant depres-
    sion: psychotherapeutic perspectives. J Clin Psychiatry 63:18–24, 2001
Thase ME, Friedman ES, Biggs MM, et al: Cognitive therapy versus medication in
    augmentation and switch strategies as second-step treatments: a STAR*D re-
    port. Am J Psychiatry 164:739–752, 2007
Uebelacker LA, Weisberg RB, Haggarty R, et al: Adapted behavior therapy for per-
    sistently depressed primary care patients: an open trial. Behav Modif 33:374–
    395, 2009
U.S. Department of Health and Human Services: Depression guideline panel:
    clinical practice guideline: depression in primary care, vol. 2: treatment of
    major depression (clinical practice guideline No 5; AHCPR Publ No 93-
    0551). Rockville, MD, U.S. Department of Health and Human Services, U.S.
    Public Health Service, Agency for Health care Policy and Research, 1993
Wang PS, Berglund P, Kessler R: Recent care of common mental disorders in the
    United States: prevalence and conformance with evidence-based recommen-
    dations. J Gen Intern Med 15:284–292, 2000
Weissman M, Markowitz JC, Klerman GL: Comprehensive Guide to Interpersonal
    Psychotherapy. New York, Basic Books, 2000

CHAPTER ELEVEN

Device-Related Neuromodulation in Treatment Resistant Depression

Stephan F. Taylor, M.D.
Mona Goldman, Ph.D.
Daniel F. Maixner, M.D.
Parag G. Patil, M.D., Ph.D.
John F. Greden, M.D.

Clinical Vignette

Mr. A, a 60-year-old married man, experienced his first depressive episode at age 42 following a divorce. His symptoms responded to fluoxetine and remained in remission until his second episode at age 50. This second episode responded only partially to fluoxetine, leaving him with residual anxiety and low-grade depression for 2 years.

At age 57, after 3 years of relative good health while taking sertraline, Mr. A began to experience a depressive episode. This episode failed to respond to three other second-generation antidepressants, to nortriptyline, or to various augmentation or combination strategies, including thyroid hormone, bupropion, buspirone, lorazepam, quetiapine, and mirtazapine. After Mr. A retired early from his job at age 59, his depression deepened, with severe ruminative anxiety, insomnia, and appetite loss. He was admitted to the hospital and had a course of unilateral electroconvulsive therapy (ECT; 6 sessions), followed by 6 more sessions of bilateral (BL) ECT, with a nearly complete remission. However, within 4 months of discharge, despite nortriptyline-lithium therapy, his depression returned. Another course of outpatient BL ECT (9 sessions) reduced his severe symptoms, but he remained mildly depressed and ruminative. Two months after the completion of that course, his severe depression returned.

This hypothetical patient shows the common presentation of a patient with Treatment Resistant Depression (TRD). Although definitions vary, the concept of TRD refers to the failure to respond to two courses of adequate antidepressant therapy. As reviewed in other chapters of this volume, approximately one-third of patients taking antidepressants fail to achieve a satisfactory remission of symptoms after three to four courses of medication therapy (Rush et al. 2006; Sackeim 2001). The concept, and the practice, of treating depression resistant to multiple therapies inevitably leads to nonpharmacological somatic therapy; yet many patients are not exposed to the benefits of device-related treatments.

Until 2005, only one device-related procedure existed for TRD: electroconvulsive therapy. At the time of this writing, two additional "neuromodulatory" therapies have been approved for the treatment of resistant depression, and several more device-based treatments are in various stages of research. The vignette shows that ECT is a very effective treatment when medications do not work, but an acute ECT course often does not lead to sustained remission. The clinician in these situations now has additional options, including maintenance ECT and new device-related neuromodulation therapies.

In this chapter, we review device-related neuromodulation, or simply neuromodulation, as these treatments are applied to patients with TRD. In the context of devices applied to the brain, *neuromodulation* refers to the use of electrical and magnetic currents to alter, or modulate, neural circuitry. The brain has its own neuromodulators, in the form of monoamines, neuropeptides, and cholinergic systems, and psychotropic drugs work at least partially by altering the functions of these endogenous neuromodulators. Device-related neuromodulation complements the pharmacological approach by modulating brain activity through brain-wide excitation, as with ECT, or through direct stimulation of specific structures, as with newer techniques (see Table 11–1 for a glossary of techniques). The U.S. Food and Drug Administration (FDA) approved vagus nerve stimulation (VNS) for TRD in 2005 and repetitive transcranial magnetic stimulation (rTMS) for patients in the early stages of treatment resistance in 2008. We review these approved treatments, including ECT, in addition to touching on new therapies at various stages of investigation (see Figure 11–1).

TABLE 11–1. Glossary of device-related neuromodulation therapies

Nonconvulsive, nonimplanted stimulation
Stimulation occurs noninvasively and can be performed in an outpatient setting without general anesthesia.

repetitive transcranial magnetic stimulation (rTMS)   An electromagnetic coil placed on the scalp generates a rapidly alternating magnetic field that passes through the skull and induces an electrical current that stimulates nerve cells in the underlying cerebral cortex.

transcranial direct current stimulation (investigational)   A direct electrical current applied to electrodes placed on the scalp passes through the scalp to modify the excitability of neurons in the underlying brain.

Convulsive therapies
These treatments stimulate the brain, causing a generalized seizure and requiring general anesthesia.

electroconvulsive therapy (ECT)   Two electrodes apply a brief electrical pulse to the scalp, causing a current to run between the electrodes, resulting in a generalized seizure, while the patient is under anesthesia.

magnetic seizure therapy (investigational)   A strong magnet is used to induce electrical current in the brain, evoking a seizure. This procedure has been called a cross between ECT and TMS. It is hypothesized that this procedure will generate more focal seizures and fewer memory side effects than ECT does.

Implantable stimulation
Surgical procedures are used to permanently implant electrodes, which deliver current to the brain.

vagus nerve stimulation (VNS)   A pacemaker-like device delivers intermittent stimulation to an electrode attached to the left vagus nerve in the neck, traveling to the brain.

deep brain stimulation (DBS; investigational)   Electrodes are implanted in the brain, directed at targets deep in the brain. The electrodes are connected to a small, programmable stimulator lying under the skin, very similar to a cardiac pacemaker, which delivers continuous stimulation.

epidural cortical stimulation (investigational)   Electrodes are surgically implanted on the surface of the dura mater over the cortex. The electrodes are attached to a pacemaker-like device under the skin to deliver intermittent stimulation.

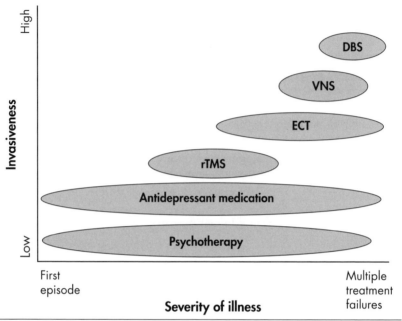

FIGURE 11–1.   Spectrum of treatments for depression.

Note. DBS = deep brain stimulation; ECT = electroconvulsive therapy; rTMS = repetitive transcranial magnetic stimulation; VNS = vagus nerve stimulation.

Electroconvulsive Therapy

Description and Possible Mechanism of Action

First used more than 70 years ago, ECT is the oldest and most effective treatment for major depression. In ECT, a brief electrical pulse is applied to the scalp while the patient is under anesthesia. This pulse excites neurons in the brain and produces a generalized seizure. The specific mechanism of action of ECT is unknown, although metaphorically it has been likened to "rebooting" the brain. ECT appears to affect many areas of brain activity, giving rise to several theories of how it works. A leading hypothesis suggests that anticonvulsant changes in brain activity induced by ECT underlie its efficacy in depression (Sackeim 1999). These changes, many of which are associated with clinical response, include an increase in seizure threshold observed over the course of ECT; postictal and interictal inhibitory processes that persist for months after treatment ends and that are characterized by an increase in electroencephalographic slow-wave (delta) activity and a decrease in cerebral blood flow; and increased transmission of inhibitory neurotransmitters and peptides. Other hypotheses suggest that ECT may work by downregulating abnormal activity in the hypothalamic-pituitary-adrenal (HPA) axis or by normalizing abnormal sleep patterns (Szuba et al. 2000). Recent studies indicate that ECT also may exert its antidepressant effect by increasing levels of neurotrophins such as brain-derived neurotrophic factor (BDNF) and by promoting neurogenesis (Taylor 2008). Combinations of mechanisms are likely. As with most treatments in psychiatry, evidence for the clinical effects of ECT has preceded an understanding of mechanisms of action, and this remains an important area of investigation.

Evidence for Effectiveness in Depression

The efficacy of ECT for treating depression was confirmed in two meta-analytic reviews of randomized clinical trials conducted more than 40 years ago (Pagnin et al. 2004; UK ECT Review Group 2003). The two reviews used different analytic approaches, but both concluded that ECT was significantly more effective than either placebo/sham ECT or antidepressant medication in treating depression. For example, an analysis of six randomized clinical trials (256 subjects) showed that real ECT was significantly more effective than sham ECT, by nearly a 10-point margin in Hamilton Rating Scale for Depression (Ham-D) scores. Another analysis combining 18 trials (1,144 subjects) found that ECT was significantly more effective than pharmacotherapy, with a mean difference of 5.2 points on the Ham-D, whereas a third analysis, combining results from 16 randomized clinical trials (892 subjects), found that the odds of response to ECT were nearly four times those of response to drug therapy.

Studies conducted in recent years have focused on remission rather than response after ECT, with *remission* typically defined as a 60% or greater reduction in the 24-item Ham-D (Ham-D-24) score and a maximum final score of 10. Remission rates for patients participating in clinical trials of ECT range from about 50% to 75% (Husain et al. 2004; Sackeim et al. 2001a). Although most of the patients in these studies had failed to respond to at least one adequate antidepressant trial, the effect of treatment resistance on response to ECT is not clear. Prudic and colleagues (1996) reported remission rates of 91% after ECT in patients with no history of treatment resistance, compared with 63% in patients who failed to respond to at least one adequate treatment trial. In contrast, Rasmussen and colleagues (2007) found no difference in ECT remission rates with similar comparison groups. In addition, remission rates in community-based studies are lower (30%–40%) than those reported in the academic-based clinical trials (Prudic et al. 2004). The lower rates have been

attributed to the inclusion of patients with more severe and complex illnesses and to greater variation in treatment practice in the community
studies. Nevertheless, remission rates after ECT, even in the community
setting, compare favorably to the 14 % remission reported for patients taking antidepressants after failing to respond to two successive medication
trials in the Sequenced Treatment Alternatives to Relieve Depression
(STAR*D) study (Rush et al. 2006).

Response to ECT is also faster than response to antidepressant medications. This is particularly important for those with life-threatening comorbidities such as suicidality or catatonia. Time to response and time to
remission were examined in 253 depressed patients receiving a course of
BL ECT during the first stage of a large multicenter study of continuation
therapy after ECT conducted by the Consortium for Research in ECT
(CORE; Husain et al. 2004). About one-third of the patients showed a sustained response (greater than 50 % reduction in baseline Ham-D-24
score) within the first week of treatment, and 75 % did so by the third
week. One-third achieved remission by the second week, and nearly two-
thirds did so by the third or fourth week. In comparison, depressed patients receiving citalopram in the first phase of the STAR*D study took an
average of 6 weeks to respond and 7 weeks to achieve remission (Rush et
al. 2006).

Data from the first phase of the CORE study also were used to prove
that ECT is a particularly fast and effective treatment for psychotic depression, a severe form of depression (Petrides et al. 2001). Of the psychotic depressed patients, 96 % (64 of 67) achieved remission after ECT
compared with 83 % (125 of 150) of those with nonpsychotic depression
($P<0.01$), and time to remission was significantly shorter for the psychot-
ically depressed group. These results suggest that ECT treatment should
be considered early in the course of psychotic depression.

Although ECT is a fast and effective treatment for depression, more
than half of remitted patients relapse within 6–12 months (Sackeim et al.
2001a), and few data exist to guide follow-up treatment to prevent relapse.
This issue was addressed in two multicenter randomized clinical trials
(Kellner et al. [CORE] 2006; Sackeim et al. 2001a). In the first phase of
both studies, patients with major depression were given an acute course
of ECT. In the Sackeim et al. study, patients who remitted with ECT
($n = 84$) were randomly assigned to receive a placebo pill, nortriptyline,
or a combination of nortriptyline and lithium. After 6 months, the relapse
rates were significantly lower with the combination therapy (39 %) than
with either nortriptyline alone (60 %) or placebo (84 %). In the CORE
group study, remitters ($n = 201$) were randomly assigned to receive continuation treatment with either BL ECT (C-ECT) or a combination of

nortriptyline and lithium. Relapse rates after 6 months were similar in the two groups (45% with C-ECT and 41% with nortriptyline-lithium) and significantly lower than the rates with placebo (84%) (Sackeim et al. 2001a). Although these studies suggest the nortriptyline-lithium combination and C-ECT are equally effective maintenance treatments for depression, one major weakness of the CORE study is of particular concern. In that trial, a rigid ECT taper was used. In real-world practice, a more flexible ECT schedule is used, often in conjunction with medications. Data are lacking to evaluate fully the effect of these factors on the relapse prevention potential of continuation ECT. Despite the efficacy of these treatments in preventing relapse, rates remain high, so new maintenance therapies are being considered for patients who remit after ECT.

Clinical Use

The American Psychiatric Association guidelines recommend electroconvulsive therapy as a treatment for depression in patients whose symptoms do not respond to, or who are intolerant of, antidepressant medications or when speed of action and a high probability of response are needed (e.g., when the risk of suicide is high; American Psychiatric Association Committee on Electroconvulsive Therapy 2001). A course of ECT typically includes 3 treatments per week, for a total of 6–12 treatments. As performed today, ECT is a safe and effective treatment for depression. The recommended procedure includes administration of general anesthesia and muscle relaxants, careful monitoring of vital signs and brain activity (with electroencephalograms), and maintenance of blood oxygen saturation. Stimulation is delivered by a precise amount of alternating, square-wave current to minimize adverse cognitive side effects. Despite its safety as now performed, misperceptions and stigma still surround treatment with ECT, based largely on past practices that are no longer used (Dowman et al. 2005), and this has limited its use in many parts of the United States. Although an estimated 100,000 patients receive ECT in the United States each year, wide regional variation is seen in use rates (Hermann et al. 1995).

Stimulus Dose and Electrode Placement

Stimulus dose (measured in millicoulombs) and the placement of electrodes are key parameters that independently and jointly affect treatment outcome and cognitive side effects of ECT (American Psychiatric Association Committee on Electroconvulsive Therapy 2001; Greenberg and Kellner 2005). To have a comparable measure across individuals, stimulus dose is usually quantified as a multiple of the threshold level of stimulation required to elicit a seizure. *Electrode placement* refers to the positioning of two handheld electrodes against the scalp. The most widely used configurations for electrode placement are right unilateral (RUL), in which one electrode is placed on the crown of the head and the other on the right temple, and bilateral (or BL), in which electrodes are placed on both temples.

The relative risks and benefits of RUL versus BL electrode placement have been studied and debated for many years. A meta-analysis of trials conducted between 1968 and 2000 (UK ECT Review Group 2003) reported that BL ECT was more effective than RUL ECT (22 trials), but BL ECT also resulted in greater impairment of retrograde memory (4 trials) and anterograde memory (7 trials) measured 1 week after ECT. However, the wide variation in dose, duration, and frequency of ECT treatment in these studies was rarely taken into account. Sackeim and colleagues (1993, 2000b) investigated the effects of electrode placement and stimulus dose on treatment outcome and cognitive side effects in two randomized clinical trials. In the 2000 study, 80 depressed patients were randomly assigned to receive RUL ECT at one of three doses (1.5, 2.5, or 6 times seizure threshold) or BL ECT at 2.5 times the seizure threshold. Symptom levels (Ham-D-24 scores) and cognitive functioning (retrograde and anterograde memory) were assessed at baseline, at the end of treatment, and 1 week post-ECT. Cognitive functioning also was assessed at 2 months after treatment. Patients who did not respond to their original treatment were switched to the BL ECT. The results showed that high-dose (6 times the seizure threshold) RUL and BL ECT were equivalent in treatment efficacy and about twice as effective as low- (1.5 times) or moderate- (2.5 times) dose RUL ECT. For example, remission rates at 1 week post-ECT were 65% for BL and 60% for high-dose RUL, 30% for moderate-dose RUL, and 35% for low-dose RUL. Furthermore, 78% of the nonresponders at any RUL dose level who switched to BL ECT responded to the new treatment. However, BL ECT produced more severe and persistent cognitive side effects than did RUL ECT at any dosage. Postictal confusion was six times more likely with BL ECT than with any RUL treatment. BL ECT compared with any RUL treatment produced greater impairment in anterograde memory (recalling new information) and retrograde memory (recalling events that occurred just prior to the course of treatment) at 1 week post-ECT and greater deficits in retrograde memory measured 2 months after ECT.

More recently, the use of bifrontal (BF) electrode placement, in which electrodes are placed on either side of the forehead, has been explored. It has been hypothesized that BF stimulation, by avoiding the temporal areas of the brain, would reduce memory impairment after ECT. Some evidence now suggests that BF ECT may be as effective as BL ECT and may produce fewer cognitive side effects (Bailine et al. 2000). However, in a larger randomized trial of BF ECT, RUL ECT, and BL ECT, all three electrode placements were similarly efficacious, but BF ECT garnered no advantage cognitively over BL ECT (Kellner et al. 2010).

In summary, these studies suggest that high-dosage RUL ECT is as effective as BL ECT for treating depression and has fewer adverse cognitive effects. However, in using high-dose (6 times the seizure threshold) RUL ECT, clinicians need to be aware that ECT has anticonvulsant effects that rise over a course of ECT and that some patients may have extremely high thresholds at the time of treatment. For many patients, to maintain a 6 times threshold dose or to achieve a suprathreshold RUL dose at the beginning of treatment may be difficult with our currently available ECT devices that have an FDA limit on the electrical dose output. In addition, some patients who receive RUL ECT may require BL ECT to obtain a response from ECT. If RUL ECT is used, a high dose at 6–8 times the seizure threshold can be used to increase effectiveness. Stimulus doses of 1.5 times the seizure threshold are effective with BL ECT, with a maximum dose of 2.5 times the seizure threshold (American Psychiatric Association Committee on Electroconvulsive Therapy 2001; Greenberg and Kellner 2005).

Side Effects

ECT today is a safe medical procedure. Treatment is performed under general anesthesia, and the mortality rate for the procedure, estimated to be 2–10 per 100,000 treatments (Shiwach et al. 2001), is similar to the mortality rate for general anesthesia alone. The most common medical complaints for ECT are related primarily to the anesthesia and the induced seizure (Greenberg and Kellner 2005) and include headache, nausea, and muscle aches. These side effects are generally treated symptomatically.

The most troubling side effects for patients are changes in cognitive functioning that relate to loss of memory. A brief postanesthesia, postictal confusion may follow a treatment and usually lasts less than a few hours. Anterograde amnesia (impairment in remembering new information) is common during the course of ECT but typically resolves within 1–3 weeks after treatment ends. Retrograde amnesia (memory loss for events that occurred just prior to a course of treatment, although it may extend back several months) is the most serious and persistent side effect of ECT. Although retrograde amnesia may improve during the first few months after treatment, patients may have some permanent memory loss (Greenberg and Kellner 2005; Lisanby et al. 2000).

The effect of ECT on other cognitive functions also has been examined. No evidence indicates that ECT results in any lasting impairment in general intelligence, executive functions, abstract thinking, visual-spatial function, creativity, semantic memory, implicit memory, or the learning of new skills (Sackeim et al. 2000a). In fact, ECT can have beneficial effects on the cognitive deficits associated with depression (e.g., increased scores on the Mini-Mental State Examination have been reported; Greenberg and Kellner 2005).

Summary

Evidence shows that ECT remains the most effective and safe treatment for depression that has not responded to antidepressant medications. Cognitive side effects, particularly retrograde amnesia, and a relapse rate of more than 50% are limitations of the treatment, but relief from severe, often life-threatening depression is a benefit that usually offsets these negative effects. Despite its established efficacy and safety, this important treatment modality is often underused (Hermann et al. 1995). Further research is needed to identify effective methods to prevent relapse after ECT and to minimize the cognitive side effects of treatment.

Vagus Nerve Stimulation

Description and Possible Mechanisms of Action

VNS involves the surgical placement of an electrode around the left vagus nerve, providing a "pipeline" to the emotional brain. It also has been referred to as a "brain pacemaker" because the implantable technology—a small, battery-powered generator placed under the skin, below the collarbone—resembles a cardiac pacemaker, and, like a pacemaker, the generator transmits electrical pulses through the electrode attached to the nerve. VNS was originally developed as a treatment for epilepsy, first approved by the FDA as an adjunctive therapy in 1997. Evidence that VNS might have a role in depression came from anecdotal observations of epilepsy patients who noted improved mood with VNS treatment. Controlled studies in epilepsy patients confirmed the clinical observations and determined that mood improvement was not simply secondary to improved seizure control (Harden et al. 2000).

The exact mechanism of VNS in the treatment of depression remains unknown, although the anatomy of the vagus nerve makes it well suited for affective neuromodulation, suggesting possible routes through which stimulation can exert effects on mood. The vagus nerve represents the major source of parasympathetic efferent nerve fibers to the abdominal viscera, but approximately 80 % of the fibers are afferents conducting information from the viscera to the brain. Also known as the tenth cranial nerve, the vagus nerve enters the brain stem and innervates the nucleus tractus solitarius. From this nucleus, fibers travel to prominent limbic centers of the brain, such as the hypothalamus and amygdala, in addition to the locus coeruleus (LC), dorsal raphe, and parabrachial nuclei, which project to limbic structures and the forebrain (Henry 2002). The raphe nuclei contain serotonergic neurons and the LC noradrenergic neurons, on which antidepressant medications exert therapeutic effects (Nemeroff and Owens 2002). In animal models (Porsolt swim test), VNS has had antidepressant effects, similar to ECT (Krahl et al. 2004). VNS also has been shown to increase monoamine turnover (Hassert et al. 2004), increase BDNF (Biggio et al. 2006), and increase firing rates in the LC (Dorr and Debonnel 2006) and the dorsal raphe (Dorr and Debonnel 2006).

Human neuroimaging studies in patients with depression have begun to elucidate effects of acute and chronic stimulation on brain activity. Although the emerging literature is somewhat heterogeneous, with small sample sizes and varying treatment parameters, evidence suggests that stimulation changes activity in the limbic regions, medial temporal lobe, thalamus, and medulla (Nemeroff et al. 2006). In a series of functional magnetic resonance imaging (fMRI) studies performed in nine subjects with VNS over a 20-month period, Nahas and colleagues (2007) showed decreasing VNS-related activity in frontal and parietal brain regions and, notably, in the ventral medial prefrontal cortex (vmPFC). A similar effect of chronic stimulation decreasing vmPFC activity also has been reported with positron emission tomography (Pardo et al. 2008) and with single-photon emission computed tomography (Zobel et al. 2005). Downregulation of activity in the vmPFC, also observed for deep brain stimulation (DBS) in depression (Lozano et al. 2008) and obsessive-compulsive disorder (Abelson et al. 2005), may be an important final common pathway of neuromodulatory techniques.

Evidence for Effectiveness in Treatment Resistant Depression

The unique mechanism by which VNS appeared to improve mood in epilepsy patients suggested that it might be effective for TRD. The therapy could be offered to patients who had exhausted standard existing treatments; given the invasiveness of surgically implanting a VNS system, the treatment would not make sense as a first-line therapy. Cyberonics, the manufacturer of a VNS device, sponsored a feasibility study in 60 patients with depression that had failed to respond to at least two adequate courses of antidepressant therapy (Rush et al. 2000; Sackeim et al. 2001b). After 10 weeks of active stimulation, 30.5% showed response (>50% decrease in Ham-D-24 scores), and 15.3% entered remission. In a larger pivotal trial (Rush et al. 2005), 235 patients received VNS implantation, and after a 2-week recovery period, 112 of 222 evaluable patients were randomly assigned to active stimulation for 10 weeks, and 110 patients were randomly assigned to "sham" stimulation for 10 weeks, in a double masked design. The patients randomly assigned to sham stimulation had the option to shift to active stimulation. At the end of the 10-week period, response rates were lower than in the feasibility study, with only 15.2% of the active stimulation patients showing a greater than 50% decrease in Ham-D-24 ratings, which was not significantly different from the sham stimulation group, in which 10% showed a response. A self-rated scale, the Inventory of Depressive Symptoms, did show a significant improvement (17.0% vs. 7.3%; $P = 0.03$; last observation carried forward), but the Ham-D-24 was the primary measure in this registration trial.

Although the results from the large pivotal trial after 10 weeks of stimulation were disappointing, additional analyses suggested that longer stimulation differentiated the VNS patients from the patients receiving usual treatment. Patients from the extension phase of the pivotal trial ($n = 205$) were compared with a group of similarly depressed patients ($n = 124$) and followed up for 1 year (George et al. 2005). Both groups had undergone a mean of 3.5 trials of adequate antidepressant therapy for their current episode, with an average length of 49.9–68.6 months (not significantly different between groups). Medication changes occurred naturalistically, except for the VNS patients during the 10-week stimulation phase. In the treatment-as-usual group, only 13% of the patients achieved a 50% decline in Ham-D-24 scores, whereas 27% in the VNS group showed a significant response ($P = 0.01$). Moreover, of the VNS patients who showed a response at 3 months, 55% (16 of 29) maintained this response at 12 months, in contrast to the treatment as usual patients, in whom only 14% (1 of 7) sustained a response over this period. The relatively robust strength of the response, also noted in the pilot study (Sackeim et al. 2001b), suggests that VNS may have cumulative antidepressant effects, in contrast to the higher relapse rates observed with ECT (Sackeim et al. 2001a).

Caution is warranted in the comparison of the VNS and treatment-as-usual groups because patients were not randomly assigned to treatment. The two groups differed on several clinical characteristics, such as the number of sites for each study, more patients with greater than 10 episodes of depression in the treatment-as-usual group, and more patients with past ECT treatment in the VNS group. Nevertheless, secondary analyses suggested that these factors could not account for differences in outcome (VNS response was best in patients with >10 episodes, a somewhat unexpected result that differed from the pilot study), and the observed response rate of 13% at 12 months for treatment-as-usual patients corresponds to the estimated response rate in other studies of TRD patients who undergo standard pharmacotherapy (Rush et al. 2006). A longer randomized study could provide important clarification about the strength of the therapeutic effect, but hiding the presence of VNS stimulation, which almost all patients detect as the device cycles on and off, makes a true placebo-controlled trial impossible. Thus, comparison with treatment-as-usual groups will remain an important method for analyzing VNS effects, and research to date provides support for the assertion that VNS therapy substantially improves TRD.

Clinical Use

In 2005, the FDA approved VNS for adjunctive treatment in patients with TRD. In the labeled indication, patients are considered to have TRD if they have had an inadequate response to four or more adequate antidepressant treatments. Although the labeled indication does not distinguish unipolar and bipolar depression, approximately 10% of the patients in the pivotal trial had bipolar depression, and this group did not have different outcomes from the unipolar depressed patients. When considering patients for VNS therapy, it is worth noting what all of the VNS trials did not include—namely, patients with psychotic, schizophrenic, or schizoaffective depressions. Thus, no data are available on the effectiveness of VNS in patients with these conditions. Similarly, few or no data exist on effectiveness in patients with comorbidities, such as personality disorders, substance abuse, or anxiety disorders. In general, one may assume that comorbidities will reduce the effectiveness of any therapy, so that patients with these conditions should be considered to have a lower rate of response than those with "uncomplicated" TRD.

Consideration of an invasive therapy such as VNS should always occur in the context of a thorough psychiatric and medical evaluation. In addition to the requirement of four adequate trials, most practitioners would require that the four trials involved at least two different classes of antidepressants, and at least one trial should include augmentation with an agent such as lithium, thyroid hormone, or bupropion. Another important consideration is ECT. As discussed earlier, in many areas, practitioners are reluctant to recommend ECT, and many patients decline ECT when it is recommended. However, any patient considering a treatment involving a surgical intervention and the implantation of a permanent device in the body needs to give serious consideration to ECT.

For patients choosing VNS, implantation and initiation of therapy are straightforward. Implantation can occur in an outpatient surgical facility, and patients are given 2 weeks to allow for tissue healing before turning on the stimulator. Initiation of therapy occurs in dose-escalating steps, beginning with a low current (typically around 25 mA) at 20–30 Hz and a duty cycle of 30 seconds of stimulation alternating with 5 minutes of rest. Over several weeks, the current is increased to a target dose of 1–1.5 mA or the highest dose tolerated. The most common side effects are directly related to local effects of stimulation: voice alteration (55 %–60 %), neck pain (15 %), dysphagia (13 %), cough (24 %), dyspnea (14 %), and laryngismus (10 %). Except for voice alteration (usually hoarseness) and dyspnea, these side effects diminish over time. They can also be managed by adjusting the stimulation parameters (e.g., reducing the pulse width or frequency of stimulation). As for the voice alteration, most patients accommodate to this and find it only a minor annoyance, at most. Patients with an implanted VNS device follow the same precautions as do patients with cardiac pacemakers (e.g., special passage or searches through airport security, avoidance of strong electrical fields that can alter the device settings, and special precautions for MRI scans). Overall, the therapy is very well tolerated.

Repetitive Transcranial Magnetic Stimulation

Description

In the modern neuroscience literature, Barker and colleagues (1985) first described in 1985 that pulses applied over the motor cortex could elicit stimulation of motor efferents and quantifiable movement. TMS has emerged in the last three decades as a flexible tool to investigate brain function and treat neuropsychiatric disorders. It involves the use of a coil, placed directly on the scalp, to generate a magnetic field that switches on and off. The changing magnetic field induces an electrical current in a conductive medium, such as a neuron. TMS coils used in practice typically evoke electrical activity at a depth of 2–3 cm, depending on the design of the coil. In addition to being completely noninvasive, the coil may be positioned anywhere over the scalp to target specific cortical regions with a precision on the order of millimeters. Single- (or paired-) pulse TMS involves the asynchronous delivery of pulses, and this technique has been used to study neural physiology. When performed during a behavioral task, stimulation with single-pulse TMS can interrupt or perturb the task, providing a valuable tool for mapping cortical function (for a review, see Paus 2005). Regular, repetitive stimulation (rTMS) has variable effects. Slow rates of stimulation (e.g., <1 Hz) are generally described as inhibitory, even after the cessation of stimulation, whereas fast rates (e.g., >5 Hz) are generally described as having long-lasting stimulatory effects. However, effects depend on many factors, including scalp location, orientation of underlying neural fibers (only fibers perpendicular to the magnetic field are excited), strength of stimulation, duration of pulse trains, and timing of pulses. Understanding the diverse effects on cortical neurocircuits is an active area of TMS research. (For a recent review of the physiology of TMS, see Bestmann 2008.)

Evidence for Effectiveness in Depression

Studies that reported prolonged effects of rTMS raised the possibility that stimulation of frontal cortex, a brain region hypofunctional in depression (Drevets 2000), may have antidepressant effects. This was confirmed in preliminary open-label studies in the 1990s (George et al. 1995; Pascual-Leone et al. 1996). Since those initial reports, more than 40 randomized controlled trials have been conducted. Effect sizes in the two recent comprehensive meta-analytic studies have been in the range of 0.39–0.48 (Lam et al. 2008; Schutter 2009), an efficacy comparable to that of pharmacotherapy (Khan and Schwart 2005). The largest randomized trial to date, sponsored by the manufacturer of an rTMS system, enrolled 301 patients. This trial provided a minimum of 4 weeks of treatment, as opposed to many of the earlier, smaller trials conducted for only 2 weeks. Patients with mild to moderate TRD were enrolled and randomly assigned to active or sham (double-blind, placebo-controlled) therapy. Responses rates (>50% symptom decrease) were 24% at 6 weeks, compared with 12% for sham stimulation, and remission rates were 16% and 6%, respectively (O'Reardon et al. 2007). These numbers represented statistically significant benefits (except for one trend-level measure), but post hoc analyses found that the mildly treatment-resistant patients—defined as having been able to tolerate no more than a single adequate medication trial—constituted the most responsive group of patients, with response rates of 54% and remission rates of 33% at 6 weeks (Lisanby et al. 2009). On the basis of the response for this group of patients, the FDA approved the rTMS system for patients who have failed a single adequate course of an antidepressant. Note that these patients had *tried,* on average, 4.6 different antidepressants, most of which they were unable to take in adequate dosages because of intolerance of medication side effects. Thus, the evidence from this large, well-controlled trial suggests that rTMS has a specific role

in moderate forms of TRD, particularly when patients have difficulty tol-
erating sufficient trials of antidepressant medications.

Delivery of Transcranial Magnetic Stimulation in the Clinical Setting

The delivery of rTMS therapy is completely noninvasive and does not require the administration of anesthesia or routine sedation; thus, rTMS can
be administered in an outpatient setting. Treatment planning involves cal-
ibration of stimulation to the patient, performed by eliciting the magnitude
of stimulation necessary to evoke a thumb twitch when the coil is placed
over the scalp location overlying the motor strip of the cerebral cortex. Establishing the "motor threshold" defines both the magnitude of power and
the location of stimulation for actual treatment, because current protocols
involve positioning the coil 5 cm in front of the motor strip. For treatment
delivery, patients come to an office 5 days per week for up to 6 weeks for a
course of therapy. Actual stimulation lasts approximately 30–40 minutes,
and a session, with positioning and setup, lasts approximately 1 hour. The
patient sits comfortably in a chair, with the coil stimulating the brain for
brief bursts (seconds) applied every 20–30 seconds. Although the delivery
of treatment over 5 days of the week has been the standard protocol, delivering the same number of pulses over 2 or 3 days of the week is safe and
possible. However, research needs to be conducted to determine whether
concentrated rTMS can provide a more convenient treatment for patients
who cannot make daily trips to the clinic for 1 month.

In general, rTMS therapy is very safe and well tolerated. At high rates of
rTMS, seizures can be induced, although within well-defined safety parameters, seizure induction is a very small, manageable risk, occurring with a frequency of less than 1 in 1,000 (Wassermann 1998). Among 325 patients and
more than 10,000 treatments, no seizures were reported in the pivotal trial
conducted by Neuronetics, a manufacturer of a TMS device. Most adverse
events were of mild to moderate severity, and the overall discontinuation rate
of 4.5% did not differ from that of sham treatment (Janicak et al. 2008). Common side effects include pain at the site of stimulation (affecting 35%–50%
of patients), which can be managed by adjusting stimulator settings or coil
placement. This was judged to be severe in only 6% of cases. Other potential
side effects occurring more frequently than in sham-stimulated patients include muscle twitching (21% of patients) and toothache (7%).

Looking Ahead

Deep Brain Stimulation

Technological developments in recent years have enabled the delivery of electrical current to modulate or stimulate very specific regions deep within the brain, a therapy known as *deep brain stimulation*. In the 1970s, therapeutic electrical stimulation was developed for chronic pain, movement disorders, and epilepsy, but not until the mid-1990s was DBS approved by the FDA for essential tremor (Benabid et al. 1996) and Parkinson's disease (Limousin et al. 1998). With the ability to reach subcortical structures and deep limbic gray matter, DBS provides a technique to modulate brain areas involved in the generation of emotion, motivation, and drive. Mayberg (2002) and colleagues took advantage of this technology and performed DBS in six depressed patients via implantation in the white matter tract adjacent to the subgenual cingulate region, because imaging studies implicated this region in depression. They found a sustained antidepressant response for 6 months in 4 of 6 patients (Mayberg et al. 2005), which was subsequently confirmed (60% responding at 6 months) in 14 additional patients (Lozano et al. 2008). Malone and colleagues (2009) used a different target in the internal capsule or ventral striatum and reported a similar response (40% responding at 6 months) in 15 patients with TRD. Although the mechanisms of these effects remain unclear, neuroimaging studies report that stimulation in both sites causes downregulation of vmPFC (Lozano et al. 2008). At this writing, the efficacy of DBS in controlled studies remains to be proved. Given the invasiveness of neurosurgical implantation and the cost of the therapy, DBS will probably never occupy a large niche in the treatment armamentarium for TRD, but it may offer the promise of another unique treatment modality for severely ill patients.

Future Developments in Neuromodulation

Neuromodulation involves a device to deliver energy to neural tissue, and diverse methods exist by which electrical or magnetic energy can modulate neural circuits. Research in the past decade has begun to develop new technologies and refine existing ones. For example, ECT causes seizures with electrical stimulation passed across one or both hemispheres of the brain, stimulating many neurons in the course of the alternating current, but a seizure also can be stimulated with magnetic energy. Whereas rTMS stimulates the cortex and avoids seizures, magnetic seizure therapy directs magnetic energy more focally to deep structures of the brain to cause a therapeutic seizure. As a convulsive therapy, magnetic seizure therapy is similar to ECT, but preliminary work suggests that it may produce fewer cognitive side effects (Lisanby et al. 2003). Other research has found that application of a simple direct current across the scalp alters perception, cognition, and mood (Been et al. 2007), and preliminary studies with transcranial direct current stimulation have reported antidepressant effects in depressed individuals (Bikson et al. 2008). Low-field magnetic stimulation—delivered at much lower intensity than with standard rTMS—has been reported to have mood-elevating effects in bipolar patients (Rohan et al. 2004). A technique that uses implanted electrodes on the surface of the brain (over the dura mater), called *epidural cortical stimulation,* has shown promising effects in a small open-label study of TRD patients (Nahas et al. 2010). However, all of these techniques have been studied in only very small samples, and larger controlled trials are necessary to establish efficacy.

The field of device-related neuromodulation will expand as the knowledge base of neuroscience opens new windows on mechanisms of brain function. Brain mapping techniques such as fMRI, near infrared imaging, and recording of brain electrical activity have begun to characterize the emergent networks of neural activity, which may define leverage points for stimulation. TMS and DBS have already translated neuroimaging findings in depression into targets of stimulation. Nevertheless, these devices have explored only a fraction of the theoretical targets in the brain, and investigators have yet to optimize the location of stimulation sites. Another avenue of research involves shaping the pulses of TMS to be in tune with intrinsic activity in neural circuits (e.g., matching theta burst activity; Huang et al. 2005). At the molecular level, "optogenetic" technology can label specific cell types in vivo to make the neurons controllable by optical signals, allowing for very precise control of very small clusters of cells (Deisseroth et al. 2006). For example, chronobiological pacemaker cells in the hypothalamus could be targeted to reset a disturbed sleep cycle. Such specific applications are only theoretical, but the growing number of opportunities for intervention suggests that neuromodulation therapies in the next few decades may yield even more specific interventions.

Conclusion

The discovery that nerves conducted electrical current actually preceded the discovery of chemical messengers, now known as *neurotransmitters,* whereas the development of therapies that exploit electromagnetic energy proceeded rather slowly after the introduction of ECT in the 1930s. It is no coincidence that with the digital age and advanced microscopic microprocessors, magnetic and electrical energy have started to find their place in the treatment of neuropsychiatric disorders in general, and TRD in particular. Whereas the mechanisms of almost all current antidepressants rely on increasing the monoaminergic tone, the addition of treatments such as VNS and TMS can provide other treatment options with very different mechanisms of action that can help when pharmacotherapy fails. Device-related neuromodulation will not help all TRD patients, but successful treatment for some gives hope to all who seek relief from the disabling symptoms of depression.

Key Clinical Concepts

■ Devices that deliver electrical or magnetic energy to the brain provide important treatment options for patients with difficult-to-treat depression.

■ Electroconvulsive therapy (ECT) is the most effective approved treatment for patients unresponsive to previous medication trials, with remission rates in the range of 50%–75% in clinical trials; for unknown reasons, its effectiveness tends to be lower in clinical practice than in the controlled trials.

■ Vagus nerve stimulation (VNS), the first device-related procedure approved for a psychiatric indication since ECT, offers potential benefits for a subset of individuals with Treatment Resistant Depression (TRD), and treatment effects appear to persist for 1–2 years after the initial response. However, large-sample randomized controlled studies are needed.

■ Repetitive transcranial magnetic stimulation (rTMS) provides a noninvasive method of stimulating brain cortex and can be conducted in an outpatient setting. rTMS has shown effectiveness in treating milder forms of TRD, with effect sizes comparable to those of pharmaceutical agents. For some individuals with TRD, the side-effect profile of rTMS may be preferable.

■ Device-related neuromodulation is an area of active research for neuropsychiatric therapy, and several newer technologies are currently under study.

References

Abelson JL, Curtis GC, Sagher O, et al: Deep brain stimulation for refractory obsessive-compulsive disorder. Biol Psychiatry 57:510–516, 2005

American Psychiatric Association Committee on Electroconvulsive Therapy: The Practice of Electroconvulsive Therapy: Recommendations for Treatment, Training, and Privileging (A Task Force Report of the American Psychiatric Association), 2nd Edition. Washington, DC, American Psychiatric Association, 2001

Bailine SH, Rifkin A, Kayne E, et al: Comparison of bifrontal and bitemporal ECT for major depression. Am J Psychiatry 157:121–123, 2000

Barker AT, Jalinous R, Freeston IL: Non-invasive magnetic stimulation of human motor cortex. Lancet 1:1106–1107, 1985

Been G, Ngo TT, Miller SM, et al: The use of tDCS and CVS as methods of non-invasive brain stimulation. Brain Res Rev 56:346–361, 2007

Benabid AL, Pollak P, Gao D: Chronic electrical stimulation of the ventralis intermedius nucleus of the thalamus as a treatment of movement disorders. J Neurosurg 84:203–214, 1996

Bestmann S: The physiological basis of transcranial magnetic stimulation. Trends Cogn Sci 12:81–83, 2008

Biggio F, Gorini G, Caria S, et al: Plastic neuronal changes in GABA(A) receptor gene expression induced by progesterone metabolites: in vitro molecular and functional studies. Pharmacol Biochem Behav 84:545–554, 2006

Bikson M, Bulow P, Stiller JW, et al: Transcranial direct current stimulation for major depression: a general system for quantifying transcranial electrotherapy dosage. Curr Treat Options Neurol 10:377–385, 2008

Deisseroth K, Feng G, Majewska AK, et al: Next-generation optical technologies for illuminating genetically targeted brain circuits. J Neurosci 26:10380–10386, 2006

Dorr AE, Debonnel G: Effect of vagus nerve stimulation on serotonergic and noradrenergic transmission. J Pharmacol Exp Ther 318:890–898, 2006

Dowman J, Patel A, Rajput K: Electroconvulsive therapy: attitudes and misconceptions. J ECT 21:84–87, 2005

Drevets WC: Functional anatomical abnormalities in limbic and prefrontal cortical structures in major depression. Prog Brain Res 126:413–431, 2000

George MS, Wassermann EM, Williams WA, et al: Daily repetitive transcranial magnetic stimulation (rTMS) improves mood in depression. Neuroreport 6:1853–1856, 1995

George MS, Rush AJ, Marangell LB, et al: A one-year comparison of vagus nerve stimulation with treatment as usual for treatment-resistant depression. Biol Psychiatry 58:364–373, 2005

Greenberg RM, Kellner CH: Electroconvulsive therapy: a selected review. Am J Geriatr Psychiatry 13:268–281, 2005

Harden CL, Pulver MC, Ravdin LD, et al: A pilot study of mood in epilepsy patients treated with vagus nerve stimulation. Epilepsy Behav 1:93–99, 2000

Hassert DL, Miyashita T, Williams CL: The effects of peripheral vagal nerve stimulation at a memory-modulating intensity on norepinephrine output in the basolateral amygdala. Behav Neurosci 118:79–88, 2004

Henry TR: Therapeutic mechanisms of vagus nerve stimulation. Neurology 59:S3–S14, 2002

Hermann RC, Dorwart RA, Hoover CW, et al: Variation in ECT use in the United States. Am J Psychiatry 152:869–875, 1995

Huang YZ, Edwards MJ, Rounis E, et al: Theta burst stimulation of the human motor cortex. Neuron 45:201–206, 2005

Husain MM, Rush AJ, Fink M, et al: Speed of response and remission in major depressive disorder with acute electroconvulsive therapy (ECT): a Consortium for Research in ECT (CORE) report. J Clin Psychiatry 65:485–491, 2004

Janicak PG, O'Reardon JP, Sampson SM, et al: Transcranial magnetic stimulation in the treatment of major depressive disorder: a comprehensive summary of safety experience from acute exposure, extended exposure, and during reintroduction treatment. J Clin Psychiatry 69:222–232, 2008

Khan A, Schwartz K: Study designs and outcomes in antidepressant clinical trials. Essent Psychopharmacol 6:221–226, 2005

Kellner CH, Knapp RG, Petrides G, et al: Continuation electroconvulsive therapy vs pharmacotherapy for relapse prevention in major depression: a multi-site study from the Consortium for Research in Electroconvulsive Therapy (CORE). Arch Gen Psychiatry 63:1337–1344, 2006

Kellner CH, Knapp R, Hussain MM, et al: Bifrontal, bitemporal and right unilateral electrode placement in ECT: randomized trial. Br J Psychiatry 196:226–234, 2010

Krahl SE, Senanayake SS, Pekary AE, et al: Vagus nerve stimulation (VNS) is effective in a rat model of antidepressant action. J Psychiatr Res 38:237–240, 2004

Lam RW, Chan P, Wilkins-Ho M, et al: Repetitive transcranial magnetic stimulation for treatment-resistant depression: a systematic review and metaanalysis. Can J Psychiatry 53:621–631, 2008

Limousin P, Krack P, Pollak P, et al: Electrical stimulation of the subthalamic nucleus in advanced Parkinson's disease. N Engl J Med 339:1105–1111, 1998

Lisanby SH, Maddox JH, Prudic J, et al: The effects of electroconvulsive therapy on memory of autobiographical and public events. Arch Gen Psychiatry 57:581–590, 2000

Lisanby SH, Luber B, Schlaepfter TE, et al: Safety and feasibility of magnetic seizure therapy (MST) in major depression: randomized within-subject comparison with electroconvulsive therapy. Neuropsychopharmacology 28:1852–1865, 2003

Lisanby SH, Husain MM, Rosenquist PB, et al: Daily left prefrontal repetitive transcranial magnetic stimulation in the acute treatment of major depression: clinical predictors of outcome in a multisite, randomized controlled clinical trial. Neuropsychopharmacology 34:522–534, 2009

Lozano AM, Mayberg HS, Giacobbe P, et al: Subcallosal cingulate gyrus deep brain stimulation for treatment-resistant depression. Biol Psychiatry 64:461–467, 2008

Malone DA Jr, Dougherty DD, Rezai AR, et al: Deep brain stimulation of the ventral capsule/ventral striatum for treatment-resistant depression. Biol Psychiatry 65:267–275, 2009

Mayberg HS: Modulating limbic-cortical circuits in depression: targets of antidepressant treatments. Semin Clin Neuropsychiatry 7:255–268, 2002

Mayberg HS, Lozano AM, Voon V, et al: Deep brain stimulation for treatment-resistant depression. Neuron 45:651–660, 2005

Nahas Z, Teneback C, Chae JH, et al: Serial vagus nerve stimulation functional MRI in treatment-resistant depression. Neuropsychopharmacology 32:1649–1660, 2007

Nahas Z, Anderson BS, Borckardt J, et al: Bilateral epidural prefrontal cortical stimulation for treatment-resistant depression. Biol Psychiatry 67:101–109, 2010

Nemeroff CB, Owens MJ: Treatment of mood disorders. Nat Neurosci 5(suppl): 1068–1070, 2002

Nemeroff CB, Mayberg HS, Krahl SE, et al: VNS therapy in treatment-resistant depression: clinical evidence and putative neurobiological mechanisms. Neuropsychopharmacology 31:1345–1355, 2006

O'Reardon JP, Solvason HB, Janicak PG, et al: Efficacy and safety of transcranial magnetic stimulation in the acute treatment of major depression: a multi-site randomized controlled trial. Biol Psychiatry 62:1208–1216, 2007

Pagnin D, de Queiroz V, Pini S, et al: Efficacy of ECT in depression: a meta-analytic review. J ECT 20:13–20, 2004

Pardo JV, Sheikh SA, Schwindt GC, et al: Chronic vagus nerve stimulation for treatment-resistant depression decreases resting ventromedial prefrontal glucose metabolism. Neuroimage 42:879–889, 2008

Pascual-Leone A, Rubio B, Pallardo F, et al: Rapid-rate transcranial magnetic stimulation of left dorsolateral prefrontal cortex in drug-resistant depression. Lancet 348:233–237, 1996

Paus T: Inferring causality in brain images: a perturbation approach. Philos Trans R Soc Lond B Biol Sci 360:1109–1114, 2005

Petrides G, Fink M, Husain MM, et al: ECT remission rates in psychotic versus nonpsychotic depressed patients: a report from CORE. J ECT 17:244–253, 2001

Prudic J, Haskett RF, Mulsant B, et al: Resistance to antidepressant medications and short-term clinical response to ECT. Am J Psychiatry 153:985–992, 1996

Prudic J, Olfson M, Marcus SC, et al: Effectiveness of electroconvulsive therapy in community settings. Biol Psychiatry 55:301–312, 2004

Rasmussen KG, Mueller M, Knapp RG, et al: Antidepressant medication treatment failure does not predict lower remission with ECT for major depressive disorder: a report from the consortium for research in electroconvulsive therapy. J Clin Psychiatry 68:1701–1706, 2007

Rohan M, Parow A, Stoll AL, et al: Low-field magnetic stimulation in bipolar depression using an MRI-based stimulator. Am J Psychiatry 161:93–98, 2004

Rush AJ, George MS, Sackeim HA, et al: Vagus nerve stimulation (VNS) for treatment-resistant depressions: a multicenter study. Biol Psychiatry 47:276–286, 2000

Rush AJ, Marangell LB, Sackeim HA, et al: Vagus nerve stimulation for treatment-resistant depression: a randomized, controlled acute phase trial. Biol Psychiatry 58:347–354, 2005

Rush AJ, Trivedi MH, Wisniewski SR, et al: Acute and longer-term outcomes in depressed outpatients requiring one or several treatment steps: a STAR*D report. Am J Psychiatry 163:1905–1917, 2006

Sackeim HA: The anticonvulsant hypothesis of the mechanisms of action of ECT: current status. J ECT 15:5–26, 1999

Sackeim HA: The definition and meaning of treatment-resistant depression. J Clin Psychiatry 62 (suppl 16):10–17, 2001

Sackeim HA, Prudic J, Devanand DP, et al: Effects of stimulus intensity and electrode placement on the efficacy and cognitive effects of electroconvulsive therapy. N Engl J Med 328:839–846, 1993

Sackeim HA, Luber B, Moeller JR, et al: Electrophysiological correlates of the adverse cognitive effects of electroconvulsive therapy. J ECT 16:110–120, 2000a

Sackeim HA, Prudic J, Devanand DP, et al: A prospective, randomized, double-blind comparison of bilateral and right unilateral electroconvulsive therapy at different stimulus intensities. Arch Gen Psychiatry 57:425–434, 2000b

Sackeim HA, Haskett RF, Mulsant BH, et al: Continuation pharmacotherapy in the prevention of relapse following electroconvulsive therapy: a randomized controlled trial. JAMA 285:1299–1307, 2001a

Sackeim HA, Rush AJ, George MS, et al: Vagus nerve stimulation (VNS) for treatment-resistant depression: efficacy, side effects, and predictors of outcome. Neuropsychopharmacology 25:713–728, 2001b

Schutter DJ: Antidepressant efficacy of high-frequency transcranial magnetic stimulation over the left dorsolateral prefrontal cortex in double-blind sham-controlled designs: a meta-analysis. Psychol Med 39:65–75, 2009

Shiwach RS, Reid WH, Carmody TJ: An analysis of reported deaths following electroconvulsive therapy in Texas, 1993–1998. Psychiatr Serv 52:1095–1097, 2001

Szuba MP, O'Reardon JP, Evans DL: Physiological effects of electroconvulsive therapy and transcranial magnetic stimulation in major depression. Depress Anxiety 12:170–177, 2000

Taylor SM: Electroconvulsive therapy, brain-derived neurotrophic factor, and possible neurorestorative benefit of the clinical application of electroconvulsive therapy. J ECT 24:160–165, 2008

UK ECT Review Group: Efficacy and safety of electroconvulsive therapy in depressive disorders: a systematic review and meta-analysis. Lancet 361:799–808, 2003

Wassermann EM: Risk and safety of repetitive transcranial magnetic stimulation: report and suggested guidelines from the International Workshop on the Safety of Repetitive Transcranial Magnetic Stimulation, June 5–7, 1996. Electroencephalogr Clin Neurophysiol 108:1–16, 1998

Zobel A, Joe A, Freymann N, et al: Changes in regional cerebral blood flow by therapeutic vagus nerve stimulation in depression: an exploratory approach. Psychiatry Res 139:165–179, 2005

CHAPTER TWELVE

Exercise, Nutrition, and Treatment Resistant Depression

Simon Evans, Ph.D.
Paul Burghardt, Ph.D.

EVIDENCE IS GROWING that lifestyle choices, especially exercise, nutrition, and sleep, play a role in the onset, treatment, and progression of depression and bipolar disorders. Emerging data indicate that specific nutrients and physical activity levels influence the course of clinical depression and bipolar disorders and may play roles in the alleviation and prevention of treatment resistance. Clinicians would do well to consider incorporating lifestyle approaches in their treatment strategies, most frequently as complementary approaches to pharmacological or cognitive therapies, and in appropriate cases as stand-alone paradigms. In this chapter, we aim to provide a primer on the fundamentals of exercise and nutrition how clinicians may use them in their evaluation and treatment of patients.

Exercise

The beneficial effects of exercise on general health have been recognized for several decades. More recent data suggest that the brain also benefits from increased physical activity. As illustrations, animal studies show increased hippocampal neurogenesis or production of new neuronal cells, a process that may be important for antidepressant action, whereas human imaging studies show increased frontal cortical volume and activity following exercise. Stated succinctly, exercise appears to be good for the brain.

Terminology

Exercise falls into two general categories, anaerobic and aerobic, depending on the intensity and duration of the activity. The distinction between the two forms concerns the use of oxygen to produce the energy that muscles use to move. In clinical settings, consideration of this distinction is relevant for two reasons. First, it is important to know whether the individual has any concurrent health problems and to plan accordingly with prior medical consultations. Second, depression and bipolar disorder both have been linked with alterations of metabolism; therefore, prevention or proper management of the metabolic syndrome (as defined by the National Cholesterol Education Program and Adult Treatment Panel ["Executive Summary" 2001]) may be vital for long-term stabilization of mood and affect. With this in mind, the timing and implementation of either type of exercise should be considered.

Very intense exercise that can be sustained for only a relatively short amount of time (seconds to a couple of minutes) requires energy very quickly and therefore relies almost entirely on anaerobic metabolism. This type of intense, brief exercise is referred to as *anaerobic exercise.* Sprinting and weightlifting are activities that fall into the category of anaerobic exercise.

During relatively prolonged and less intense exercise, oxygen is used to break down stored forms of energy more completely into immediately usable forms. This type of exercise is commonly known as *aerobic* exercise. Examples include activities such as jogging or running, biking, and swimming, during which muscles have access to oxygen. Aerobic activities can be sustained for at least 10 minutes. Many activities actually fall somewhere between these metabolic definitions because they incorporate varying intensities that require muscles to work under both anaerobic and aerobic conditions.

Exercise, Neurogenesis, and Brain Changes

Exercise has been consistently shown to increase the rate of neurogenesis and probably induces structural changes in the adult brain. Patients may not understand how this effect of exercise is possible, so clinicians may benefit from incorporating a simple explanation if recommending an exercise program as part of their clinical program. The common vehicles of the changes are brain neurotrophins or growth factors, which affect neurogenesis and neuroplasticity.

Growth factors are proteins containing several different subfamilies, are expressed in the brain, and are involved in an array of processes affecting brain growth and plasticity. Changes in levels of growth factor messenger ribonucleic acid (mRNA) (Evans et al. 2004) have been identified in the brains of people with depression. Intriguingly, exercise has the capacity to change growth factor expression (Gomez-Pinilla et al. 1997; Russo-Neustadt et al. 1999), brain structure (Pereira et al. 2007), and behavior (Burghardt et al. 2004) in preclinical models.

Brain-derived neurotrophic factor (BDNF) was one of the first growth factors reported to be increased after exercise in the brains of animals (Russo-Neustadt et al. 1999); however, several other families of growth factors also respond to exercise, including the insulin-like (IGF), vascular endothelial (VEGF), and fibroblast (FGF) growth factors (Cotman et al. 2007). These molecules are also increased after exposure to an enriched environment (Turner and Lewis 2003) and antidepressant treatment (Berton and Nestler 2006) and may be a necessary part of the cellular machinery for response to antidepressant drugs (Adachi et al. 2008).

Increased levels of neurogenesis in rodents also have been reported after exposure to exercise, an "enriched (complex) environment," and antidepressant treatment (Cotman et al. 2007; Duman 2004; van Praag et al. 1999), indicating that changes in mood that occur after pharmacological treatment might have some biological commonality with exercise and environmental enrichment. Although the work on neurogenesis has been relegated to preclinical models, Pereira et al. (2007) recently used functional magnetic resonance imaging (fMRI) in mice to correlate changes in blood flow with (direct) histological determinants of neurogenesis. By establishing this association in rodents, the investigators were able to estimate the viability of neurogenesis in humans by using fMRI measurements of blood flow as a proxy for neurogenesis.

With these data in mind, it becomes apparent that exercise has the ability to alter the brain physically, particularly in areas such as the hippocampus that are known to decrease in size in individuals with depression (Sheline et al. 1996). Therefore, the biological plausibility of exercise counteracting the deleterious effects associated with depression is high, and exercise arguably should be considered as an integral part of treatment programs for those who are medically capable of increasing their physical activity.

Exercise for Treatment and Prevention of Depression

On average, individuals who exercise regularly or who maintain physically active lives have better mood than do sedentary individuals (Brosse et al. 2002). Low levels of physical activity are associated with elevations in depressive mood, whereas people who are more physically active have lower levels of depressive feelings. In addition, decreases in physical activity over the preceding year predicted higher levels of depressive symptoms in elderly individuals (Lindwall et al. 2007). Whether the physiological adaptations that accompany prolonged exercise are necessary for reducing the risk of depression remains an issue of contention; however, the benefits of exercise on mood are clear even if the underlying mechanism is not.

Improvements in mood occur after a single session of either aerobic or anaerobic exercise (Lane et al. 2002). Individuals who exercise regularly also experience greater elevations in mood after a single session of exercise compared with sedentary individuals (Hoffman and Hoffman 2008).

Taken together, physical activity or exercise appears to have benefit in reducing the risk for developing depression and improving mood in individuals without mood disorders. However, it is apparent that the maintenance of physical activity is as important as the implementation, and efforts should be made to prioritize and sustain physical activity.

Clinical Potential

Clinicians considering how to implement exercise programs in people with major depressive disorder (MDD) of mild to moderate severity also have additional basis to guide them. Age is not a barrier; exercise is effective in reducing depressive symptoms in older adults and younger individuals (Blumenthal et al. 1999; Petty et al. 2009). Blumenthal et al. (1999) reported decreases in scores on both the Beck Depression Inventory and the Hamilton Rating Scale for Depression (Ham-D) after 16 weeks of treatment with sertraline, aerobic exercise three times per week, or the combination. All three interventions had comparable effects (Blumenthal et al. 1999). In a later study, Blumenthal and colleagues (2007) compared the effects of group-based exercise, home-based exercise, sertraline treatment, and placebo. The exercise and sertraline groups had remission rates significantly higher than those in the placebo group. Reports indicate that both aerobic and anaerobic exercise are effective in reducing depressive symptoms (Martinsen 1990), and thus there are multiple options for implementing exercise as a treatment strategy for people with depression.

Intriguingly, the ability of exercise to decrease depressive symptoms appears to follow a dose-response relation (Dunn et al. 2005). A dose of exercise analogous to that recommended for general public health (energy expenditure of 17.5 kcal/kg/week) was more effective in reducing depression scores than was a stretching control group or a low dose of exercise (7.0 kcal/kg/week) after 12 weeks. This has two important implications. First, exercise is arguably indicated whenever possible for individuals with mild to moderate MDD. Second, doses are important; exercise rates that are lower than those recommended for general public health benefit are equivalent to placebo.

Exercise in Relation to Treatment Resistant Depression and Bipolar Disorder

The use of exercise as a means for addressing Treatment Resistant Depression (TRD) has not been a major research focus to date. However, two studies have reported positive effects of exercise in patients with TRD. Exercise was added as an adjunctive treatment to pharmacotherapy and produced decreases in depressive symptoms over 8 months not seen in individuals who received pharmacotherapy but no exercise (Pilu et al. 2007). TRD patients given the combination therapy showed a substantial decline in Ham-D scores, from approximately 20 at baseline to 8 after 8 months of supervised exercise. In comparison, the group that did not exercise had a baseline Ham-D score of 19 and an 8-month score of approximately 17. Assessed improvements in global functioning (Global Assessment of Functioning Scale) and psychopathology (Clinical Global Impression Scale) also were seen after 8 months of supervised exercise. The small study by Pilu and colleagues (2007) also suggested that exercise may have utility as an adjunctive treatment for individuals with TRD. In a follow-up study, women with TRD who exercised in addition to receiving pharmacotherapy showed increases in measured quality of life that were not experienced by women receiving pharmacotherapy without exercise (Carta et al. 2008). It has not been determined whether exercise could serve as a stand-alone treatment for TRD. In summary, although evidence for the use of exercise as a strategy for addressing TRD is still emerging, initial indications are promising.

At this point, it cannot be stated with confidence whether reductions in measures of depression were the result of social interaction in a treatment setting or solely an effect of exercise. We could speculate from other research in nondepressed and MDD populations that exercise likely has an effect that may be bolstered by the social interaction provided during the exercise training sessions. From an academic perspective, "the jury is still out" regarding the exact contribution of exercise to managing TRD. The potential for exercise to be efficacious in managing TRD in clinical populations is very promising. Furthermore, the additional benefits of exercise on general health can be of great value because of the robust link between mood disorders and dysfunction of metabolism, which results in a high co-occurrence of mood disorders, cardiovascular disease, diabetes, and metabolic syndrome. Because of the potential benefit, low cost, and low risk of side effects, increasing physical activity and exercise should be considered as routine parts of the treatment program for all patients with TRD who are medically capable of participating in such programs.

Specific Exercise Regimens for Individuals to Follow

The physical condition, in terms of both fitness and preexisting medical conditions, should be considered before an individual increases physical activity or begins an exercise regimen. Monitoring and adapting the physical activity or exercise regimens to provide variety also are critical to promote long-term adherence.

As a preventive application, the American College of Sports Medicine and the American Heart Association have suggested that individuals engage in moderate physical activity for 30 minutes on most days of the week or intense physical activity for 30–60 minutes on 3 days per week. The target of 17.5 kcal/kg/week has been shown to be effective in improving mood in patients with depression (Dunn et al. 2005) and is in agreement with levels recommended for general public health.

A major concern for the implementation and maintenance of exercise in patients with depression and related disorders is that these individuals are, by definition, depressed. The general population shows very low adherence to physical activity recommendations, and it is expected that the barriers that must be overcome to promote adherence in individuals with mood disorders will be greater than those in the general public. Although benefits may be clear, adherence barriers are likely to be substantial. However, involving exercise professionals in the treatment process may aid in surmounting such barriers.

Clinical Vignette 1

Mr. M, a 40-year-old man, has TRD. After consulting with his private physician, he actively sought help from a psychiatrist because of his concerns over work stress and death of his parent. Mr. M has had two major episodes of depression, the first in his mid-20s and the second in his late 30s, neither of which responded completely to antidepressant treatment. He is currently taking sertraline. Mr. M is overweight and has a family history of diabetes. Recent blood panels indicated that Mr. M had an elevated fasting blood glucose level (105 mg/dL), which is not at the threshold for diabetes. His high-density lipoprotein level was 28 (considered low), and he had elevated triglyceride levels. During the interview with the psychiatrist, Mr. M mentioned that he and his family have made an effort over the past year to "eat better" and that he lost a couple of pounds, but his weight had not changed for several months. Although he enjoys walking, he has not been joining his family for their evening walks around their neighborhood over the past couple of months because of his increasingly low mood.

Because of Mr. M's unresponsiveness to antidepressant treatment and his metabolic status, the psychiatrist brought in family members and suggested that they all commit to evening walks. Furthermore, the psychiatrist recommended that Mr. M start working with a personal trainer twice a week while continuing his current treatment with sertraline.

After 2 months, Mr. M reported feeling less depressed and mentioned that he enjoys and values his evening walks with his family; the "walking talks" appear to have helped his marital relationship. In addition, a follow-up blood panel indicated that although Mr. M's low-density lipoprotein and cholesterol levels have dropped only a modest amount, his fasting blood glucose level is now 80 mg/dL, and his high-density lipoprotein level has increased to 41. He also has lost 8 pounds. The psychiatrist recommended that Mr. M continue his walking routine and personal training sessions and suggested that it may be possible to reduce his dose of sertraline if his mood remains stable.

Nutrition

Nutritional factors affect brain function. The simple concept of "you are what you eat" applies. The macro- and micronutrients that we consume become the raw materials for the constant activity and remodeling that occurs in our neural circuitry in several ways. First, the brain is approximately 60 % fat by dry weight, and approximately 25 % of that fat is optimally the omega-3 fatty acid docosahexaenoic acid (DHA). Omega-3 and omega-6 fatty acids cannot be synthesized de novo and must come from dietary sources. Furthermore, the dietary ratios of these and other polyunsaturated fatty acids (PUFAs) are reflected in neuronal membrane concentrations

(Chalon et al. 1998). This is important because fatty acid membrane composition controls membrane fluidity and receptor kinetics (Grossfield et al. 2006), which can affect all neurotransmitter systems. Second, the protein sources we choose to eat also affect brain function. Eight of the 20 amino acids are essential and must be obtained from the diet, some of which are precursors to neurotransmitter synthesis. For example, diet influences the local concentrations of tryptophan in the brain, which controls the synthesis rate of serotonin (Fernstrom and Fernstrom 2007) and can have functional consequences on mood (Smith et al. 1997). Third, the supply of glucose, the brain's primary energy source, from food carbohydrates also controls the temporal rates of metabolic activity in the brain, and this has multifarious effects. Eating high-glycemic carbohydrates that elevate blood sugar levels quickly can alter mood and cognitive function (Benton and Nabb 2003). Placing this type of eating against a backdrop of depression, in which glucose regulation may already be compromised as a result of glucocorticoid (cortisol) dysregulation, can further exacerbate the effect. In summary, the amount and type of dietary fats, proteins, and carbohydrates can control several aspects of brain function and mood.

In addition, micronutrients, including vitamins, minerals, and a plethora of other phytonutrients, exert their own control over brain function. For example, vitamin B_{12} and folate are involved in monoamine synthesis, and low levels can affect the efficiency of monoamine activity in the brain (Bottiglieri 1996). Several nutrients, including coenzyme Q10, lipoic acid, and acetyl-L-carnitine, also affect the efficiency of mitochondrial function (Liu 2008). Given that the brain is responsible for 10 % – 20 % of the body's total energy expenditure, adequate mitochondrial support for efficient energy production is crucial for many aspects of brain function. Minerals are also key in brain function, which should be no surprise given the success of lithium at "normalizing" mood. Adequate calcium intake is crucial for many aspects of our physiology, including cardiovascular, muscular, skeletal, and nervous system function. Related to that, and problematic in today's society, is the effect of insufficient vitamin D intake on calcium absorption through the gut and calcium transport throughout the body. This is an important consideration because emerging data indicate that vitamin D deficiency is rather widespread in the United States, making this a major current issue for public health policy. Deficiencies of other minerals, notably selenium, zinc, chromium, magnesium, and iron, have been associated with mood disorders including depression and aggressive behavior, highlighting the importance of the diet in brain function.

Today much of this is taken for granted and forgotten because of the success of public health policies and food fortifications to minimize nutrient deficiencies. However, clinical and subclinical nutrient deficiencies are still present and potentially becoming more common with recent dietary trends and should be considered by the clinician as a factor in mood disorder etiology.

Nutrition for Prevention

Our understanding of the role of nutrition in health dates back a couple of millennia. Hippocrates is quoted as having said, "Leave your drugs in the chemist's pot if you can heal the patient with food," underscoring an opinion that nutrients were of value in medical practice. In the early 1900s it was a common belief that food played a role in brain health. Dr. T.J. Ritter's (1910) popular *The People's Home Medical Book* cited "imperfect nutrition" as a cause for "temporary insanity." The current lack of focus on nutritional factors as major contributors to mental health status is a relatively new direction. The discovery of lithium as a mood stabilizer and the subsequent partial characterization of the molecular mechanisms of current antidepressants effectively withdrew focus on nutritional factors as direct contributors to mood regulation. Pharmacological studies gained momentum and contributed greatly to our understanding of the neurochemistry of mood-controlling circuits and approaches to normalize them but unfortunately diverted our attention from nutritional factors. Recent work has redirected some attention to the role of nutrients in contributing to neurochemical activity. We now know that several nutrients can alter neurotransmitter activity, including activity in monoaminergic systems, which clearly play a role in mood disorders. In a sense, research on this topic has come full circle. We started with an understanding that nutrition contributes to mood through anecdotal evidence, gained insight into the molecular nature of mood through pharmacological studies, and are now returning to the role of nutrition in controlling these molecular mechanisms.

Nutrition for Treatment

The strongest focus of recent years has been on the role of dietary omega-3 fatty acids and dietary ratio of omega-3 to omega-6 fatty acids. These two classes of fatty acids play essential and often opposing roles in several aspects of physiology. They compete with each other for incorporation into cellular membranes, including neurons, where they influence the dynamics of the microenvironment and interact with receptors to control rates of signaling and turnover. The omega-3 fatty acid DHA increases fluidity and receptor kinetics, whereas the omega-6 arachidonic acid

(AA), by competition, has an opposing effect. Omega-6 fatty acids are converted to inflammatory eicosanoids, whereas omega-3 fatty acids compete with omega-6 fatty acids for enzymatic processing to convey an antiinflammatory signal. Therefore, these two fatty acid classes must be kept in balance for optimal physiological performance. This translates to a dietary ratio of omega-3 to omega-6 fatty acids of approximately 1:4. However, today's Western diet has deviated from this ratio, which was maintained for most of human evolution, to a current ratio of approximately 1:17 in favor of omega-6 fatty acids (Simopoulos 2006). This change affects metabolism in general, including neurochemical signaling related to depression.

Animal experiments have shown that manipulating dietary omega-3 and omega-6 concentrations alters neurochemical signaling in limbic structures that control mood. Monoamine systems have proven especially sensitive to fluctuations in omega-3 dietary intake. Several studies have documented alterations in dopamine and serotonin activity in brain frontal cortex, hippocampus, striatum, and nucleus accumbens after dietary omega-3 manipulation (Acar et al. 2003; Kodas et al. 2004). To state this differently, omega-3-deficient animals have a decrease in dopamine and serotonin in frontal cortex that is reversed by omega-3 supplementation.

In humans, many observational studies connect dietary omega-3 intake to various aspects of mood and depression. In general, societies that eat more fish, the primary source of the omega-3 fatty acids eicosapentaenoic acid (EPA) and DHA, have lower rates of depression, but this does not prove causality (Hibbeln 1998). Seasonal variations in suicidal behavior correlate with fish intake (De Vriese et al. 2004) as well. In Scandinavian countries, during times of the year when fish intake is lower, violent suicides increase. In some studies, people who attempted suicide had lower blood levels of omega-3 fatty acids (Huan et al. 2004), and in other studies, people with less fish intake more frequently admitted to considering suicide (Sublette et. al. 2006). Additionally, dietary omega-3 to omega-6 ratios affect cardiovascular physiology and insulin sensitivity and thus are important factors in heart disease and diabetes. Given the co-occurrence of these metabolic disorders and depression, it behooves clinicians to consider lifestyle factors, among which omega-3 fatty acids are clearly included, that contribute to physiological and mood disorders. Clinical trials testing the efficacy of omega-3 fatty acids in treating depression are ongoing and have reported mixed results. Although larger randomized studies are still required, small studies are suggesting benefit, at least in some patient populations (Owen et al. 2008).

Other nutrient levels that have been consistently inversely correlated with depression are those of several of the B vitamins. Folic acid (also called folate or vitamin B_9) and vitamin B_{12} have been the subjects of numerous studies related to nutrition and mood regulation. Data associate low levels of vitamin B_{12} and folate in the blood with depression. Conversely, increasing folate and vitamin B_{12} seems to help treat depression (Folstein et al. 2007; Mischoulon and Raab 2007). This is likely because folate and vitamin B_{12} are involved in the synthesis of dopamine, serotonin, and norepinephrine. Low dietary intake of folate and B_{12} seem to contribute to lowering the levels of these important mood-regulating molecules. Conversely, adequate dietary intake of the B vitamins seems to normalize their levels in the brain.

Nutrition and Treatment Resistant Depression

Among nutritional approaches to TRD, folate has the most data. Patients with low folate levels (<2.5 pg/mL) preceding antidepressant treatment are significantly less likely to respond to selective serotonin reuptake inhibitors and achieve recovery (Morris et al. 2008). Furthermore, a review of clinical trials suggests that supplementation with folate in combination with antidepressant therapy significantly improves the number of patients who respond to treatment, regardless of whether they were hypofolemic at baseline (Morris et al. 2008). Even if baseline folate assays are completed and show deficiencies, folate supplementation is not always recommended, and it is probably rarely given for patients who do not have clinical deficiency. However, clinicians would do well to consider this as an adjunctive treatment, especially because of the low cost and low toxicity of folate supplementation.

Data on the use of omega-3 fatty acids as adjunctive therapy for the treatment of depression have not yet reached critical mass. However, several small studies suggest a benefit. For example, Nemets et al. (2002) showed that among depressed patients taking an antidepressant in combination with EPA supplementation, a greater number attained a reduction of 50% or more in depressive symptoms compared with those taking an antidepressant plus placebo oil. Similarly, Su et al. (2003) showed that medicated depressed patients who took a fish oil supplement had a greater reduction in symptoms than did those taking medication plus a placebo oil. The use of omega-3 fatty acids as either monotherapy or adjunctive therapy is an active area of research that should lend itself to large-scale meta-analyses and large-scale studies in emerging depression networks such as the National Network of Depression Centers (www.NNDC.org). Meanwhile, even with the preliminary nature of this research, the low side effects and low cost of omega-3 supplementation suggest it should be considered by clinicians as an augmenting approach for those with TRD and bipolar disorder. The largest drawback of omega-3 supplementation as a therapeutic tool is the time delay in possible benefits. Several weeks are required for dietary changes to be fully reflected in neuronal membrane fatty acid composition, as may be required for any effects on mood regulation.

Beyond individual nutrients, a general approach to control or influence the diet of depressed patients is likely to have beneficial effects in combination with standard therapies. A recent review raised the question of whether depression should be classified as metabolic syndrome type II (McIntyre et al. 2007). This may be an extreme suggestion, but the link between mood and physiology is becoming undeniable. Given that diet plays a primary role in insulin regulation and metabolic health, a significant role for diet in mood regulation should not be a stretch of the imagination. Patients would likely benefit from interaction with nutritional consultants as a standard component of depression therapy.

Clinical Vignette 2

Ms. J, a 40-year-old woman, has had sustained depression for several years and is approximately 20 pounds overweight but had no any other signs of metabolic problems following a blood workup. She has struggled with her mood since her mid-20s but never felt as though she needed clinical help until recently.

After a careful psychiatric evaluation, the psychiatrist decided that Ms. J was a good candidate for antidepressant therapy and recommended 30 mg/day of citalopram. After a month of treatment, Ms. J's symptoms did not seem to be responding to the medication. On further consultation, Ms. J disclosed that she had started a low-carbohydrate diet a few months ago to attempt to lose the extra weight she has been carrying around for the last decade. Until this point, Ms. J had eaten a lot of cereal and bread products, which she stopped abruptly. Ms. J also does not like many leafy-green vegetables and had never eaten these as a regular part of her diet, and she was not currently taking any vitamin supplements. Even though Ms. J did not have a positive test result for a folic acid deficiency, the psychiatrist suspected a sudden decline in folate intake caused by the removal of fortified breads and cereals from her diet and the absence of other foods high in folate. Instead of trying another antidepressant, the psychiatrist recommended that Ms. J take a daily multivitamin supplement with 400 µg of folic acid, in addition to maintaining her current antidepressant therapy. The psychiatrist also recommended that Ms. J see a nutritionist to ensure that she is obtaining the appropriate B-complex vitamins, which are involved in the synthesis and proper balance of monoamines.

After another month, Ms. J has become responsive to the treatment. The psychiatrist continues to work with Ms. J and her nutritionist to minimize the dose of antidepressants and the need for extensive pharmacotherapy.

Summary

Exercise and nutritional approaches for the treatment and prevention of depression and related disorders show considerable promise of efficacy. Although additional evidence from well-designed clinical studies is still needed, how long should clinicians wait for more data before incorporating lifestyle approaches as a primary tool in their practices? Given the general health benefits, relatively low occurrence of side effects, and low cost of these strategies, increasing physical activity and exercise along with a focus on quality nutrition appear to warrant inclusion in most treatment strategies for individuals with all depressions, and especially those with TRD and bipolar disorder.

Key Clinical Concepts

- ▮ Exercise and nutrition can have significant effects on the brain neurochemistry controlling mood behaviors.

- ▮ Exercise increases neurogenesis in the hippocampus and growth factor expression in various brain regions; these processes are also mechanisms of antidepressant action.

- ▮ Exercise improves cardiovascular tone, which relates to neurovascular health.

- ▮ Acute exercise (anaerobic) can improve mood after a single session, and extended exercise (aerobic) can reduce symptoms of depression.

- ▮ Omega-3 fatty acids, folate, and vitamin B_{12} are all involved in monoamine activity, which controls mood circuitry.

- ▮ Deficiencies of omega-3 fatty acids, folate, or vitamin B_{12} are associated with depressive syndromes and probably with Treatment Resistant Depression and bipolar disorder; supplementation can improve the success of standard medication and psychotherapy programs.

References

Acar N, Chardigny JM, Darbois M, et al: Modification of the dopaminergic neurotransmitters in striatum, frontal cortex and hippocampus of rats fed for 21 months with trans isomers of alpha-linolenic acid. Neurosci Res 45:375–382, 2003

Adachi M, Barrot M, Autry AE, et al: Selective loss of brain-derived neurotrophic factor in the dentate gyrus attenuates antidepressant efficacy. Biol Psychiatry 63:642–649, 2008

Benton D, Nabb S: Carbohydrate, memory, and mood. Nutr Rev 61:S61–S67, 2003

Berton O, Nestler EJ: New approaches to antidepressant drug discovery: beyond monoamines. Nat Rev Neurosci 7:137–151, 2006

Blumenthal JA, Babyak MA, Moore KA, et al: Effects of exercise training on older patients with major depression. Arch Intern Med 159:2349–2356, 1999

Blumenthal JA, Babyak MA, Doraiswamy PM, et al: Exercise and pharmacotherapy in the treatment of major depressive disorder. Psychosom Med 69:587–596, 2007

Bottiglieri T: Folate, vitamin B12, and neuropsychiatric disorders. Nutr Rev 54:382–390, 1996

Brosse AL, Sheets ES, Lett HS, et al: Exercise and the treatment of clinical depression in adults: recent findings and future directions. Sports Med 32:741–760, 2002

Burghardt PR, Fulk LJ, Hand GA, et al: The effects of chronic treadmill and wheel running on behavior in rats. Brain Res 1019:84–96, 2004

Carta MG, Hardoy MC, Pilu A, et al: Improving physical quality of life with group physical activity in the adjunctive treatment of major depressive disorder. Clin Pract Epidemiol Ment Health 4:1, 2008

Chalon S, Delion-Vancassel S, Belzung C, et al: Dietary fish oil affects monoaminergic neurotransmission and behavior in rats. J Nutr 128:2512–2519, 1998

Cotman CW, Berchtold NC, Christie LA: Exercise builds brain health: key roles of growth factor cascades and inflammation. Trends Neurosci 30:464–472, 2007

De Vriese SR, Christophe AB, Maes M: In humans, the seasonal variation in poly unsaturated fatty acids is related to the seasonal variation in violent suicide and serotonergic markers of violent suicide. Prostaglandins Leukot Essent Fatty Acids 71:13–18, 2004

Duman RS: Depression: a case of neuronal life and death? Biol Psychiatry 56:140–145, 2004

Dunn AL, Trivedi MH, Kampert JB, et al: Exercise treatment for depression: efficacy and dose response. Am J Prev Med 28:1–8, 2005

Evans SJ, Choudary PV, Neal CR, et al: Dysregulation of the fibroblast growth factor system in major depression. Proc Natl Acad Sci USA 101:15506–15511, 2004

Executive Summary of The Third Report of The National Cholesterol Education Program (NCEP) Expert Panel on Detection, Evaluation, And Treatment of High Blood Cholesterol In Adults (Adult Treatment Panel III). JAMA 285:2486–2497, 2001

Fernstrom JD, Fernstrom MH: Tyrosine, phenylalanine, and catecholamine synthesis and function in the brain. J Nutr 137:1539S–1547S; discussion 1548S, 2007

Folstein M, Liu T, Peter I, et al: The homocysteine hypothesis of depression. Am J Psychiatry 164:861–867, 2007

Gomez-Pinilla F, Dao L, So V: Physical exercise induces FGF-2 and its mRNA in the hippocampus. Brain Res 764:1–8, 1997

Grossfield A, Feller SE, Pitman MC: A role for direct interactions in the modulation of rhodopsin by omega-3 polyunsaturated lipids. Proc Natl Acad Sci U S A 103:4888–4893, 2006

Hibbeln JR: Fish consumption and major depression. Lancet 351:1213, 1998

Hoffman MD, Hoffman DR: Exercisers achieve greater acute exercise-induced mood enhancement than nonexercisers. Arch Phys Med Rehabil 89:358–363, 2008

Huan M, Hamazaki K, Sun Y, et al: Suicide attempt and n-3 fatty acid levels in red blood cells: a case control study in China. Biol Psychiatry 56:490–496, 2004

Kodas E, Galineau L, Bodard S, et al: Serotoninergic neurotransmission is affected by n-3 polyunsaturated fatty acids in the rat. J Neurochem 89:695–702, 2004

Lane AM, Crone-Grant D, Lane H: Mood changes following exercise. Percept Mot Skills 94:732–734, 2002

Lindwall M, Rennemark M, Halling A: Depression and exercise in elderly men and women: findings from the Swedish national study on aging and care. J Aging Phys Act 15:41–55, 2007

Liu J: The effects and mechanisms of mitochondrial nutrient alpha-lipoic acid on improving age-associated mitochondrial and cognitive dysfunction: an overview. Neurochem Res 33:194–203, 2008

Martinsen EW: Benefits of exercise for the treatment of depression. Sports Med 9:380–389, 1990

McIntyre RS, Soczynska JK, Konarski JZ, et al: Should depressive syndromes be reclassified as "metabolic syndrome type II"? Ann Clin Psychiatry 19:257–264, 2007

Mischoulon D, Raab MF: The role of folate in depression and dementia. J Clin Psychiatry 68 (suppl 10):28–33, 2007

Morris DW, Trivedi MH, Rush AJ: Folate and unipolar depression. J Altern Complement Med 14:277–285, 2008

Nemets B, Stahl Z, Belmaker RH: Addition of omega-3 fatty acid to maintenance medication treatment for recurrent unipolar depressive disorder. Am J Psychiatry 159:477–479, 2002

Owen C, Rees AM, Parker G: The role of fatty acids in the development and treatment of mood disorders. Curr Opin Psychiatry 21:19–24, 2008

Pereira AC, Huddleston DE, Brickman AM, et al: An in vivo correlate of exercise-induced neurogenesis in the adult dentate gyrus. Proc Natl Acad Sci USA 104:5638–5643, 2007

Petty KH, Davis CL, Tkacz J, et al: Exercise effects on depressive symptoms and self-worth in overweight children: a randomized controlled trial. J Pediatr Psychol 34:929–939, 2009

Pilu A, Sorba M, Hardoy MC, et al: Efficacy of physical activity in the adjunctive treatment of major depressive disorders: preliminary results. Clin Pract Epidemol Ment Health 3:8, 2007

Ritter TJ: The People's Home Medical Book. Cleveland, OH, RC Barnum, 1910

Russo-Neustadt A, Beard RC, Cotman CW: Exercise, antidepressant medications, and enhanced brain derived neurotrophic factor expression. Neuropsychopharmacology 21:679–682, 1999

Sheline YI, Wang PW, Gado MH, et al: Hippocampal atrophy in recurrent major
    depression. Proc Natl Acad Sci USA 93:3908–3913, 1996

Simopoulos AP: Evolutionary aspects of diet, the omega-6/omega-3 ratio and ge-
    netic variation: nutritional implications for chronic diseases. Biomed Phar-
    macother 60:502–507, 2006

Smith KA, Fairburn CG, Cowen PJ: Relapse of depression after rapid depletion of
    tryptophan. Lancet 349:915–919, 1997

Su KP, Huang SY, Chiu CC, et al: Omega-3 fatty acids in major depressive disorder:
    a preliminary double-blind, placebo-controlled trial. Eur Neuropsychophar-
    macol 13:267–271, 2003

Sublette ME, Hibbeln JR, Galfalvy H, et al: Omega-3 polyunsaturated essential fatty
    acid status as a predictor of future suicide risk. Am J Psychiatry 163:1100–
    1102, 2006

Turner CA, Lewis MH: Environmental enrichment: effects on stereotyped behav-
    ior and neurotrophin levels. Physiol Behav 80:259–266, 2003

van Praag H, Kempermann G, Gage FH: Running increases cell proliferation and
    neurogenesis in the adult mouse dentate gyrus. Nat Neurosci 2:266–270,
    1999

CHAPTER THIRTEEN

The Bipolar Disorder Medical Care Model

A Collaborative Approach for Reducing Disparities in Medical Care Among Patients With Bipolar Disorder

Amy M. Kilbourne, Ph.D., M.P.H.
David E. Goodrich, M.S., M.A., Ed.D.

BIPOLAR DISORDER is a chronic condition associated with substantial functional impairment and poor quality of life. Medical comorbidities, particularly cardiovascular disease (CVD) risk factors, are more common among patients with bipolar disorder than in the general population. Individuals with bipolar disorder are especially prone to the adverse effects of CVD because of behaviors and unstable treatment course stemming from the condition's cyclical nature of manic and depressive episodes and multiple medication use. These complexities can contribute to poor adherence and unstable treatment course, ultimately resulting in disparities in health outcomes. These disparities are further exacerbated by the organizational separation of physical and mental health care that inhibits coordination and communication between primary care and mental health care providers.

In this chapter, we review the current knowledge about integrated medical and psychiatric care for bipolar disorder. We then provide the rationale for the development and implementation of a collaborative care treatment model entitled the Bipolar Disorder Medical Care Model (BCM). The BCM aims to address health disparities by 1) promoting coordinated care management, 2) empowering patients to self-manage mental and physical risk factors, and 3) enhancing decision support to clinicians that promotes guideline-concordant patient care. Collaborative care models like the BCM provide clinicians and policy makers with a clear framework to implement quality improvements in organizational and patient-level processes of care. Moreover, quality improvements can be implemented in a cost-effective manner that permits customization for factors such as clinic size, resources, and patient characteristics that ensure long-term adoption of these practices.

The Need for a Bipolar Medical Treatment Model

Burden of Bipolar Disorder on the Health Care System

Bipolar disorders (I, II) are complex and chronic conditions that affect up to 5.5 % of the population and are associated with significant personal and societal costs (Bauer et al. 2002). The World Health Organization's Global Burden of Disease Report ranks bipolar disorder as the sixth most disabling health condition (Murray and Lopez 1996). This burden affects not only patients but also family, friends, and employers who feel the effect of the condition's increased risk for homelessness, incarceration, suicide, and unemployment (Hawton et al. 2005; Post 2005). Coexisting psychiatric conditions such as anxiety disorders, substance abuse disorders, and suicidal thoughts are ubiquitous (Merikangas et al. 2007; Post 2005), frequently complicating treatment and increasing health care costs (Simon and Unützer 1999). According to some estimations, bipolar disorder incurs the most health care costs of any mental illness (Peele et al. 2003; Simon and Unutzer 1999). It is estimated that 40 %–70 % of these costs may be associated with care for general medical conditions (Bryant-Comstock et al. 2002; Peele et al. 2003). Among some private health insurance plans, analyses have shown that patients with bipolar disorder generate a disproportionate percentage of health care plans' total direct medical costs (25%–40%), with up to 70% of these costs occurring in non–mental health settings such as primary care clinics (Bryant-Comstock et al. 2002; Simon and Unutzer 1999).

Risk for Excess Medical Morbidity and Mortality

The burden of general medical conditions among persons with bipolar disorder is significant, but evidence suggests that patients with the illness are particularly susceptible to CVD. CVD is the leading cause of mortality in patients with bipolar disorder (Osby et al. 2001; Roshanaei-Moghaddam and Katon 2009), with a 1.5- to 2.5-fold increase in risk for CVD mortality (Osby et al. 2001; Weeke et al. 1987). The reasons for increased CVD mortality risk are multifactorial and occur simultaneously at the patient, treatment, and organizational levels of care. The prevalence rates of diabetes, dyslipidemia, hypertension, heart disease, obesity, and obstructive sleep apnea are significantly higher among patients with bipolar disorder than among the general population (Goldstein et al. 2009b; Kilbourne et al. 2004; Sharafkhaneh et al. 2005). CVD risk appears to be similar across all of the bipolar spectrum disorders (Kilbourne et al. 2004; Kupfer 2005). However, patients with bipolar disorder are 15%–20% more likely to have CVD-related risk factors than are patients with schizophrenia (Kilbourne et al. 2007a). Onset of these CVD risk factors may occur 4–6 years earlier than in patients with major depressive disorder and up to 14 years earlier than in the general population (Goldstein et al. 2009a; Kilbourne et al. 2004), thus hastening premature mortality.

Untreated CVD morbidity in persons with bipolar disorder imposes a tremendous burden on the health care system. Greater physical impairment and symptoms are positively associated with increased depression and anxiety symptoms and can lead to reduced health-related quality of life over time (Kilbourne et al. 2009; Pirraglia et al. 2008). As persons with bipolar disorder age, their health care costs rise significantly compared with non-psychiatric populations because they increasingly use both primary and mental health services (Bartels et al. 2000; Sajatovic et al. 2004).

Increased Morbidity Due to Interaction Between Psychiatric Symptoms and Health Behaviors

Unhealthy lifestyle behaviors are modifiable risk factors that not only increase medical morbidity but also exacerbate psychiatric symptoms, leading to suboptimal mental and physical health outcomes (Fagiolini et al. 2003). Compared with other serious mental illnesses, bipolar disorder is uniquely characterized by alternating periods of manic, depressive, mixed, or euthymic episodes that may lead to impaired psychosocial functioning (Huxley and Baldessarini 2007). Impaired social contact can lead to job loss, social instability, poor medication adherence, and unstable treatment course, which increase medical comorbidity (Keck 2006) (see Table 13–1). For example, depression can decrease motivation to seek medical care when needed (Kilbourne et al. 2005). Furthermore, depressed mood not only increases production of neuroendocrine factors (i.e., glucocorticoids, catecholamines) that promote inflammation conducive to CVD progression but also may increase risk for type 2 diabetes through a behavioral pathway of physical inactivity, poor diet, and subsequent weight gain (Goldstein et al. 2009b; Kilbourne et al. 2005). Manic and premanic episodes also are associated with poor lifestyle behaviors, such as binge eating, which can contribute to obesity (Wildes et al. 2008). Manic episodes are associated with social behaviors that elevate risk for infectious diseases (e.g., hepatitis C, HIV) acquired through sexual indiscretion or illicit substance use, which have long-term consequences for medical management (el-Serag et al. 2002; Kilbourne et al. 2004).

Increased Cardiovascular Risk Due to Pharmacological Treatments

Medication side effects caused by the pharmacological treatments used to manage psychiatric symptoms further elevate the risk for CVD morbidity in patients with bipolar disorder (Newcomer 2007). Compared with patients with schizophrenia, patients with bipolar disorder are also more likely to be exposed to different classes of psychotropic medications (notably, anticonvulsants, antidepressants, and atypical antipsychotics), all of which have side effects that can lead to adverse health outcomes (Post 2005). In 2009, the International Society for Bipolar Disorder released consensus guidelines for safety monitoring to minimize adverse side effects from the treatments (Ng et al. 2009).

One impetus for these guidelines may have been the growing awareness of the adverse medical risks associated with second-generation atypical antipsychotics. It has become increasingly common for patients with bipolar disorder to be prescribed atypical antipsychotics to manage psychiatric symptoms. However, these medications may cause rapid weight gain and adverse cardiometabolic changes (i.e., dyslipidemia, hyperglycemia, and hypertension) in some patients (Newcomer 2007). Consequently, consensus guidelines were created and disseminated in 2004 by the American Diabetes Association (American Diabetes Association et al. 2004) to provide clinicians with guidance regarding how to monitor and minimize the cardiometabolic risks associated with these medications. Follow-up studies

TABLE 13–1. Behavioral health risk factors associated with changes in bipolar disorder episodes

Episode	Consequent health risk factors
Manic or premanic	Binge eating[a]
	Unstable social behavior
	Risk-taking behaviors (gambling, unprotected sexual intercourse)
	Substance abuse
	Injury
Depressive	Sedentary lifestyle
	Overeating or undereating[a]
	Suicidal ideation
	Anxiety
Psychotic	Hallucinations
	Violence or injury
	Tobacco abuse
	Need for atypical antipsychotic drugs
Euthymic	Nonadherence

[a]Weight gain related to high consumption of sweetened beverages is a dietary behavior common among patients with bipolar disorder and may be a coping strategy for dry-mouth symptoms caused by some medications.

found that fewer than half of the patients prescribed these drugs were appropriately monitored and screened for medication side effects as outlined in the guidelines (Kilbourne et al. 2007c; Morrato et al. 2009), resulting in little effect on patient health outcomes. Clinicians must weigh the benefit of these medications (i.e., improved symptom management and improved function) with their negative effects (increased CVD morbidity and mortality). However, few behavioral interventions have been developed to adequately address these risks by changing organizational behavior with respect to cardiometabolic screening, coordination of care between a patient's providers, and use of risk factor modification programs that help patients implement health-promoting lifestyle changes.

Undertreatment of General Medical Conditions Due to Fragmented Health Care

Chronic medical conditions in patients with bipolar disorder are often missed because patients are primarily seen in the mental health setting, and management of CVD risk factors most often occurs in general medical

settings (Druss and Rosenheck 2000; Kupfer 2005). In the mental health
setting, CVD or diabetes may be overlooked, in part because psychiatrists
lack the time or resources to manage these conditions in routine care (Fagiolini 2008). Moreover, recent studies that evaluated psychiatrists' compliance with the 2004 guidelines for monitoring health risks associated
with atypical antipsychotics indicate that psychiatrists are often uncertain as to who is responsible for monitoring risks, lack confidence to in-
terpret abnormal screening results, and do not believe that atypical
antipsychotics are strongly associated with metabolic risks (Fagiolini
2008). Similar studies have not been performed with primary care physicians, who often prescribe these drugs.

The societal costs of bipolar disorder often exceed those of other serious mental illnesses because individuals with bipolar illness tend to be
higher functioning, with many individuals being productive members of
society (Wells et al. 2002). Undertreated CVD-related conditions can exacerbate this problem and lead to further economic costs as a result of
missed work, preventable hospitalizations, or overuse of emergency department services (Kupfer 2005). Patients with serious mental illnesses
such as bipolar disorder also face barriers to accessing general medical
care, including lack of insurance, difficulty navigating medical care services, and dismissal of somatic complaints by medical providers (Horvitz-
Lennon et al. 2006; Wells et al. 2002). Many older patients also have
health care needs that span several locations (e.g., medicine, rehabilitation) but have trouble accessing care at these locations because of functional limitations and transportation barriers (Kilbourne et al. 2008b).

Paucity of Integrated Models in the Psychiatric Literature

Only a limited number of medical treatment models have been proposed
in the psychiatric literature to address the disparities in medical care for
patients with serious mental illness, and none were designed specifically
for bipolar disorder. One strategy to improve medical outcomes has been
to improve the coordination of patient care via existing treatment models
created for patients with serious mental illness, such as Assertive Community Treatment (ACT; Drake et al. 1998) and intensive case management (ICM; Druss et al. 2001; Quinlivan et al. 1995). However, ACT and
ICM were designed to treat substance use disorders among patients with
schizophrenia but were not intended to manage patients able to function
independently, who represent the vast majority of patients with bipolar
disorder. In addition, the high startup costs associated with hiring addi-

tional personnel to integrate ACT and ICM into routine care limit the feasibility of adapting these models to general medical settings (Horvitz-Lennon et al. 2006).

Another model of treatment has been to improve access to medical care by either co-locating medical providers in mental health settings or creating multidisciplinary treatment teams to provide comprehensive, integrated care. Although this model has the potential to be successful in large staff-model health systems (e.g., Department of Veterans Affairs, Kaiser Permanente) in which medical and psychiatric care are provided by the same health plan, this model may be too costly to implement for smaller, geographically dispersed clinics that operate within network models of care (Horvitz-Lennon et al. 2006). Without the economies of scale of a health system, these networks would find it infeasible to hire medical providers for each clinic. Alternatively, some have proposed training psychiatrists to provide general medical care for such situations (Golomb et al. 2000), yet psychiatrists often lack the time, resources, and incentives to treat their patients' medical conditions (Druss and Rosenheck 2000).

A Framework to Target Disparities in Health Care

The significant gaps in the delivery of quality medical care for patients with bipolar disorder combined with the chronic and episodic nature of the illness require a treatment model that can improve coordination and continuity of care among various health care providers. One treatment model that is ideally suited for this task is Wagner's Chronic Care Model (CCM; Wagner et al. 1996). The CCM is an evidence-based framework to guide systemic improvement in the quality of treatment that consumers receive for chronic conditions. The model has proved to be versatile and cost-effective when implemented to enhance existing services in several treatment settings and to significantly improve patient outcomes for chronic conditions such as asthma, diabetes, and major depressive disorder (Simon 2009). The CCM offers the potential to improve the quality of medical care for patients with bipolar disorder as well, because it involves organizational changes in health care delivery that transform the focus from acute care to chronic disease management and promote health care coordination and collaboration among multiple providers. The six major components of the CCM are summarized in Table 13–2.

The CCM is a particularly effective integrated care model because it combines use of nonphysician staff (i.e., care managers) to enhance communication among different providers, activate patient self-management,

TABLE 13–2. Components of the Chronic Care Model

Component	Role
Community	Mobilize community resources to meet needs of consumers
Health system	Create a culture, organization, and mechanisms that promote safe, high-quality care
Self-management support	Empower and prepare consumers to manage their health and health care
Delivery system design	Ensure the delivery of effective and efficient clinical care
Decision support	Promote clinical care that is consistent with scientific evidence and consumer preferences
Clinical information systems	Organize consumer and population data to facilitate efficient and effective care

implement evidence-based guidelines, and provide ongoing monitoring of patient status through an electronic consumer registry that does not require a sophisticated information system. The manual-based framework of the CCM also facilitates its customization and adaptability to different settings and levels of consumer care. Personnel from a variety of backgrounds (e.g., registered nurses, social workers) can implement the model's elements and track consumer progress as part of ongoing clinical care (Druss et al. 2001). A multicomponent approach is necessary because guideline dissemination alone has proven ineffective in improving quality of care or patient outcomes. Moreover, effective behavioral interventions targeting patient self-management are more likely to be sustained when supported by ongoing care management.

Preliminary Use of the Chronic Care Model for Bipolar Disorder

The CCM was eventually adapted for bipolar disorders and tested as the Bipolar Collaborative CCM, with the aim of improving psychiatric symptoms and psychosocial functioning through coordinated care. Patients in the intervention group received a patient workbook based on a modular psychoeducational curriculum for bipolar disorder entitled Life Goals (Bauer and McBride 2003). In three randomized controlled trials (RCTs) that included more than 750 consumers who had bipolar disorder diagnoses (Bauer et al. 2006b; Kilbourne et al. 2008a; Simon et al. 2005), the integrated care management program that used the Life Goals patient workbook improved functioning, quality of life, and satisfaction with care, as well as reduced affective symptom burden, compared with usual care. Moreover, Life Goals was designed and tested in settings that resembled real-world procedures and populations. Bauer and colleagues conducted the RCT of the Life Goals intervention compared with usual care across 11 Veterans Affairs sites. The RCT ($N = 306$) found that, compared with usual care, the Life Goals intervention reduced the number of consumer weeks in affective episodes, improved overall function, and improved mental health–related quality of life. Life Goals was also cost-neutral, meaning that it did not result in additional costs to the providers who implemented the model in the studies. Although the Bipolar Collaborative CCM confirmed that the CCM could be applied to improve mental health outcomes, the model did not address medical issues for patients with bipolar disorder because no linkages were established between care managers and general medical providers.

Bipolar Disorder Medical Care Model

Program Overview

The BCM was created (Kilbourne et al. 2008a) to extend the Bipolar Disorder CCM developed by Bauer et al. (2006a) and Simon et al. (2005) to reduce the risks for CVD in patients with bipolar disorder by placing greater emphasis on facilitating access to medical care and helping patients adopt healthier lifestyle habits. In a recent study, the BCM, adapted to address medical care and CVD risk, improved physical health outcomes among patients with bipolar disorder (Kilbourne et al. 2008a). The BCM is based on three core intervention components from the original CCM: patient self-management, care management, and decision support (Figure 13–1). The BCM is implemented by a care manager and involves the use of individual or group sessions, provider engagement (i.e., with each patient's primary physical and mental health providers), and innovative follow-up care contacts (Figure 13–2). It brings the patient into partnership with his or her providers by empowering self-management, improving care management, and building a decision support system for providers.

These core components are unified by a central belief that psychiatric symptoms, if not managed within the context of behavior change, can impede progress toward adopting healthier lifestyles and adhering to treatment plans (Kilbourne et al. 2008b). At the same time, the model acknowledges that health behavior change strategies need to be tailored to

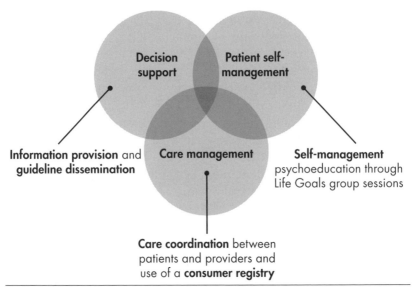

Information provision and   Care management   Self-management
guideline dissemination   psychoeducation through
                                                   Life Goals group sessions

Care coordination between
patients and providers and
use of a consumer registry

FIGURE 13–1.   Bipolar Disorder Medical Care Model.

patients within the context of waxing and waning of residual psychiatric symptoms (e.g., increased physical activity in depressed patients might improve mood). Moreover, patient self-efficacy and self-management skills are developed over time by regular contacts between the patient and the care manager that reinforce symptom control and attainment of patient-centered health behavior goals (e.g., diet, exercise, smoking cessation) (Figure 13–3).

Core Intervention Elements

Core elements are components of the BCM that are critical to the fidelity of this evidence-based intervention (Kilbourne et al. 2007b). These must be implemented and maintained to ensure the effectiveness of the intervention. In other words, core elements cannot be changed, omitted, or added to. The BCM's core elements are meant to influence the organization of care for bipolar disorder and activate consumers to collaborate with providers (see Table 13–3). Each element of the BCM is described briefly in the following subsections.

Self-Management

The BCM defines *self-management* as the belief that patients are the leaders of their treatment teams and therefore need to be knowledgeable about their illness and care. The BCM self-management program was adapted from the

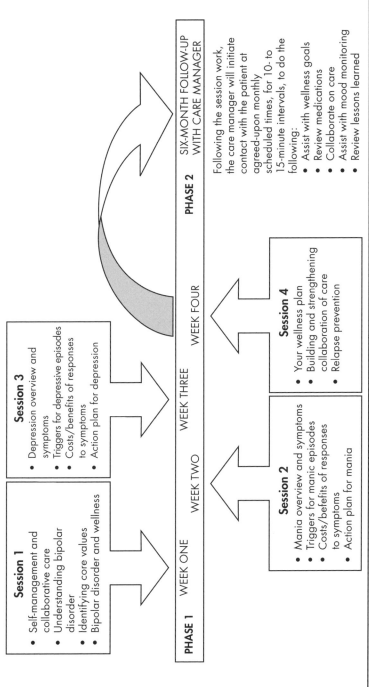

Session 1
- Self-management and collaborative care
- Understanding bipolar disorder
- Identifying core values
- Bipolar disorder and wellness

Session 3
- Depression overview and symptoms
- Triggers for depressive episodes
- Costs/benefits of responses to symptoms
- Action plan for depression

Session 2
- Mania overview and symptoms
- Triggers for manic episodes
- Costs/befefits of responses to symptoms
- Action plan for mania

Session 4
- Your wellness plan
- Building and strengthening collaboration of care
- Relapse prevention

PHASE 1

WEEK ONE   WEEK TWO   WEEK THREE   WEEK FOUR

PHASE 2

SIX-MONTH FOLLOW-UP WITH CARE MANAGER

Following the session work, the care manager will initiate contact with the patient at agreed-upon monthly scheduled times, for 10- to 15-minute intervals, to do the following:
- Assist with wellness goals
- Review medications
- Collaborate on care
- Assist with mood monitoring
- Review lessons learned

FIGURE 13–2.   Bipolar Disorder Medical Care Model: timeline and overview.

TABLE 13–3.   Summary of core intervention elements in the Bipolar Disorder Medical Care Model (BCM)

BCM domain	Core elements	Menu option examples
Patient self-management	Four group sessions Bipolar disorder facts Setting personal goals Active discussions of symptom coping strategies and management Provider engagement and communication tips	Makeup sessions—telephone or in-person Family involvement
Care management	Ongoing patient contacts to reinforce lessons from self-management and facilitate provider communication (at least one per month) Provider contacts (cues) regarding medication side effects, symptoms, or urgent health concerns Crisis management Registry tracking Community resources	Crisis intervention protocols Provider communication preferences Link to existing services and resources
Decision support	Summary information on bipolar disorder treatment and health issues (e.g., cardiometabolic risk monitoring)	Mode of delivery

Life Goals Program (Bauer and McBride 2003), a group-based psychoeducational program for bipolar disorder delivered in two phases (see Figure 13–2). The program uses an updated patient workbook featuring modules on wellness (e.g., sleep, exercise) and mental health comorbidities (e.g., anxiety, substance abuse) (Bauer et al. 2008). Phase 1 consists of convening four 2-hour group sessions led by the care manager with the aim of raising awareness of steps to manage mental and physical health conditions, activating consumer motivation for change, developing skills and knowledge to manage health conditions, and increasing self-confidence to sustain and adhere to changes. Participation in active group discussions is considered a critical element of this phase, but patients may make up sessions via one-on-one contacts as long as they attend at least one of the sessions in person. Phase 2 aims to reinforce Phase 1 lessons and to support patient personal goals through at least six monthly care manager contacts with patients. Each phase emphasizes materials tailored to bipolar disorder that address CVD risk, strategies to modify lifestyle behaviors, and tips for engaging medical providers for patients with medical issues (see Table 13–4).

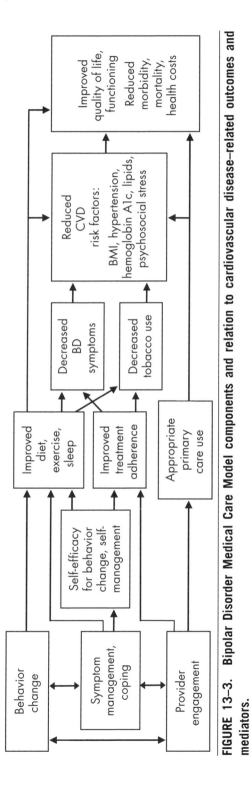

FIGURE 13–3. Bipolar Disorder Medical Care Model components and relation to cardiovascular disease–related outcomes and mediators.

BD = bipolar disorder; BMI = body mass index; CVD = cardiovascular disease.

TABLE 13–4. **Self-management topics covered in the Bipolar Disorder Medical Care Model to improve medical care and reduce cardiovascular disease risk**

Phase/Session	Wellness self-management discussion topics
Phase 1	
Session 1: Orientation	Effect of bipolar disease on health and symptoms
	Effect of stigma on health care access
	Identification of patients' collaborative health care "team"
	Awareness and cause of cardiovascular disease risk for persons with bipolar disorder
	Linking personal life goals or values to health
	"Small steps" approach to lifestyle change for better mental and physical health
Session 2: Mania	Physical health triggers for mania
	Medical and behavioral consequences of mania
	Alternative coping behaviors for mania that also reduce cardiovascular disease risk (e.g., diet, exercise, sleep, stress)
	Setting and measuring personal wellness goals
Session 3: Depression	Physical health triggers for depression
	Medical and behavioral consequences of depression
	Alternative coping behaviors for depression that also reduce medical risks
	Strategies to enhance maintenance of wellness goals (portion control, using a pedometer, contingency planning for high-risk situations)
Session 4: Goal adherence, provider engagement	Identifying barriers to wellness goals
	Coping with relapses
	Identifying and accessing community wellness resources
	Communicating and coordinating care with providers
	–Preparing for visits (list of personal concerns)
	–Understanding medical and psychiatric treatments to make informed decisions
	–Informing providers of medication side effects
	–Obtaining regular screening for cardiometabolic risks

TABLE 13–4. Self-management topics covered in the Bipolar Disorder Medical Care Model to improve medical care and reduce cardiovascular disease risk *(continued)*

Phase/Session	Wellness self-management discussion topics
Phase 2	
Follow-up contacts with care manager	Problem-solving barriers to goals and self-management
	Reinforcing shared decision making and provider engagement
	Monitoring of emergent issues and medication side effects
	Seeking help for comorbidities (e.g., smoking, substance abuse, stress, anxiety, sleep disorders)
	Providing medical information tailored to patients' context

Care Management

Care management is a core element completed by the care manager to encourage and support a collaborative relationship between patients and their providers. The care manager practices care management by educating patients on how to come prepared for medical visits with providers, monitoring both patient treatment adherence and response, and providing feedback to providers about patient progress so that any needed changes in a patient's management plan can be made in a timely manner. Care managers facilitate patient-provider communication by relaying pertinent bipolar symptom issues or co-occurring conditions (e.g., cardiometabolic symptoms, anxiety disorder) to providers. This role is expedited by using an electronic registry to track patients' clinical progress (e.g., symptoms, health outcomes) over time, with regular documentation of patient status and provider contacts. A registry helps make this information accessible and allows for more timely updates and feedback for providers.

Decision Support

Decision support aims to improve providers' knowledge about evidence-based care for persons with bipolar disorder. Care managers build a decision support system by facilitating access to bipolar disorder treatment information. The care manager effectively serves as an informationist, listening to the needs of providers and then locating and distributing the requested information. The care manager may provide information or references on health topics related to bipolar disorder, such as pregnancy or comorbid conditions, depending on the provider's needs and interests.

Evidence

To date, only one clinical trial has been published on the efficacy of the BCM (Kilbourne et al. 2008b) for improving both medical and psychiatric outcomes in bipolar patients. However, as of 2010, publication of results was expected soon from two randomized clinical trials testing the efficacy of the BCM for 1) improving physiological markers related to cardiovascular disease risk in veterans with bipolar disorder and 2) improving patient outcomes in community mental health clinics. A large multisite clinical trial was also started in 2009 to determine which implementation strategy is best to disseminate the BCM to a variety of community mental health settings that vary according to clinic size and patient sociodemographic characteristics.

Summary

Coordination of care between mental and physical health care providers is currently fragmented for individuals with bipolar disorder. Patients with bipolar disorder often receive fragmented care that results in underdiagnosis and undertreatment of preventable medical conditions. These gaps in care translate into significant disparities in medical morbidity and mortality from conditions such as cardiovascular disease. The Bipolar Disorder Medical Care Model specifically aims to reduce these medical disparities by improving processes of care that help providers remain informed of the many medical risks common to patients with bipolar disorder. The BCM also emphasizes empowering patients to take a more active role in their care by managing physical and mental health risks and by working with providers to make treatment decisions that will enhance long-term adherence and subsequent outcomes. This manual-based intervention implemented by a care manager provides a versatile approach that enables the model to be integrated into existing services in several settings more cost-effectively than are alternative treatment models. Some large multisite trials are currently testing the BCM in a variety of settings, including Department of Veterans Affairs mental health clinics and community-based mental health organizations. It is hoped that these trials will not only provide greater insight into the specific aspects of the model that provide benefit to patients and health care organizations but also shed light on ways to disseminate the program to diverse contexts without losing program fidelity or effectiveness.

Key Clinical Concepts

■ Medical comorbidities, particularly cardiovascular disease (CVD) risk factors, are more common among patients with bipolar disorder than among the general population, resulting in a tremendous burden on the health care system.

■ CVD is the leading cause of mortality among patients with bipolar disorder, with onset of diagnosed CVD risk factors occurring up to 14 years earlier than in patients without a mental health condition.

■ Individuals with bipolar disorder are especially susceptible to the adverse effects of CVD because of unhealthy lifestyle behaviors, multiple medication use, and unstable treatment course stemming from the condition's cyclical nature of manic and depressive episodes.

■ The traditional separation of physical and mental health care has exacerbated disparities in health outcomes for patients with bipolar disorder, but new models of integrated patient care are being tested that recognize the complexity of treating chronic, serious conditions by facilitating greater communication between the patient and his or her medical treatment team.

■ Collaborative care treatment models such as the Bipolar Disorder Medical Care Model (BCM) provide clinicians and policy makers with a clear framework to implement quality improvements in organizational and patient-level processes of care to address physical health disparities.

■ The BCM provides a flexible approach to improve overall patient outcomes by promoting coordinated care management, educating patients to self-manage mental and physical risk factors, and enhancing decision support to clinicians that maintains guideline-concordant patient care.

References

American Diabetes Association, American Psychiatric Association, American Association of Clinical Endocrinologists, et al: Consensus development conference on antipsychotic drugs and obesity and diabetes. Diabetes Care 27:596–601, 2004

Bartels SJ, Forester B, Miles KM, et al: Mental health service use by elderly patients with bipolar disorder and unipolar major depression. Am J Geriatr Psychiatry 8:160–166, 2000

Bauer MS, McBride L: Structured Group Psychotherapy for Bipolar Disorder: The Life Goals Program, 2nd Edition. New York, Springer, 2003

Bauer MS, Unützer J, Pincus HA, et al: Bipolar disorder. Ment Health Serv Res 4:225–229, 2002

Bauer MS, McBride L, Williford WO, et al: Collaborative care for bipolar disorder, part I: intervention and implementation in a randomized effectiveness trial. Psychiatr Serv 57:927–936, 2006a

Bauer MS, McBride L, Williford WO, et al: Collaborative care for bipolar disorder, part II: impact on clinical outcome, function, and costs. Psychiatr Serv 57:937–945, 2006b

Bauer MS, Kilbourne AM, Greenwald DE, et al: Overcoming Bipolar Disorder: A Comprehensive Workbook for Managing Your Symptoms and Achieving Your Life Goals. Oakland, CA, New Harbinger Publications, 2008

Bryant-Comstock L, Stender M, Devercelli G: Health care utilization and costs among privately insured patients with bipolar I disorder. Bipolar Disord 4:398–405, 2002

Drake RE, McHugo GJ, Clark RE, et al: Assertive community treatment for patients with co-occurring severe mental illness and substance use disorder: a clinical trial. Am J Orthopsychiatry 68:201–215, 1998

Druss BG, Rosenheck RA: Locus of mental health treatment in an integrated service system. Psychiatr Serv 51:890–892, 2000

Druss BG, Rohrbaugh RM, Levinson CM, et al: Integrated medical care for patients with serious psychiatric illness: a randomized trial. Arch Gen Psychiatry 58:861–868, 2001

el-Serag HB, Kunik M, Richardson P, et al: Psychiatric disorders among veterans with hepatitis C infection. Gastroenterology 123:476–482, 2002

Fagiolini A: Overcoming hurdles to achieving good physical health in patients treated with atypical antipsychotics. Eur Neuropsychopharmacol 18 (suppl 2): S102–S107, 2008

Fagiolini A, Kupfer DJ, Houck PR, et al: Obesity as a correlate of outcome in patients with bipolar I disorder. Am J Psychiatry 160:112–117, 2003

Goldstein BI, Fagiolini A, Houck P, et al: Cardiovascular disease and hypertension among adults with bipolar I disorder in the United States. Bipolar Disord 11:657–662, 2009a

Goldstein BI, Kemp DE, Soczynska JK, et al: Inflammation and the phenomenology, pathophysiology, comorbidity, and treatment of bipolar disorder: a systematic review of the literature. J Clin Psychiatry 70:1078–1090, 2009b

Golomb BA, Pyne JM, Wright B, et al: The role of psychiatrists in primary care of patients with severe mental illness. Psychiatr Serv 51:766–773, 2000

Hawton K, Sutton L, Haw C, et al: Suicide and attempted suicide in bipolar disorder: a systematic review of risk factors. J Clin Psychiatry 66:693–704, 2005

Horvitz-Lennon M, Kilbourne AM, Pincus HA: From silos to bridges: meeting the general health care needs of adults with severe mental illnesses. Health Aff (Millwood) 25:659–669, 2006

Huxley N, Baldessarini RJ: Disability and its treatment in bipolar disorder patients. Bipolar Disord 9:183–196, 2007

Keck PE: Long-term management strategies to achieve optimal function in patients with bipolar disorder. J Clin Psychiatry 67:E17, 2006

Kilbourne AM, Cornelius JR, Han X, et al: Burden of general medical conditions among individuals with bipolar disorder. Bipolar Disord 6:368–373, 2004

Kilbourne AM, Reynolds CF 3rd, Good CB, et al: How does depression influence diabetes medication adherence in older patients? Am J Geriatr Psychiatry 13:202–210, 2005

Kilbourne AM, Brar JS, Drayer RA, et al: Cardiovascular disease and metabolic risk factors in male patients with schizophrenia, schizoaffective disorder, and bipolar disorder. Psychosomatics 48:412–417, 2007a

Kilbourne AM, Neumann MS, Pincus HA, et al: Implementing evidence-based interventions in health care: application of the replicating effective programs framework. Implement Sci 2:42, 2007b

Kilbourne AM, Post EP, Bauer MS, et al: Therapeutic drug and cardiovascular disease risk monitoring in patients with bipolar disorder. J Affect Disord 102:145–151, 2007c

Kilbourne AM, Post EP, Nossek A, et al: Improving medical and psychiatric outcomes among individuals with bipolar disorder: a randomized controlled trial. Psychiatr Serv 59:760–768, 2008a

Kilbourne AM, Post EP, Nossek A, et al: Service delivery in older patients with bipolar disorder: a review and development of a medical care model. Bipolar Disord 10:672–683, 2008b

Kilbourne AM, Perron BE, Mezuk B, et al: Co-occurring conditions and health-related quality of life in patients with bipolar disorder. Psychosom Med 71:894–900, 2009

Kupfer DJ: The increasing medical burden in bipolar disorder. JAMA 293:2528–2530, 2005

Merikangas KR, Akiskal HS, Angst J, et al: Lifetime and 12-month prevalence of bipolar spectrum disorder in the National Comorbidity Survey replication. Arch Gen Psychiatry 64:543–552, 2007

Morrato EH, Newcomer JW, Kamat S, et al: Metabolic screening after the American Diabetes Association's consensus statement on antipsychotic drugs and diabetes. Diabetes Care 32:1037–1042, 2009

Murray CJ, Lopez AD: Evidence-based health policy—lessons from the Global Burden of Disease Study. Science 274:740–743, 1996

Newcomer JW: Antipsychotic medications: metabolic and cardiovascular risk. J Clin Psychiatry 68 (suppl 4):8–13, 2007

Ng F, Mammen OK, Wilting I, et al: The International Society for Bipolar Disorders (ISBD) consensus guidelines for the safety monitoring of bipolar disorder treatments. Bipolar Disord 11:559–595, 2009

Osby U, Brandt L, Correia N, et al: Excess mortality in bipolar and unipolar disorder in Sweden. Arch Gen Psychiatry 58:844–850, 2001

Peele PB, Xu Y, Kupfer DJ: Insurance expenditures on bipolar disorder: clinical and parity implications. Am J Psychiatry 160:1286–1290, 2003

Pirraglia PA, Biswas K, Kilbourne AM, et al: A prospective study of the impact of comorbid medical disease on bipolar disorder outcomes. J Affect Disord 115:355–359, 2008

Post RM: The impact of bipolar depression. J Clin Psychiatry 66 (suppl 5):5–10, 2005

Quinlivan R, Hough R, Crowell A, et al: Service utilization and costs of care for severely mentally ill clients in an intensive case management program. Psychiatr Serv 46:365–371, 1995

Roshanaei-Moghaddam B, Katon W: Premature mortality from general medical illnesses among persons with bipolar disorder: a review. Psychiatr Serv 60:147–156, 2009

Sajatovic M, Blow FC, Ignacio RV, et al: Age-related modifiers of clinical presentation and health service use among veterans with bipolar disorder. Psychiatr Serv 55:1014–1021, 2004

Sharafkhaneh A, Giray N, Richardson P, et al: Association of psychiatric disorders and sleep apnea in a large cohort. Sleep 28:1405–1411, 2005

Simon G: Collaborative care for mood disorders. Curr Opin Psychiatry 22:37–41, 2009

Simon GE, Unützer J: Health care utilization and costs among patients treated for bipolar disorder in an insured population. Psychiatr Serv 50:1303–1308, 1999

Simon GE, Ludman EJ, Unützer J, et al: Randomized trial of a population-based care program for people with bipolar disorder. Psychol Med 35:13–24, 2005

Wagner EH, Austin BT, Von Korff M: Organizing care for patients with chronic illness. Milbank Q 74:511–544, 1996

Weeke A, Juel K, Vaeth M: Cardiovascular death and manic-depressive psychosis. J Affect Disord 13:287–292, 1987

Wells KB, Miranda J, Bauer MS, et al: Overcoming barriers to reducing the burden of affective disorders. Biol Psychiatry 52:655–675, 2002

Wildes JE, Marcus MD, Fagiolini A: Prevalence and correlates of eating disorder co-morbidity in patients with bipolar disorder. Psychiatry Res 161:51–58, 2008

CHAPTER FOURTEEN

Expanding Services for Patients With Treatment Resistant Depression

The Role of Peer Support

Kathryn Roeder, B.S.
Jamie Travis, B.A.
Heather Walters, M.S.
Claire Stano, M.A.
Marcia Valenstein, M.D., M.S.
Paul Pfeiffer, M.D., M.S.

PATIENTS WITH DEPRESSION that resists treatment may need proactive, frequent, and supportive contacts to remain in treatment and maintain the motivation and skills necessary to manage their symptoms, increase functional capacity, and achieve valued life goals. Between 1987 and 1997, the prevalence of depression treatment increased threefold in the United States; however, treated patients were less likely to receive psychotherapy, and the average number of visits per user declined (Olfson

273

et al. 2002). One way to supply frequent supportive contacts for patients coping with longer-term depressive symptoms is the provision of peer support services. Peer support services bring together nonprofessionals with similar stressors or health problems for the purpose of providing mutual support. Supportive peer interactions can occur at varying frequencies, take place through a variety of modalities, and supplement existing evidence-based health services.

Two conceptual frameworks, the Chronic Care Model and the Recovery Model, provide a basis for developing peer support programs for patients with chronic depression. The Chronic Care Model emphasizes a systematic, organized, and proactive approach to the treatment and management of chronic medical conditions. Supporting patients' self-management skills, often through care management or supportive peer relationships, is an essential element of this model (Wagner et al. 2001a). Collaborative care strategies that incorporate several elements of the Chronic Care Model have been shown to improve the outcomes of depressed patients in primary care (Katon et al. 1997, 1999).

The Recovery Model is also relevant in developing interventions for patients with continuing depressive symptoms. The Substance Abuse and Mental Health Services Administration (SAMHSA) National Consensus Statement on recovery included peer support as one of the fundamental components of recovery-oriented services. Other components of recovery-oriented services related to peer support include self-direction in defining and reaching life goals; individualized and person-centered services; empowerment; and responsibility of consumers for their own self-care and recovery (Substance Abuse and Mental Health Services Administration 2006). These recovery principles have been most often applied to persons with serious mental illness; however, they are clearly relevant to patients with longer-term depressive symptoms.

Peer support programs for patients with chronic depression or Treatment Resistant Depression (TRD) have the potential to fulfill several elements of the Chronic Care and Recovery Models. Peer support services vary widely in structure, but all programs are rooted in the idea that individuals with similar health problems or stressors can come together to support one another effectively and promote healthy coping strategies. The collaborative, supportive nature of such programs can foster a sense of community, empowerment, and self-determination; provide a forum for the sharing of knowledge and skills, as recommended by the SAMHSA Recovery Model; and encourage self-management behaviors, in accordance with the Chronic Care Model. The following clinical vignettes, taken from a pilot study of a mutual peer support program, illustrate how these concepts may function for patients with continuing depression.

The following case illustrates the potential of mutual support programs to facilitate supportive, lasting relationships and the advantages these relationships provide to augment standard depression treatment.

Clinical Vignette 1

Two women receiving treatment at a university depression clinic participated in a telephone-based mutual support program.

Ms. H, a 52-year-old married woman, has a long-standing history of major depression and dysthymia. She reported a history of childhood physical abuse and sexual assault as a young adult, as well as significant stress related to her son's severe behavior problems. For the past decade, she had received sporadic treatment for depression with little success, including several antidepressant trials that were discontinued because of side effects. Ms. H continued to have experience depressive symptoms and received individual cognitive-behavioral therapy at a university depression clinic.

Ms. E, a 54-year-old married woman, reported difficulties with depression and mood stability that had been present for much of her adult life. These difficulties included depressive episodes with mixed or manic features, two of which resulted in psychiatric hospitalization. At age 48, she began to experience seizures and short-term memory difficulties and subsequently received valproic acid. Around the same time, her depressive symptoms worsened and she began taking venlafaxine, which was later augmented with lithium. For the past 2 years, Ms. E has received individual psychotherapy in addition to medication management at a university depression clinic.

Both Ms. H and Ms. E were mothers of teenagers, were not currently employed outside the home, and reported mild to moderate depressive symptoms at baseline. The program staff paired Ms. H and Ms. E because of these similarities in demographic variables and treatment history.

During the beginning weeks of their mutual support work, both Ms. H and Ms. E disclosed that they were mothers of adopted children. This shared experience served to form an immediate connection between the two participants, and the pair went on to talk several times per week for the duration of the 12-week program. Both patients greatly appreciated the opportunity to speak with someone who understood both the difficulties of depression and the challenges of adoptive parenting. The pair seemed to develop a strong, supportive bond and even referred to each other as "husbands who listen." At the end of the 12-week program, neither participant reported clinical levels of depression, and both reported increased motivation to engage in daily mood management activities.

The following case illustrates some of the potential barriers to successful peer support interactions.

Clinical Vignette 2

Two male veterans receiving mental health treatment at a Midwestern Department of Veterans Affairs (VA) facility participated in a 12-week telephone-based mutual support program.

Mr. B, a 61-year-old unemployed divorced veteran, regularly attended a depression treatment group at the VA mental health clinic. He had been in and out of psychiatric care for primarily depressive symptoms since receiving the diagnosis of bipolar II disorder at age 14. Mr. B decided to participate in a mutual support program because he appreciated the value of the social support he had received while attending his depression treatment group and wanted to help someone else in a similar manner.

Mr. J, a 56-year-old single disabled veteran with major depressive disorder, lived with his sister, with whom he had a supportive yet sometimes tumultuous relationship. Mr. J was wheelchair bound and usually left his home only to come to VA appointments. His psychiatrist had recommended that he participate in the peer support program to combat his increasing social isolation.

Mr. B and Mr. J were paired together by the program staff because of similar demographics and treatment history. Although both participants had experienced chronic depression, Mr. B had difficulty finding common ground with Mr. J. Mr. J was dealing with chronic pain in addition to depression, whereas Mr. B was recovering from substance dependence. The two had discussed Mr. J's chronic pain in detail; however, Mr. B had never experienced chronic pain and therefore felt that he would never be able to truly understand Mr. J's feelings. Mr. B struggled to find ways to support Mr. J and questioned further participation in the program because he saw their problems as being very different.

Program staff worked with the pair and emphasized that they could provide meaningful support to each other by listening attentively and providing empathy, even when one person did not have personal experience with a specific problem. Additionally, Mr. B and Mr. J were encouraged to use part of their conversation time to discuss steps each person could take to work toward personal goals and to keep each other accountable regarding the completion of each step.

With encouragement, Mr. B was eventually able to help Mr. J open up and even relied on Mr. J when he was dealing with a difficult situation and needed advice. Mr. J, previously isolated at home much of the time, began to schedule time each week to leave his house and find a quiet location from which he could phone Mr. B. By the end of the program, only modest gains were made in improving either participant's depression symptoms; however, both Mr. B and Mr. J reported an improved sense of social connectedness and valued their participation in the program.

What Is Peer Support?

By definition, *peer support services* bring together individuals with similar stressors or health problems for the purpose of providing additional support, but these programs can vary widely in structure and can involve a wide range of modalities. Peer support participants may assume a variety of roles, including educator, mentor, mentee, or reciprocal peer (both a provider and

TABLE 14–1. Variations in the provision of peer support

Structural component	Variations
Persons involved	Peers only
	Peers and professional staff
	Peers and paraprofessionals
Degree of professional involvement	None
	Modest involvement, mostly facilitating peer interactions
	Major role in structuring and moderating peer interactions
Relationships of peers	Reciprocal • Peers are givers and receivers of support
	Peer mentor • A designated peer primarily "gives support" and serves as a positive role model
	Peer staff • A designated peer is a full member of mental health staff
Content/focus of interactions	Expressive or supportive
	Psychoeducational
	Skill- or task-oriented
	Psychotherapeutic
Degree of connection to health system	No connection; operate in parallel
	Modest cooperation
	Extensive cooperation between health system and peer support efforts (partnership model)
Mode of interaction	In-person (dyadic or group)
	Telephone (usually dyadic)
	Internet (usually group)
Other logistics	Frequency of interactions
	Duration of interactions
	Flexibility of interactions

a recipient of support). The frequency, structure, and scope of peer support contacts can differ, and interventions can take place independently or in conjunction with current evidence-based treatments. Programs can include in-person, telephone-based, or Internet-based peer interactions, and these interactions may or may not be facilitated by professional staff. The structural variation in peer support interventions is outlined in Table 14–1.

Peer support interventions generally follow one of the following models: mutual self-help, professional treatment, mentor or paraprofessional, or reciprocal.

Mutual Self-Help Groups

Mutual self-help refers to an organized process in which "individuals who share a common condition or interest assist themselves rather than relying exclusively on the assistance of professionalized others" (van Tosh and del Vecchio 2000, p. 4). Mutual self-help groups are often voluntary gatherings of people with the same health condition. Such groups are typically led by peers who are currently living with the chronic illness. In these settings, peers share their experiences of managing their illness, navigating the health care system, and working with health care providers. These groups provide the opportunity for members to develop friendships and build social networks, both of which are important to the well-being of individuals with depression (Kilpatrick et al. 2007; Mofidi et al. 2007; Sacco and Yanover 2006).

Professional Treatment Groups

Professional treatment groups bring together patients who share a common health condition in a group setting moderated by professional health care providers. During group visits, professional care providers facilitate group discussion on specific topics related to the medical illness or self-care management skills. The facilitators then ask participants to discuss issues they are facing related to the topic. This process allows patients to receive support from their peers while also sharing their experiences and offering support to other group members. Professional treatment groups give patients additional contacts with health care providers without greatly increasing the workload of the provider (Trento et al. 2001).

Peer Mentor or Paraprofessional

Peer mentors or paraprofessionals are patients who have made significant progress toward recovery and are working to assist other people with their recovery. Some peers may have training that is part of a certification program, whereas others may not. Peer mentors provide flexible services that are personalized to the needs of the individual and that allow the peer mentor to act as a role model for recovery. Such mentors can share effective coping strategies and self-management skills learned during their own recovery processes. Peer mentors can also teach others how to incorporate treatment recommendations into their daily routines and can draw on their own experiences to help others address resistance, fears, and uncertainties.

Reciprocal Peer Interactions

Reciprocal peer support programs pair two or more individuals who have made similar progress toward recovery. Because both peers have personal experience with the same health condition, the reciprocal model incorporates many aspects of the mentorship model, such as the opportunity to share coping strategies and self-management skills. Unlike mentorship programs, reciprocal support programs provide an arena in which participants can both provide and receive support. The opportunity to provide support may be especially pertinent to patients with depression, because studies suggest that contributing to the welfare of others may be associated with improved well-being, decreased depressive symptoms, and improved quality of life (Krause and Shaw 2000; Krause et al. 1992; Musick et al. 1999; Schwartz and Sendor 1999; van Willigen 2000; Wheeler et al. 1998).

Existing Peer Support Organizations

The various forms of peer support have a long history in mental health and substance abuse treatment. One of the most commonly used mutual self-help groups is the substance abuse recovery program Alcoholics Anonymous (AA). Founded in 1935, AA is a self-help group designed to help individuals in alcohol recovery maintain sobriety through its emphasis on spirituality, social support, and its progressive 12 steps (Groh et al. 2008). Similar to other peer support groups, AA is run by members, rather than professionals, and is often used in conjunction with clinical treatments.

GROW is an international mutual self-help organization founded by former psychiatric patients in the 1950s. The founders were inspired by the techniques used by AA. Like AA, GROW is peer-directed and uses a 12-step framework (Rappaport et al. 1985). GROW's treatment materials were developed as members recorded what helped them manage or overcome their problems. Meetings are structured around a form of "layman's cognitive-behavioral therapy," which uses nontechnical language to frame cognitive-behavioral therapy strategies. In addition to attending formal meetings, members are encouraged to network with one another by telephone and to participate in training and social activities as a means of enhancing social and communication skills (Finn et al. 2007).

Another mutual help group, Recovery International (formerly Recovery, Inc.), was founded by psychiatrist Abraham Low in 1937 and has been member-managed since the 1950s. Low's Recovery International method involves techniques similar to cognitive-behavioral therapy principles. In meetings, members learn to "identify self-defeating illness-promoting thoughts and impulses and counter them with self-endorsing thoughts and wellness-promoting actions" (Murray 1996, p. 1378). Recovery International is intended to serve as an adjunct to traditional mental health treatments such as psychotherapy and medication. Groups are lead by trained volunteers who have personally experienced emotional problems and used the Recovery International method of self-help.

Like Recovery International, the Depression and Bipolar Support Alliance (DBSA; formerly National Depressive and Manic-Depressive Association) is a patient-directed mutual help organization intended to be an adjunct to traditional mental health treatment (Depression and Bipolar Support Alliance 2008). DBSA's mission is to provide hope, help, and support to improve the lives of people living with depression and bipolar disorder through the provision of peer-based, recovery-oriented, empowering services and resources. Mutual help groups are led by trained and certified peer specialists who have personal experience with depression and/or bipolar disorder. The specific selection of services offered varies across chapters according to members' needs; however, most groups follow a "share and care" format, in which all members are encouraged to participate (Depression and Bipolar Support Alliance 2008).

How Peer Support Might Benefit Patients: Conceptual Models

Several conceptual models exist to explain how mutual support programs might function to produce positive outcomes for mental health patients, including those with chronic depression or TRD. In a concept analysis of peer support within a health care context, Dennis (2003b) described three overlapping models of the salutary effects of peer support: direct effects, buffering effects, and mediating effects.

In the direct effects model, Dennis posited that peer support could influence health outcomes by enhancing social integration and reducing feelings of isolation, both of which are directly related to negative affect and symptoms of depression. Additionally, peer support interactions can directly benefit patients by encouraging appropriate help-seeking behaviors, providing additional sources of health information, and increasing motivation for self-care (Dennis 2003b).

Peer support programs also have the potential to benefit depressed patients indirectly. According to the buffering effects model, peer support can protect patients from some of the deleterious effects of stressful life events (Dennis 2003b). Peer support participants have more opportunities to reassess initial appraisals of major stressors and engage in problem-solving techniques, which could limit the depressogenic effects of stressful events.

In the mediating effects model, Dennis (2003b) proposed that peer support can indirectly influence health through its effects on cognitive, emotional, and/or behavioral processes. For example, successful social interactions in the context of peer support can bolster self-efficacy, reinforce positive social behaviors, provide positive role modeling, and encourage cognitive restructuring. Such indirect pathways have the potential to influence the individual experience of depression.

Other authors have proposed additional models to explain how peer support may benefit patients with depression. As mentioned earlier, contributing to the welfare of others, in addition to receiving support, is associated with improved psychological well-being (Maton 1988; Riessman 1965; Roberts et al. 1999). Reciprocal peer support programs may benefit depressed patients by giving them the opportunity to help others and experience the resulting feelings of competence, independence, and increased social value. In a similar vein, Rogers and colleagues (2007) posited that peer support programs allow patients to play a more active role in their self-care and that this sense of empowerment may decrease symptoms of depression. Yalom (2005) presented an additional model and hypothesized that nonprofessional peer support may provide many of the elements central to symptom improvement in formal group psychotherapy, such as opportunities for emotional catharsis and the mobilization of feelings such as hope and cohesiveness.

Figure 14–1 summarizes the mechanisms through which peer support may enhance important outcomes for patients with depressive disorders.

Effect of Peer Support on Mental Health Outcomes

Encouragement for the use of mutual peer support programs has grown in recent years. Peer support initiatives have been recommended specifically by the President's New Freedom Commission on Mental Health (2003) and may be one way to provide frequent, supportive contacts to individuals with depression. Numerous studies have documented the relations between social support and better outcomes among patients with a variety of medical conditions, including depressive disorders, and social support has been shown to buffer individuals against the development of depression when facing severe stressors (Kilpatrick et al. 2007; Mofidi et al. 2007; Musick and Wilson 2003; Sacco and Yanover 2006). Additionally, several observational studies reported that providing social support to others is associated with improvements in health that are comparable to or even greater than those associated with receiving support. Individuals who provide social support through volunteering experience less depression and improved quality of life (Krause and Shaw 2000; Krause et al. 1992; Musick et al. 1999; Schwartz and Sendor 1999; van Willigen 2000; Wheeler et al. 1998). These findings suggest that increased social support for patients with depression, especially in the form of mutual self-help programs, may be important to recovery from depressive episodes and ongoing relapse prevention.

There is also a growing literature on the efficacy of bringing patients with the same chronic medical conditions and self-management challenges together for interactive group visits. These interventions have led to improved outcomes in chronic medical conditions and improved self-efficacy and satisfaction (Clancy et al. 2003; Lorig et al. 2001a, 2001b; Trento et al. 2001; Wagner et al. 2001b). Although many of these groups are facilitated by professionals, much peer-to-peer interaction occurs in the context of these groups. These professionally led groups also have given rise to peer-led self-help groups that incorporate many of the same self-management principles used in the professionally led groups.

Several studies indicate that participation in peer support organizations is associated with positive health outcomes. Past correlational meta-analyses have found links between AA participation and positive drinking outcomes, as well as modest relations with better psychological health, social functioning, employment, and legal status (Emrick et al. 1993; Tonigan et al. 1996). Studies have shown that involvement in AA is associated with sustaining a consistent number of friendships through the recovery process, larger friendship networks, and higher friendship quality (Humphreys 1999; Humphreys and Noke 1997; Humphreys and Rappaport 1994). Like studies of other mutual help groups, studies of AA suggest that both the receipt and the provision of help within the program can aid in recovery (Galanter 1988; Sheeren 1988).

Research on participation in formal mutual self-help groups for individuals with mental health conditions also has yielded encouraging results. In a controlled study, Galanter (1988) found that membership in Recovery International was associated with decreased distress over time. Several studies suggested that involvement with a peer support group is associated with increased psychological well-being (Finn et al. 2007; Galanter 1988; Raiff 1982) and improved coping (Depression and Bipolar Support Alliance 2008; Finn et al. 2007; Kurtz 1988; Raiff 1982). Participation in mutual help groups may have a protective effect; studies of members of DBSA and GROW found that patients were less likely to be

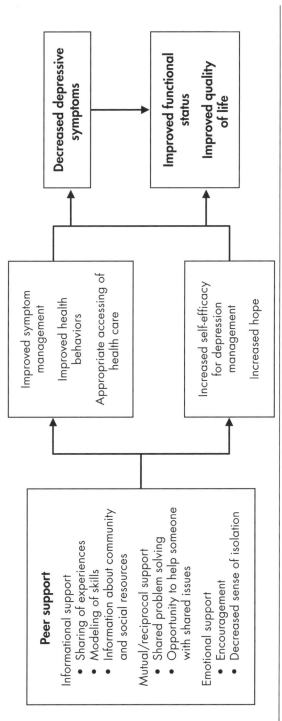

FIGURE 14–1. Proposed mechanisms of action for peer support.

hospitalized for psychiatric reasons after participating in those groups (Depression and Bipolar Support Alliance 2008; Finn et al. 2007). Additional research suggested that Recovery International and DBSA are successful in their goal to serve as a positive adjunct to traditional mental health treatments; patients report more consistent treatment adherence and medication use after receiving mutual self-help (Depression and Bipolar Support Alliance 2008; Kurtz 1988). In addition, Finn et al. (2007) found that greater length and extent of involvement in GROW activities were associated with improved self-esteem and autonomy.

These data indicate that patients who participate in peer support organizations for a range of mental health and substance use concerns sustain improvements in general well-being and quality of life. Although significantly fewer studies have systematically investigated the effect of peer support on depressive disorders, the existing literature indicates that mutual peer support interventions may have a positive effect on depressive symptoms and social support.

In a systematic review of the literature on mutual peer support interventions for patients with depression, 10 of 11 studies showed improvement in depressive symptoms following a peer support intervention (Bright et al. 1999; Chen et al. 2000; Dennis 2003a; Evans and Connis 1995; Fleming et al. 1992; Hunkeler et al. 2000; Kelly et al. 1993; Ludman et al. 2007; Onozawa et al. 2001; Verduyn et al. 2003). Of the 7 studies that compared peer support alone (i.e., without care management from a professional) with a no-intervention control condition, 4 showed statistically superior improvements in depression with the peer support intervention (Chen et al. 2000; Dennis 2003a; Evans and Connis 1995; Kelly et al. 1993). Four of the 11 studies reviewed compared peer support groups to group cognitive-behavioral therapy. Three of these 4 studies found peer support to be as effective as group cognitive-behavioral therapy in improving depression symptoms, although one study showed a specialized group cognitive-behavioral therapy designed specifically for women to be superior to a peer support group (Maynard 1993).

These results, although not conclusive, suggest that the efficacy of peer support in reducing depressive symptoms may be on par with other current psychosocial treatment options. Importantly, these findings also alleviate concerns that loosely controlled interactions between depressed individuals might result in reinforced hopelessness or negative self-image and thereby worsen depression; currently, no evidence suggests that this happens in practice. Further research is warranted, but these preliminary findings indicate that mutual support programs may represent a safe, efficacious way to provide additional support to patients with ongoing depression.

Other Advantages of Peer Support

In addition to having positive effects on mental health outcomes, mutual support services can contribute importantly to depression treatment within existing health care systems by addressing the key elements of access to health care—affordability, acceptability, accommodation, and availability (Penchansky and Thomas 1981).

Affordability

Cost of treatment is a significant barrier to the use of current mental health services (McCarthy et al. 2007; Simon et al. 1996; Steele et al. 2007). As suggested by the Chronic Care Model, patients with chronic health conditions, including TRD, may need frequent, ongoing support to maintain necessary self-management skills. However, many insurance policies limit the number of covered mental health visits. Additionally, patients with TRD are more likely to experience job loss and financial stressors, which may further limit their ability to access ongoing treatment (Amital et al. 2008). Volunteer-based peer support programs represent a promising adjunct to standard clinical treatment for patients with TRD because they can provide patients with additional supportive interactions to promote recovery without exacerbating financial difficulties.

Peer support programs are likely to be affordable for the health care system as well. Initial costs for peer support programs tend to be minimal. Peer support interventions examined in prior studies often included training elements such as role-playing, sharing of coping skills, providing emotional support, and knowing when to refer to professional services. In some cases, this training was delivered in as little as 4 hours. The success of these studies suggests that brief training can effectively prepare volunteers to provide meaningful mutual support, without requiring substantial additional effort on the part of professional staff (Dennis 2003a; Hunkeler et al. 2000).

The maintenance of peer support services is also inherently low cost because such programs rely on the voluntary efforts of nonprofessionals. Because patients also act as service providers in peer support interventions, the ability to scale services is increased, even among larger clinical populations. By facilitating peer support interventions, health care systems have the potential to expand their reach without overtaxing existing resources (Glasgow et al. 2001).

Acceptability

The extension of peer support services into depression treatments is also likely to be acceptable to many patients: approximately 25 million Americans already have used some form of a self-help group outside of the professional mental health community (Kessler 1997). The acceptability of peer support services may have pronounced benefits among individuals who are reluctant to seek formal mental health services because of fear of stigma. Such patients might feel comfortable engaging in more anonymous peer support programs, which can act as a "bridge" to the formal mental health care network. In these situations, promoting peer support services in addition to existing mental health services can facilitate the eventual engagement of traditionally underserved populations into more comprehensive mental health care.

Accommodation and Availability

As discussed earlier, patients with chronic depression likely need proactive, frequent, and supportive contacts to maintain the motivation and skills necessary to best manage their symptoms, increase their functional capacity, and maintain a focus on valued life goals. An innate benefit of peer support interventions is the increased access to social and psychological support. Although it is not feasible for professionals to provide daily, off-hours support for their entire caseloads, mutual support partners can be available between mental health visits for as-needed support. The additional interactions provided by peer support programs can supplement existing mental health services and reinforce self-management skills between formal clinic visits.

As previously discussed, peer support interventions can be delivered in a variety of models with the ability to reach different populations. The current mental health system is not meeting the needs of a large portion of patients (Rush et al. 2006), and several programs have turned to telephone- or Internet-based mutual support services to address this service gap and expand the range of treatment options. Pilot studies of supplemental telephone- or Internet-based support for patients with chronic health conditions have reported positive results, with participants reporting high levels of satisfaction, increased motivation for self-management, and improved self-confidence (Heisler et al. 2005; Zrebiec 2005).

Such programs also might be effective in reaching subsets of the depressed population who have fewer opportunities for face-to-face contacts with mental health clinicians. For example, rural, low-income, or physically disabled populations with depression may be unable to participate in frequent, in-person clinic visits. In these cases, telephone- or Internet-based peer support programs can provide supportive contacts and encourage self-management skills between clinic appointments.

Future Directions

The President's New Freedom Commission on Mental Health advocates re-aligning mental health care to be recovery-oriented and to engage consumers at various levels of service delivery. Peer support services are consistent with those goals, and several theoretical frameworks and preliminary studies support the use of peer support services among patients with depression. However, the systematic implementation and evaluation of such services among patients with depression is limited by a lack of large, well-controlled studies in this treatment population. To maximize the potential benefits of mutual support programs, significant advances will be required to determine the efficacy and optimal delivery of these services.

Most important, larger studies must determine overall efficacy of peer support interventions for patients with TRD, as well as predictors of individual response. Additionally, future trials of peer support programs should consider whether group interventions or peer partnerships are more effective and whether peer support is best delivered in person, over the telephone, or via the Internet. Such research is crucial to understanding the mechanisms by which peer support may improve symptom outcomes.

Future research also must investigate the successful integration of peer support programs into traditional mental health care. This integration of professional and peer-led services is common in substance dependence treatment, in which participation in peer programs (i.e., 12-step programs) is a common component of formal treatment. However, this approach is not yet common in depression treatment; indeed, one survey found that only one-third of psychiatrists discussed self-help groups with their mood disorder patients (Powell et al. 2000). More research is needed to determine how peer support programs can be developed and successfully integrated into existing mental health care networks. Such research will optimally lead to a standardization of peer support service development and operation to ease dissemination and adoption.

Key Clinical Concepts

■ Peer support services bring together nonprofessionals with similar stressors or health problems for the purpose of providing mutual support.

■ A growing body of literature suggests that participation in peer-based organizations (e.g., Alcoholics Anonymous, Depression and

Bipolar Support Alliance) or mutual self-help groups for patients with chronic health conditions can lead to improved health outcomes and increased self-efficacy.

■ Less is known about the effect of such groups on psychiatric conditions, but preliminary evidence suggests that participation in a mutual support intervention may be associated with improvement in depressive symptoms among mental health patients.

■ Peer support services confer additional advantages because such programs are likely to be acceptable to and affordable for patients, cost-effective for the health care system, and capable of providing expanded services to underserved populations.

■ Peer support programs may represent an efficacious adjunct to standard clinical treatment for patients with continuing depressive symptoms. However, future research, especially in the form of large, controlled studies, is needed to maximize the benefits and facilitate the implementation of peer support programs.

References

Amital D, Fostick L, Silberman A, et al: Serious life events among resistant and non-resistant MDD patients. J Affect Disord 110:260–264, 2008

Bright JI, Baker KD, Neimeyer RA: Professional and paraprofessional group treatments for depression: a comparison of cognitive-behavioral and mutual support interventions. J Consult Clin Psychol 67:491–501, 1999

Chen CH, Tseng YF, Chou FH, et al: Effects of support group intervention in postnatally distressed women: a controlled study in Taiwan. J Psychosom Res 49:395–399, 2000

Clancy DE, Cope DW, Magruder KM, et al: Evaluating group visits in an uninsured or inadequately insured patient population with uncontrolled type 2 diabetes. Diabetes Educ 29:292–302, 2003

Dennis CL: The effect of peer support on postpartum depression: a pilot randomized controlled trial. Can J Psychiatry 48:115–124, 2003a

Dennis CL: Peer support within a health care context: a concept analysis. Int J Nurs Stud 40:321–332, 2003b

Depression and Bipolar Support Alliance: DBSA Support Groups: An Important Step on the Road to Recovery. Chicago, IL, Depression and Bipolar Support Alliance, 2008

Emrick CD, Tonigan JS, Montgomery H, et al: Alcoholics Anonymous: what is currently known?, in Research on Alcoholics Anonymous: Opportunities and Alternatives. Edited by McCrady BS, Miller WR. Piscataway, NJ, Rutgers Center of Alcohol Studies, 1993, pp 41–76

Evans RL, Connis RT: Comparison of brief group therapies for depressed cancer patients receiving radiation treatment. Public Health Rep 110:306–311, 1995

Finn LD, Bishop B, Sparrow NH: Mutual help groups: an important gateway to wellbeing and mental health. Aust Health Rev 31:246–255, 2007

Fleming AS, Klein E, Corter C: The effects of a social support group on depression, maternal attitudes and behavior in new mothers. J Child Psychol Psychiatry 33:685–698, 1992

Galanter M: Zealous self-help groups as adjuncts to psychiatric treatment: a study of Recovery, Inc. Am J Psychiatry 145:1248–1253, 1988

Glasgow RE, McKay HG, Piette JD, et al: The RE-AIM framework for evaluating interventions: what can it tell us about approaches to chronic illness management? Patient Educ Couns 44:119–127, 2001

Groh DR, Jason LA, Keys CB: Social network variables in Alcoholics Anonymous: a literature review. Clin Psychol Rev 28:430–450, 2008

Heisler M, Piette JD, Heisler M, et al: "I help you, and you help me": facilitated telephone peer support among patients with diabetes. Diabetes Educ 31:869–879, 2005

Humphreys K: Professional interventions that facilitate 12-step self-help group involvement. Alcohol Res Health 23:93–98, 1999

Humphreys K, Noke JM: The influence of posttreatment mutual help group participation on the friendship networks of substance abuse patients. Am J Community Psychol 25:1–16, 1997

Humphreys K, Rappaport J: Researching self-help mutual aid groups and organizations: many roads, one journey. Appl Prev Psychol 3:217–231, 1994

Hunkeler EM, Meresman JF, Hargreaves WA, et al: Efficacy of nurse telehealth care and peer support in augmenting treatment of depression in primary care. Arch Fam Med 9:700–708, 2000

Katon W, Von Korff M, Lin E, et al: Collaborative management to achieve depression treatment guidelines. J Clin Psychiatry 58:20–23, 1997

Katon W, Ludman E, Russo J, et al: Stepped collaborative care for primary care patients with persistent symptoms of depression: a randomized trial. Arch Gen Psychiatry 56:1109–1115, 1999

Kelly JA, Murphy DA, Bahr GR, et al: Outcome of cognitive-behavioral and support group brief therapies for depressed, HIV-infected persons. Am J Psychiatry 150:1679–1686, 1993

Kessler RC, Mickelson KD, Zhao S: Patterns and correlates of self-help group membership in the United States. Soc Policy 27:27–46, 1997

Kilpatrick D, Koenen K, Ruggiero K, et al: The serotonin transporter genotype and social support and moderation of posttraumatic stress disorder and depression in hurricane-exposed adults. Am J Psychiatry 164:1693–1699, 2007

Krause N, Shaw BA: Giving social support to others, socioeconomic status, and changes in self-esteem in late life. J Gerontol B Psychol Sci Soc Sci 55:S323–S333, 2000

Krause N, Herzog AR, Baker E: Providing support to others and well-being in later life. J Gerontol 47:300–311, 1992

Kurtz LF: Mutual aid for affective disorders: the manic depressive and depressive association. Am J Orthopsychiatry 58:152–155, 1988

Lorig KR, Sobel DS, Ritter PL, et al: Effect of a self-management program on patients with chronic disease. Eff Clin Pract 4:256–262, 2001a

Lorig KR, Ritter P, Stewart AL, et al: Chronic disease self-management program: 2-year health status and health care utilization outcomes. Med Care 39:1217–1223, 2001b

Ludman EJ, Simon GE, Grothaus LC, et al: A pilot study of telephone care management and structured disease self-management groups for chronic depression. Psychiatr Serv 58:1065–1072, 2007

Maton KI: Social support, organizational characteristics, psychological well-being, and group appraisal in three self-help group populations. Am J Community Psychol 16:53–77, 1988

Maynard CK: Comparison of effectiveness of group interventions for depression in women. Arch Psychiatr Nurs 7:277–283, 1993

McCarthy JF, Blow FC, Valenstein M, et al: Veterans Affairs Health System and mental health treatment retention among patients with serious mental illness: evaluating accessibility and availability barriers. Health Serv Res 42:1042–1060, 2007

Mofidi M, DeVellis RF, DeVellis BM, et al: The relationship between spirituality and depressive symptoms: testing psychosocial mechanisms. J Nerv Ment Dis 195:681–688, 2007

Murray P: Recovery, Inc., as an adjunct to treatment in an era of managed care. Psychiatr Serv 47:1378–1381, 1996

Musick MA, Wilson J: Volunteering and depression: the role of psychological and social resources in different age groups. Soc Sci Med 56:259–269, 2003

Musick MA, Herzog AR, House JS: Volunteering and mortality among older adults: findings from a national sample. J Gerontol B Psychol Sci Soc Sci 54:S173–S180, 1999

Olfson M, Pincus H, Tanielian T, et al: National trends in the outpatient treatment of depression. JAMA 287:203–209, 2002

Onozawa K, Glover V, Adams D, et al: Infant massage improves mother-infant interaction for mothers with postnatal depression. J Affect Disord 63:201–207, 2001

Penchansky R, Thomas JW: The concept of access: definition and relationship to consumer satisfaction. Med Care 19:127–140, 1981

Powell TJ, Silk KR, Albeck JH: Psychiatrists' referrals to self-help groups for people with mood disorders. Psychiatr Serv 51:809–811, 2000

President's New Freedom Commission on Mental Health: Achieving the promise: transforming mental health care in America. Final report (DHHS Publ No SMA-03-3832). Rockville, MD, U.S. Department of Health and Human Services, 2003

Raiff NR: Self-help participation and quality of life: a study of the staff of Recovery, Inc. Prev Hum Serv 1:79–89, 1982

Rappaport J, Seidman E, Toro PA, et al: Collaborative research with a mutual help organization. Soc Policy 15:12–24, 1985

Riessman F: The "helper" therapy principle. Soc Work 10:27–32, 1965

Roberts LJ, Salem D, Rappaport J, et al: Giving and receiving help: interpersonal transactions in mutual-help meetings and psychosocial adjustment of members. Am J Community Psychol 27:841–868, 1999

Rogers ES, Teague GB, Lichenstein C, et al: Effects of participation in consumer-operated service programs on both personal and organizationally mediated empowerment: results of multisite study. J Rehabil Res Dev 47:785–799, 2007

Rush AJ, Trivedi MH, Wisniewski SR, et al: Acute and longer-term outcomes in depressed outpatients requiring one or several treatment steps: a STAR*D report. Am J Psychiatry 163:1905–1917, 2006

Sacco WP, Yanover T: Diabetes and depression: the role of social support and medical symptoms. J Behav Med 29:523–532, 2006

Schwartz CE, Sendor M: Helping others helps oneself: response shift effects in peer support. Soc Sci Med 48:1563–1575, 1999

Sheeren M: The relationship between relapse and involvement in Alcoholics Anonymous. J Stud Alcohol 49:104–106, 1988

Simon GE, Grothaus L, Durham ML, et al: Impact of visit copayments on outpatient mental health utilization by members of a health maintenance organization. Am J Psychiatry 153:331–338, 1996

Steele L, Dewa C, Lee K: Socioeconomic status and self-reported barriers to mental health service use. Can J Psychiatry 52:201–206, 2007

Substance Abuse and Mental Health Services Administration: National Consensus Statement on Mental Health Recovery. Rockville, MD, U.S. Department of Health and Human Services, 2006

Tonigan JS, Toscova R, Miller WR: Meta-analysis of the literature on alcoholics anonymous: Sample and study characteristics moderate findings. J Stud Alcohol 57:65–72, 1996

Trento M, Passera P, Tomalino M, et al: Group visits improve metabolic control in type 2 diabetes: a 2-year follow-up. Diabetes Care 24:995–1000, 2001

van Tosh L, del Vecchio P: Consumer/Survivor-Operated Self-Help Programs: A Technical Report. Rockville, MD, U.S. Center for Mental Health Services, 2000

van Willigen M: Differential benefits of volunteering across the life course. J Gerontol B Psychol Sci Soc Sci 55:S308–S318, 2000

Verduyn C, Barrowclough C, Roberts J, et al: Maternal depression and child behaviour problems: randomised placebo-controlled trial of a cognitive-behavioural group intervention. Br J Psychiatry 183:342–348, 2003

Wagner EH, Austin BT, Davis C, et al: Improving chronic illness care: translating evidence into action. Health Aff (Millwood) 20:64–78, 2001a

Wagner EH, Grothaus LC, Sandhu N, et al: Chronic care clinics for diabetes in primary care: a system-wide randomized trial. Diabetes Care 24:695–700, 2001b

Wheeler JA, Gorey KM, Greenblatt B: The beneficial effects of volunteering for older volunteers and the people they serve: a meta-analysis. Int J Aging Hum Dev 47:69–79, 1998

Yalom ID: Theory and Practice of Group Psychotherapy, 5th Edition. New York, Basic Books, 2005

Zrebiec JF: Internet communities: do they improve coping with diabetes? Diabetes Educ 31:825–836, 2005

CHAPTER FIFTEEN

Genetics of Mood Disorders

General Principles and Potential Applications for Treatment Resistant Depression

Masoud Kamali, M.D.
Melvin G. McInnis, M.D.

> Such as the temperature of the father is, such is the son's, and look what disease the father had when he begot him, his son will have after him.
>
> Robert Burton, *The Anatomy of Melancholy*, 1621

Clinical Vignette (Part 1)

Mr. F, a 54-year-old engineer, reported struggling with recurrent episodes of clinical depression for the past 24 years, with five well-confirmed episodes. Careful history documented that for the first three episodes, he had received treatment in separate stages with fluoxetine, paroxetine, and bupropion for intervals of 7 weeks, 8 weeks, and 6 weeks, respectively, and then fluoxetine plus bupropion for another 11 weeks. Doses were in therapeutic ranges. Mr. F subsequently resisted treatments with antidepressants, maintaining that he "had tried them and none of them worked." He denied having any side effects and observed that after 6–8 months, he seemed to cycle out of the episode spontaneously. No linkage with seasonality was reported.

His current episode, however, has become progressively more severe, lasting 1 year, and is now preventing him from working. Mr. F has recently read on the Internet about genetic tests and wonders whether the physician has any suggestions about future options.

Background

Observations of individuals with clinical depression or bipolar illness have long noted genetic influences and consistently indicated an increased risk of occurrence in relatives of affected probands (an individual or member of a family being studied in a genetic investigation). Although advances in genomics (the study of the genomes of organisms) and pharmacogenetics (the study or clinical testing of genetic variations that underlie divergent responses to medications) of depression and bipolar disorder have been relatively rapid and promising, little is known, or has been specifically studied, about the genetics of Treatment Resistant Depression (TRD). Nevertheless, treatment and prevention advances almost certainly will incorporate genetic strategies, so clinicians and academicians are well advised to stay abreast of fundamental principles and emerging developments.

The historical aspects of the genetics of depressive disorders are often confusing to the casual reader in this field because early investigators in the field followed the tradition of Kraepelin and assumed that manic-depressive illness was a unitary condition. Reported risks were thus based on both manic and depressive episodes (Stenstedt 1952). In the 1960s, Perris (1966) and Angst (1966) suggested that there were in fact two distinct disorders, bipolar and unipolar disorder, and each tended to "breed true." Later studies, however, found considerable overlap in the risk for bipolar disorder and major depressive disorder (MDD) (Gershon et al. 1982). Environmental and other factors contribute strongly to the clinical manifestation of depressed moods, which in many respects are the "fevers" of psychiatric illnesses. Major depression and bipolar disorder depression episodes are ubiquitous, with lifetime risks in the range of 25% of the population (Kessler et al. 2003), and considerable comorbidity exists with other psychiatric disorders.

MDD is a syndrome rather than a clear-cut disease entity and, indeed, may be best considered in the plural, as MDD*s;* it has several subtypes, some of which may occur with greater prevalence in certain families (Winokur

1997) and are considered familial subtypes. Although no universal agreement exists, such familial subtypes are generally reported to have an earlier age at onset and more frequent melancholic and vegetative symptoms than nonfamilial MDD, but otherwise few distinguishing features.

General Genetic Principles

In considering the genetics of MDD and bipolar disorder, often referred to collectively as *mood disorders,* it is useful to review, in broad terms, the principles of genetics. Mood disorders, like most psychiatric disorders, do not conform to the classic traditions of genetics that practicing clinicians learned in their training. No one genetic variant definitively predisposes to mood disorders. It is highly likely, and in fact generally accepted, that many genes and genetic systems of neurotransmitter pathways and neuronal circuitry will be components of the etiology of disruptions of moods and contribute to the complexity of the treatment-resistant form of the illness. However, the serious student of mood disorders must be familiar with the basic genetic concepts because the genes and genetic systems conform to the rules and logic inherent in human genetics and the genome.

The observed clinical manifestation (*phenotype*) of major depression is an integral component of biological systems, of which genes, stress systems, neuronal circuits, sleep mechanisms, and other variables are all critical components, and these clearly interact with the environment. Unlike conditions such as Huntington's disease or cystic fibrosis, in mood disorders the observed clinical phenotype does not conform to any of the three primary Mendelian inheritance patterns (autosomal dominant, autosomal recessive, or X-linked inheritance); however, there may be related physiological states or endophenotypes (e.g., cortisol levels in the stress response) that are driven by a limited number of genes that conform to classic genetics.

The reader is referred to Online Mendelian Inheritance in Man (www.ncbi.nlm.nih.gov/omim) for a catalog and discussion of single-gene disorders. It becomes readily apparent that even single-gene disorders are heavily influenced by additional modifying genes.

Complex Genetics

In contrast to the examples of classic Mendelian genetics, most common human traits and illnesses are inherited in a multifactorial manner, and the term *disorders of complex inheritance* is generously adapted in the descriptive sense. It has been used to distinguish these diseases from "monogenic" disorders—those that are caused by mutations in single genes. The observed phenotype is considered to be the combination of a multitude of genetic and environmental interactions. Some genetic variants are thought to increase the risk, and others will likely have protective or "resilient" effects. In essence, it is by no means clear why illness develops. A threshold of certain environmental factors in combination with genetic contributions may lead to illness. Most common medical conditions are believed to be multifactorial. Such conditions include cardiovascular diseases, diabetes, arthritis, cancers, obesity, and depression and bipolar illnesses.

How Do We know That Mood Disorders Are Genetic?

In *The Anatomy of Melancholy,* Burton (1932) commented on the predisposition for mood disorders to "run in families"; Kraepelin observed the same in the family members with manic depression (Trede et al. 2005). However, language patterns such as speaking English or French also "run in families" but are not genetically determined. In the absence of knowledge of a definitive underlying molecular genetic mechanism, we are left with the study of inheritance patterns among families.

Family, Twin, and Adoption Studies

The heritability of any disorder may be estimated by epidemiological inquiry. In a typical family study, the rate of the disorder in family members of probands with the disorder (cases) is compared with the rate of the disorder in family members of unaffected control subjects. The latter are chosen to be similar in all aspects to the cases but do not have the disorder. If the observed rate of the disorder is higher in the cases than in the controls, then it is deduced that the disorder runs in families and is heritable. Family studies have consistently reported elevated rates of depression among family members of probands with MDDs (Perris et al. 1982). However, family studies alone will not determine whether the disorder has a genetic etiology because the higher rate of disorder in the cases could be a result of the shared environment in the family and not necessarily shared genes.

By controlling to a greater degree for the shared environment, twin and adoption studies address this matter. Twin studies compare the level of *concordance* of a trait in monozygotic twins and dizygotic twins (twins are concordant for a trait when they both share that trait). Adoption studies compare disease rates in the adopted and biological relatives of individuals with the disorder. Twin and adoption studies generally have supported the genetic basis of various mood disorders (McGuffin et al. 1996; Wender et al. 1986), particularly if the proband has an early age at onset (Kendler et al. 2009).

Molecular Genetics of Major Depression

Evidence from family, adoption, and twin studies hypothesizes that genetic variants contribute to the biological basis of depression. Methods of molecular genetics have yielded several proposed risk variants. Earlier studies used linkage analysis, whereas the current approaches are primarily population based and use association methods. The characteristics of each method are summarized in Tables 15-1 and 15-2.

The study of the variation in genetic markers along the genome is the basis for molecular genetic inquiry into the etiology of diseases such as major depression. The genetic polymorphism that is the current standard in modern genetic analysis is the single-nucleotide polymorphism (SNP), characterized by variation at a single specific locus (e.g., a shift from a C to a T in the genetic code). SNPs are reported as the frequency of each variant (*allele*) in a specific population.

These techniques are now being applied to clinical questions. There have been several genome-wide linkage analyses and genome-wide association studies of major depression or directly related personality traits such as neuroticism. Sample sizes for the linkage studies vary from 81 pedigrees to 5,069 sib pairs. Some studies have included bipolar or anxiety disorder subjects, and others have primarily examined recurrent major depression with early age at onset. Two genome-wide association studies of MDD with large sample sizes (more than 1,300 individuals with MDD and 1,700 control subjects) have not identified SNPs that reached statistical significance (Muglia et al. 2010; Sullivan et al. 2009). Large samples almost certainly will be required when current strategies are used. The overall results (Boomsma et al. 2008; Figure 15–1) have not been consistent because large samples are lacking. Some areas, such as the short arm of chromosome 8 and the long arm of chromosomes 12 and 15, have shown suggestive evidence of linkage, and one genome-wide association study found a clustering of SNPs on chromosome 7. No single SNP difference reached statistical significance, however.

TABLE 15–1. Features of linkage analysis

- Includes:
  1. Identification of families in which some members have the trait of interest
  2. Analysis of their DNA and mapping of the chromosomes using genetic markers (for genome-wide linkage, roughly 400–500 markers)
  3. Identification of the genetic marker that is "linked" to the trait of interest (i.e. family members who have the trait of interest also have the genetic marker on their chromosomes).
- Does not identify the gene for the trait but, rather, suggests an area on the chromosome that may locate the genes for the trait of interest
- Is evaluated using the statistical formula, the LOD score (logarithm of the odds of linkage). A LOD score of 3 and above will indicate linkage while lower numbers may be suggestive.
- Is most successful in identifying conditions with classical Mendelian inheritance (e.g., Huntington's disease)

TABLE 15–2. Features of association studies

- Include:
  1. Identification of cases with the trait of interest and matched controls from a population and
  2. Analysis of their DNA
     - For GWAS, mapping of their entire genome using multiple genetic markers (sometimes more than 500,000 SNPs)
     - For candidate gene studies, examining the gene of interest that has been identified from the literature or scientific theory
- Examine the statistical association between the genetic marker and the trait of interest in cases vs. controls
- Identify a gene (in candidate gene studies) or SNP (in GWAS) that has a statistically significant association with the trait of interest
- Set a much higher level for statistical significance in GWAS, due to the extreme number of statistical comparisons
- Have more power than linkage studies in detecting genes that have modest effects, which includes many of the complex human diseases such as psychiatric disorders

Note. GWAS = genome-wide association studies; SNP = single-nucleotide polymorphism.

Meta-Analysis

Along with technological advances in the field of genetics, developments in statistics and the systematic review of research have aided investigators who study the genetics of complex diseases. Meta-analysis is a statistical

TABLE 15–3. Steps in conducting a meta-analysis

1. Clear definition of goals of the review

2. Systematic review of literature with detailed description of search methods and inclusion and exclusion criteria to reduce potential sources of bias

3. Presentation of data in a standardized format (e.g., odds ratios or relative risk and their confidence intervals, means and standard deviations)

4. Use of statistical models to combine data

   ∎ Fixed-effects models assume that the source of variation between the studies is random chance alone.

   ∎ Random-effects models assume that there are other unknown sources of variation and heterogeneity between the studies.

5. Exploration and investigation of the sources of heterogeneity between studies

method of combining data from different studies. This approach has the benefit of increasing power and reducing type II errors (false negatives) (Akobeng 2005; Zwahlen et al. 2008). This method has been used frequently in genetic association studies because at times the sample sizes are small, which leads to statistical power that is inadequate to provide reliable projections about the value of observed differences and contradictory results. Table 15–3 describes the steps in conducting a meta-analysis.

Clinical Vignette (Part 2)

The treating clinician, working with Mr. F, performs a reevaluation with a more detailed focus on treatment history in family members and investigates other comorbidities in Mr. F and his family members that may be affecting his treatment outcome (e.g., undiagnosed comorbid symptoms of obsessive-compulsive disorder or a family history of bipolar disorder). No new significant findings emerge. His lack of response to trials of adequate duration and dosage could indicate a predisposition to more rapid metabolism of medications, particularly because he has not reported significant side effects. In these instances, higher doses of medications may be required to achieve therapeutic levels.

Pharmacogenetics

The study of response to medication based on the genetic background of the individual has focused primarily on genetic variations in the common enzymes that regulate metabolism. Variants in certain cytochrome P450 (CYP) enzymes (CYP2D6, CYP2C19, and several others) may be typed commercially in panels that capture the bulk of the considerable variability. Currently, no firm evidence-based recommendations are available to guide the clinician with regard to testing of genetic variants of metabolizing enzymes. While awaiting larger-sample assessments to enable firm future

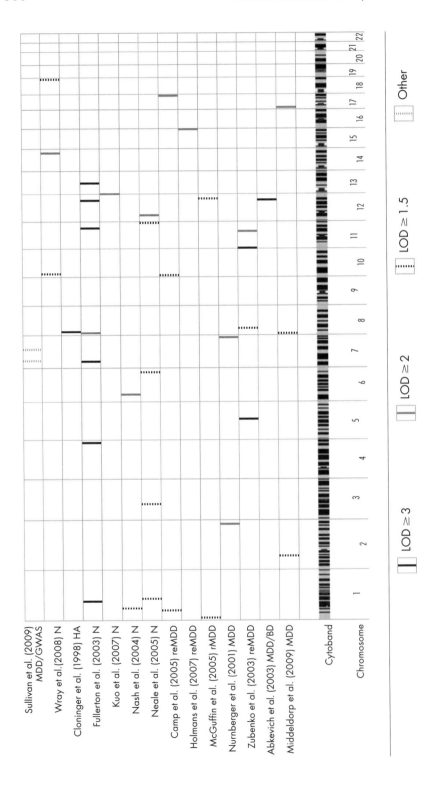

FIGURE 15–1. Summary of genome-wide association and linkage findings.

Summary findings from a genome-wide association study (GWAS) of major depressive disorder (MDD) and several genome-wide linkage scans of MDD and related personality traits including neuroticism (N) and harm avoidance (HA). Results are presented as patterned bars in each row, with the bars indicating the approximate location and strength of the findings. The GWAS findings include the highest-ranked statistical findings with a P value of at least 1.2×10^{-6} using the Cochran-Armitage trend test.

LOD = logarithm of odds for genetic linkage; reMDD = recurrent early-onset MDD; rMDD = recurrent MDD; BD = bipolar disorder.

Source. Adapted, by permission from Macmillan Publishers Ltd, from Boomsma DI, Willemsen G, Sullivan PF, et al.: "Genome-Wide Association of Major Depression: Description of Samples for the GAIN Major Depressive Disorder Study: NTR and NESDA Biobank Projects." *European Journal of Human Genetics* 16:335–342, © 2008.

TABLE 15–4.   Considerations in pharmacogenetics

Pharmacogenetics tests for variants at cytochrome P450 2D6 and 2C19.

*   "Ultrarapid" and "poor" metabolizers make up 5%–15% of the population
*   Should be considered in medication nonresponders and medically complex patients
*   Is not currently recommended in routine care
*   Is not covered as part of standard insurance benefits

recommendations, clinical prudence would suggest (as summarized in Table 15–4) that patients with a personal or family history of aberrant drug response patterns (e.g., the patient who never responds, potentially an ultrarapid metabolizer, or someone who experiences side effects at the lowest medication doses, possibly a poor metabolizer) and medically complex patients who take numerous medications (increasing the possibility of drug interactions mediated through inhibition of the metabolizing enzymes) would be strong candidates for testing. Although clinicians have differences of opinion, it is not currently standard practice to routinely perform pharmacogenetic testing. Costs of pharmacogenetic tests are not yet reimbursed routinely, which is another barrier. This is, of course, balanced against the costs of unresolved treatment resistance, which rapidly overwhelm the costs and inconveniences of the tests (Steimer 2010). The wise clinician will be familiar with a well-maintained Web site that catalogues and monitors the literature and presents the information in an accessible and easily understood manner (for one such site, see Flockhart 2009).

It is critical to appreciate that the inhibitory effects of several medications may render an enzyme functionally inactive. For example, a patient taking a therapeutic dose of paroxetine, fluoxetine, or bupropion will have effectively no available enzymatic activity at CYP2D6. Although drug metabolism accounts for considerable variability in clinical effect, the variability found in drug transporter molecules (e.g., serotonin transporter, p-glycoprotein) and neuroreceptors (dopamine and serotonin) will ultimately contribute to biological variability in drug response.

Clinical Vignette (Part 3)

After a discussion about the pros and cons of genetic testing, Mr. F and his treating clinician agree to a trial of an antidepressant (nortriptyline) with readily measurable and well-defined blood levels at given dosages. Testing is currently available to determine whether Mr. F's CYP2D6 activity is higher than the general population average (ultrarapid metabolizer), but they agree to withhold this test at least until they have attempted a trial with a medication that enables measuring therapeutic blood levels.

TABLE 15–5. Clinical implications of genetic factors

A family history that is as detailed as possible should be obtained from the patient and, if available, other family members.

- Presence of a family history of bipolar disorder, psychosis, suicide, substance use, attention-deficit/hyperactivity disorder, obsessive-compulsive disorder, or other anxiety disorders can point to possible comorbidity or misdiagnosis in the patient with Treatment Resistant Depression.

- Obtaining a history of successful treatment in family members may assist in choice of treatment options.

- Inquiring about a family history of poor response to treatments or side effects from treatment modalities may potentially reduce rates of adverse effects or treatment failures.

- Attention should be paid to the limitations of obtaining a family history (e.g., limited specificity and sensitivity, memory lapses).

- Clinicians should be aware of the legal and confidentiality issues with documenting other subjects' protected health information in the patient's medical records (this can be addressed by describing the relationship rather than using names).

Pharmacogenetic tests can assist in choice of treatment modality and reduce risk of adverse events.

Clinical Implications

There have been major technological advancements in the pharmacogenetics field, but the strength of the findings is low and the clinical implications (Table 15–5) are currently modest. Areas of further investigation include the interactions between genes and the environment, epigenetics, and the more detailed examination of various phenotypes of the disease. Our growing knowledge of the genomic substrates of mood disorders will guide the clinician in making decisions about diagnosis and treatment.

Personal Genetic Testing: Guidelines for Clinicians

In this era of growing emphasis on personalized medicine, it is understandable that personal genetic testing kits are being commercialized. Examples are saliva swab kits that are purported to predict vulnerability or response to prescribed medications. Some testing kits are priced as low as $20, while others approach $1,000. A common approach is to receive the kit by mail, swab the inside of the cheek, and mail the DNA sample to the company where the genetic or pharmacogenetic analyses are conducted.

Results are returned by e-mail. The utility of information provided by such laboratories is often greatly compromised by the absence of professional genetic and other clinical counseling and may be compromised further by the risk of providing misleading information.

In 1988, Congress passed the Clinical Laboratory Improvement Amendments (CLIA) to promote quality standards, accuracy, reliability, and timeliness of laboratory test results. The Centers for Medicare and Medicaid Services (CMS) oversees and accredits providers. CMS has had essentially no oversight over personalized genetic test kits, however, and recently intervened to deter more widespread marketing of such tests. Patients and families are generally unaware of the lack of regulatory authority over these tests. Clinicians, patients, and families will likely increasingly request these services, given the publicity and marketing.

As the research database grows, we hope that clinicians and counselors will be able to provide optimal advice about how genetic and pharmacogenetic test results can be best interpreted. The primary problem is that most individuals (including physicians) have a limited understanding of risk and probability.

While clinicians await more conclusive results and "genetic roadmaps," all pharmacogenetic test results should be viewed with interest but as exploratory data and in the context of comprehensive clinical information about the patient and his or her course of illness.

Future of Psychiatric Genetics Research and Treatment Resistant Depression

There have been suggestions of genetic overlap between schizophrenia and mood disorders (Craddock and Forty 2006). These are, in part, the impetus behind the efforts of the Psychiatric Genome-Wide Association Studies Consortium (Cichon et al. 2009). The aim is to integrate all available genomic data from the major psychiatric disorders and perform meta-analyses that involve the following components:

- Within-disorder meta-analyses of all available studies on a specific disorder; several data sets are emerging for each disorder, which must be pooled and reanalyzed
- Cross-disorder analyses that include all phenotypes, combinations of phenotypes, and other exploratory analyses
- Analysis of comorbidities such as alcohol or other substance use disorders that are common among the major psychiatric disorders

Although these approaches are sure to identify several interesting loci, several shortcomings are inherent in the data sets. The extant data sets focus primarily on the one-time assessments of affected individuals and recording of the categorical diagnosis. Data are limited on additional phenotypic features such as neurophysiology, neuroimaging, and other biological parameters as well as course and outcome of disease. In addition to the clinical limitations, significant methodological limitations remain in the genetic analyses. Not all variants are assayed, and no method is available to evaluate gene-environment effects. It can be anticipated that the ability to perform whole-genome deep resequencing of the individual will be an important but not definitive step in the process of integrating knowledge of the genomic structure with the clinical manifestations of the disorders and affiliated syndromes.

Few genetic studies have maintained an engaged cohort of subjects who are available for ongoing participative research. Such studies can build a dataset that includes a depth of clinical and physiological data, sufficient to study intermediate phenotypes and coexisting conditions and the genetic effects on these phenotypes. It will be necessary to generate large datasets to identify variants of modest effect, but it will be critical to have access to well-studied cohorts to understand the implications of these variants at the individual level.

The student of clinical depressive, bipolar, and related disorders can expect to be exposed to progressively more information about genes, gene families, and integrated genetic pathways that have been found to predispose to these prevalent and serious disorders. It is clear that no single gene will be responsible for the illness. We are instead dealing with a symphony of genetic mechanisms that interact with the internal and external environment, resulting in disease. The clinician of the future can anticipate that applications of rapidly emerging knowledge will play a role in diagnosis, treatment, and even prevention of the burdensome and disabling set of illnesses known as Treatment Resistant Depression.

Key Clinical Concepts

- The etiology of major depressive disorder, like that of many other chronic medical conditions, is multifactorial and includes a significant familial and genetic component.

- Our current understanding of the genetic underpinnings of major depressive disorder is limited, and future research will likely require larger sample sizes, more detailed evaluations of the clinical phenotype, and longitudinal assessments.

■ When evaluating individuals with Treatment Resistant Depression (TRD), it is important to obtain a detailed family history. The presence of psychiatric diagnoses such as bipolar disorder, anxiety disorder, and psychotic disorders in family members can help identify undiagnosed comorbid conditions in the individual with TRD.

■ In choosing medications, the clinician also might consider the pattern of response to medications and adverse effects in biologically related family members of the individual with TRD.

■ In certain clinical situations, pharmacogenetic testing can guide the clinician in prescribing medications.

References

Abkevich V, Camp NJ, Hensel CH, et al: Predisposition locus for major depression at chromosome 12q22–12q23.2. Am J Hum Genet 73:1271–1281, 2003

Akobeng AK: Understanding systematic reviews and meta-analysis. Arch Dis Child 90:845–848, 2005

Angst J: [On the etiology and nosology of endogenous depressive psychoses: a genetic, sociologic and clinical study]. Monogr Gesamtgeb Neurol Psychiatr 112:1–118, 1966

Boomsma DI, Willemsen G, Sullivan PF, et al: Genome-wide association of major depression: description of samples for the GAIN Major Depressive Disorder Study: NTR and NESDA biobank projects. Eur J Hum Genet 16:335–342, 2008

Burton R: The Anatomy of Melancholy. Edited with an introduction by Jackson H. London, Dent, 1932, 1st partition, p 211

Camp NJ, Lowry MR, Richards RL, et al: Genome-wide linkage analyses of extended Utah pedigrees identifies loci that influence recurrent, early onset major depression and anxiety disorders. Am J Med Genet B Neuropsychiatr Genet 135B:85–93, 2005

Cichon S, Craddock N, Daly M, et al: Genomewide association studies: history, rationale, and prospects for psychiatric disorders. Am J Psychiatry 166:540–556, 2009

Cloninger CR, Van Eerdewegh P, Goate A, et al: Anxiety proneness linked to epistatic loci in genome scan of human personality traits. Am J Med Genet 81:313–317, 1998

Craddock N, Forty L: Genetics of affective (mood) disorders. Eur J Hum Genet 14:660–668, 2006

Flockhart DA: Drug Interactions: Defining Genetic Influences on Pharmacologic Responses. Cytochrome P450 Drug Interaction Table, Version 5.0 (released January 12, 2009). Indianapolis, Indiana University School of Medicine, Department of Medicine, Division of Clinical Pharmacology. Available at: http://medicine.iupui.edu/clinpharm/ddis/table.asp. Accessed January 26, 2011.

Fullerton J, Cubin M, Tiwari H, et al: Linkage analysis of extremely discordant and concordant sibling pairs identifies quantitative-trait loci that influence variation in the human personality trait neuroticism. Am J Hum Genet 72:879–890, 2003

Gershon ES, Hamovit J, Guroff JJ, et al: A family study of schizoaffective, bipolar I, bipolar II, unipolar, and normal control probands. Arch Gen Psychiatry 39:1157–1167, 1982

Holmans P, Weissman MM, Zubenko GS, et al: Genetics of recurrent early onset major depression (GenRED): final genome scan report. Am J Psychiatry 164:248–258, 2007

Kendler KS, Fiske A, Gardner CO, et al: Delineation of two genetic pathways to major depression. Biol Psychiatry 65:808–811, 2009

Kessler RC, Berglund P, Demler O, et al: The epidemiology of major depressive disorder: results from the National Comorbidity Survey Replication (NCS-R). JAMA 289:3095–3105, 2003

Kuo PH, Neale M, Riley B, et al: A genome-wide linkage analysis for the personality trait neuroticism in the Irish affected sib-pair study of alcohol dependence. Am J Med Genet B Neuropsychiatr Genet 144B:463–468, 2007

McGuffin P, Katz R, Watkins S, et al: A hospital-based twin register of the heritability of DSM-IV unipolar depression. Arch Gen Psychiatry 53:129–136, 1996

McGuffin P, Knight J, Breen G, et al: Whole genome linkage scan of recurrent depressive disorder from the depression network study. Hum Mol Genet 14:3337–3345, 2005

Middeldorp CM, Sullivan PF, Wray NR, et al: Suggestive linkage on chromosome 2, 8, and 17 for lifetime major depression. Am J Med Genet B Neuropsychiatr Genet 150B:352–358, 2009

Muglia P, Tozzi F, Galewer NW, et al: Genome-wide association study of recurrent major depressive disorder in two European case-control cohorts. Mol Psychiatry 15:589–601, 2010

Nash MW, Huezo-Diaz P, Williamson RJ, et al: Genome-wide linkage analysis of a composite index of neuroticism and mood-related scales in extreme selected sibships. Hum Mol Genet 13:2173–2182, 2004

Neale BM, Sullivan PF, Kendler KS: A genome scan of neuroticism in nicotine dependent smokers. Am J Med Genet B Neuropsychiatr Genet 132B:65–69, 2005

Nurnberger JI Jr, Foroud T, Flury L, et al: Evidence for a locus on chromosome 1 that influences vulnerability to alcoholism and affective disorder. Am J Psychiatry 158:718–724, 2001

Perris C: A study of bipolar (manic-depressive) and unipolar recurrent depressive psychoses, VII: studies in perception. B) flicker- and fusion threshold. Acta Psychiatr Scand Suppl 194:102–117, 1966

Perris C, Perris H, Ericsson U, et al: The genetics of depression: a family study of unipolar and neurotic-reactive depressed patients. Arch Psychiatr Nervenkr 232:137–155, 1982

Steimer W: Pharmacogenetics and psychoactive drug therapy: ready for the patient? Ther Drug Monit 32:381–386, 2010

Stenstedt A: A study in manic-depressive psychosis; clinical, social and genetic investigations. Acta Psychiatr Neurol Scand 28:1–111, 1952

Sullivan PF, de Geus EJ, Willemsen G, et al: Genome-wide association for major depressive disorder: A possible role for the presynaptic protein piccolo. Mol Psychiatry 14:359–375, 2009

Trede K, Salvatore P, Baethge C, et al: Manic-depressive illness: evolution in Kraepelin's Textbook, 1883–1926. Harv Rev Psychiatry 13:155–178, 2005

Wender PH, Kety SS, Rosenthal D, et al: Psychiatric disorders in the biological and adoptive families of adopted individuals with affective disorders. Arch Gen Psychiatry 43:923–929, 1986

Winokur G: All roads lead to depression: clinically homogeneous, etiologically heterogeneous. J Affect Disord 45:97–108, 1997

Wray NR, Middeldorp CM, Birley AJ, et al: Genome-wide linkage analysis of multiple measures of neuroticism of 2 large cohorts from Australia and the Netherlands. Arch Gen Psychiatry 65:649–658, 2008

Zubenko GS, Maher B, Hughes HB III, et al: Genome-wide linkage survey for genetic loci that influence the development of depressive disorders in families with recurrent, early onset, major depression. Am J Med Genet B Neuropsychiatr Genet 123B:1–18, 2003

Zwahlen M, Renehan A, Egger M: Meta-analysis in medical research: potentials and limitations. Urol Oncol 26:320–329, 2008

Index

Page numbers printed in **boldface** type refer to tables or figures.

combined with
pharmacotherapy, 20, 53,
54, 60
goals of, 54
for cancer patients, 147, 149
for college students, 78
combined with pharmacotherapy,
18, 28, 37–38
for adolescents, 20, 53, 54, 60
for relapse prevention, 200–201
depression-specific, 194, 195, 206–
207
duration of treatment with, 204
effectiveness of, 195, 197, 201
in GROW meetings, 279
for insomnia, 188, 189, 198
for late-life depression with
anxiety, 132
in nontraditional settings, 203–
204
online modules for, 18
in pregnancy, 90, 109
simplifying treatment strategies
for, 204
STAR*D study of effectiveness of,
6
for substance use disorders, 176
therapist training and competence
for, 202, 204
College Screening Project, 82
College students, 77–87
campus health and counseling
services for, 78, 80–81
case identification, interventions
and treatment of, 81–85
clinical vignettes of mood
disorders in, 78–79
epidemiology of mood disorders
in, 79–80
future research directions related
to, 85–86
in graduate and professional
schools, 80–81
key clinical concepts related to, 87

parents' relationships with, 81,
84–85
Treatment Resistant Depression
in, 85
Columbia Suicide-Severity Rating
Scale (C-SSRS), **16**
Compliance. *See* Adherence to
treatment
Comprehensive treatment approach, 19
Computed tomography, 64, 130
Concise Health Risk Tracking
(CHRT) scale, **16**
Conduct disorder, 63
Congenital malformations
antidepressants and, 100–101, **103**
antipsychotics and, **105,** 106
benzodiazepines and, 106
carbamazepine and, 102
in infants of epileptic women, 102
lamotrigine and, **105,** 106
lithium and, 102, **104**
valproate and, 102, **104,** 106
Consortium for Research in ECT, 218
Consultation, 23
Contingency management, for
substance use disorders, 176
Continuous positive airway pressure,
for sleep apnea, 17
Corticotropin-releasing factor
antagonists, **46**
Costs. *See* Economic issues
Counseling services for college
students, 78, 80–81
CRAFFT Screening Test, 161
Crisis intervention, for cancer
patients, 149
CSK-3 inhibitors, **46**
C-SSRS (Columbia Suicide-Severity
Rating Scale), **16**
CVD. *See* Cardiovascular disease
Cytochrome P450 (CYP) enzyme
system, 299, 302
drug interactions related to, 142,
148, 151, 299